EUTHANASIA EXAMINED

Whether euthanasia or assisted suicide should be legalised is one of the most pressing and profound questions facing legislators, health care professionals, their patients and indeed all members of society. Regrettably, the debate is too often characterised by rhetoric rather than reason. This book aims to inform the debate by acquainting anyone interested in this vital question with some of the major ethical, clinical, legal and theological issues involved. The essays it contains are authoritative, balanced and readable: authoritative in that they have been commissioned from some of the world's leading experts; balanced in that they reflect divergent viewpoints (including a vigorous debate between two eminent philosophers); and readable in that they should be readily intelligible to the general reader. This accessible, fair and learned collection should enlighten all who wish to be better informed about the debate surrounding this momentous issue.

EUTHANASIA EXAMINED

Ethical, clinical and legal perspectives

Edited by

JOHN KEOWN

Lecturer in the Law and Ethics of Medicine,
Faculty of Law, University of Cambridge;
Fellow and Tutor, Queens' College, Cambridge

CAMBRIDGE
UNIVERSITY PRESS

PUBLISHED BY THE PRESS SYNDICATE OF THE UNIVERSITY OF CAMBRIDGE
The Pitt Building, Trumpington Street, Cambridge, United Kingdom

CAMBRIDGE UNIVERSITY PRESS
The Edinburgh Building, Cambridge CB2 2RU, UK www.cup.cam.ac.uk
40 West 20th Street, New York, NY 10011-4211, USA www.cup.org
10 Stamford Road, Oakleigh, Melbourne 3166, Australia
Ruiz de Alarcón 13, 28014 Madrid, Spain

First published 1995
Reprinted 1996 (twice)
First paperback edition with revisions 1997
Reprinted 1999

Printed in the United Kingdom at the University Press, Cambridge

Typeset in Sabon 10/12 pt [VN]

A catalogue record for this book is available from the British Library

Library of Congress cataloguing in publication data

Euthanasia examined: ethical, clinical and legal perspectives / edited by John Keown.
p. cm.
Includes index
ISBN 0 521 45141 8 (hc)
1. Euthanasia – Moral and ethical aspects. I. Keown, John.
R726.E96 1995
179'.7–dc20 95-17900 CIP

ISBN 0 521 45141 8 hardback
ISBN 0 521 58613 5 paperback

To the late Professor Dieter Giesen

Contents

Contributors

REV DR KENNETH BOYD
Research Director, Institute of Medical Ethics, University of Edinburgh, Edinburgh EH3 9YW, UK

JOSEPH BOYLE
Principal and Professor, St Michael's College, University of Toronto, 81 St Mary Stret, Toronto, Ontario M5S 1J4, Canada

DANIEL CALLAHAN
President, Hastings Center, 255 Elm Road, Briarcliff Manor, New York, NY 10501, USA

JEAN DAVIES
Voluntary Euthanasia Society, 13 Prince of Wales Terrace, London W8 5TG, UK

JOHN FINNIS
Professor of Law and Legal Philosophy, University of Oxford; Fellow, University College, Oxford OX1 4BH, UK

REV DR ANTHONY FISHER OP
Lecturer in Ethics and Moral Theology, Australian Catholic University, 412 Mt Alexander Road, Ascot Vale (Melbourne), VIC 3032, Australia

DIETER GIESEN
Professor of Private and Comparative Law, Law Department, Free University of Berlin, Bolzmannstrasse 3, D-14195, Berlin (Dahlem), Germany

LUKE GORMALLY
Director, Linacre Centre for Health Care Ethics, London NW8 9NH, UK

JOHN HARRIS
Professor of Bioethics and Applied Philosophy, Centre for Social Ethics and Policy, University of Manchester, Oxford Road, Manchester M13 9PL, UK

STUART HORNETT
29 Bedford Row Chambers, London WC1R 4HE, UK

BRYAN JENNETT
Emeritus Professor of Neurosurgery, University of Glasgow; Department of Neurological Science, Southern General Hospital, Glasgow G12 9XN, UK

YALE KAMISAR
Clarence Darrow Distinguished University Professor, Law School, University of Michigan, Ann Arbor, MI 48109–1215, USA

JOHN KEOWN
Lecturer in the Law and Ethics of Medicine, Faculty of Law, University of Cambridge; Fellow and Tutor, Queens' College, Cambridge CB3 9ET, UK

ROBERT TWYCROSS
Macmillan Clinical Reader in Palliative Medicine, University of Oxford; Consultant Physician, Sir Michael Sobell House, Churchill Hospital, Oxford, OX3 7LJ, UK

Acknowledgements

I should like to record my appreciation to the contributors for their efforts and their unfailing punctuality, and to Richard Barling and Peter Silver of Cambridge University Press. Thanks are also due to Jane Farrell for her expert copy-editing. I am also grateful to the British Academy for research funding essential to the compilation of this book.

John Keown

Foreword

Euthanasia and physician-assisted suicide are hardly new subjects on the human agenda. Though the profession of medicine has long condemned such practices – all the way back to Hippocrates – and even though opposition to them has been ratified time and again in different eras and in diverse societies, they have persistently lurked behind the scenes. Physicians have probably always, to some slight degree, practiced both of them – at least there have always been rumors to that effect – and, from time to time, public debate has broken out. In Great Britain, one can find efforts to change the law and medical practice going back over half a century, and in the United States legislation was pursued in various states as long as 50 years ago to change the laws that forbid euthanasia and physician-assisted suicide. Despite those efforts, and despite a long-standing minority of physicians and lay people interested to see a legal change, nothing much happened as a result of the earlier skirmishes. The laws remained unchanged and the medical profession continued to condemn such practices.

This time the agitation is different. Public opinion polls in the United States and Great Britain indicate a growing willingness on the part of both physicians and lay people to see a change in the law. Holland has already made euthanasia legally acceptable, and the state of Oregon, on the basis of a voter initiative referendum, has now legalized physician-assisted suicide (though not euthanasia). A voluntary euthanasia Bill was recently passed in Northern Territory, Australia. No longer are the agitators a small minority, the usual reformist suspects, but a larger, more influential group of academics, physicians, legislators, judges, and well-placed and well-organized lay people.

Dr Jack Kevorkian may seem a bizarre figure to many, but to others he became a hero, perhaps a strange kind of hero but one credited with having the nerve to make the issues visible and unavoidable. Most importantly, perhaps, his extremism has been the basis for a widespread movement to find a middle way, casting the traditional opposition to any and all euthanasia as itself a form of extremism, and offering (at least in the United States) physician-assisted suicide as the moderate, compromise solution.

What has happened? Why has there been a sea change on these issues? There is no clear and obvious explanation, but some plausible candidates are easy to find: a growing fear of a long, lingering death, the consequence of changes in the way people die occasioned by more chronic illness and more death in old age; the publicity given to a number of cases where seemingly conservative resistance kept people alive longer than most people found tolerable (for instance, the Quinlan and Cruzan cases in the United States); the AIDS epidemic, with its well-publicized cases of young people dying miserable deaths from a particularly noxious and degrading disease and often turning to suicide to relieve their misery; the potent Anglo-American movement toward greater personal self-determination and autonomy – fostered most explicitly on the political left but implicitly abetted, I am convinced, by the libertarian strains so prominently espoused by conservatives for free market solutions to social problems; and perhaps a diminished willingness on the part of many to accept the pain and suffering of dying as an acceptable fact of life. As one prominent advocate of euthanasia in the Netherlands once remarked to me when I asked why euthanasia had been so easily accepted in that country, 'the Dutch are no longer willing to suffer.' Perhaps his language was hyperbolic, but then perhaps not.

At the same time, some old anxieties seem to have less purchase than they did earlier. Arguments that the practice of euthanasia and physician-assisted suicide would betray the ethic of physicians appear less persuasive to many (including a large number of physicians) than in the past. 'Slippery slope' risks strike some as far-fetched but in any case worth running, and the proclaimed right to do as one pleases with one's own body has a more powerful grip on the public imagination than was earlier the case. Where claims in the past that physicians were already practicing euthanasia or helping patients commit suicide were sometimes taken as scandalous revelations, they are now held up more favorably to suggest that doctors have already taken a private vote on the matter and bravely practice a new, more kindly medicine.

In short, explanations and interpretations of the present situation, increasingly friendly toward euthanasia and physician-assisted suicide, are not hard to find, and all of them have considerable plausibility. The kindly rationales (urged by proponents) note the pervasive public fear of a bad death and the desire of people to have some final control over their life and fate in the face of unbearable and unredeemable suffering. The proponents hold out the promise of a more humane medicine, now able to go all the way in helping patients. The more skeptical interpretations (pressed by opponents) of the change in public opinion focus on the modern unwillingness to see personal choice thwarted, the recklessness of those who want a quiet death no matter what the risk to their neighbor by the unleashing of euthanasia or physician-assisted suicide, and the naivete of those who think that those practices can be nicely regulated by well-formulated laws.

Yet apart from Holland, Oregon and Northern Territory, most of the debate is still that: a battle of words and some minor court skirmishes. If the momentum seems at the moment on the side of those who would legalize euthanasia and physician-assisted suicide, that momentum has yet to carry the legislative or juridical day. There still remains considerable time for public and professional argument. Western society has reached a critical moment, being asked whether in the name of mercy and self-determination one of the oldest of medicine's prohibitions should be overturned, or whether in the name of protecting medicine's good name and its traditional role of only healing life not taking it, the prohibitions should be upheld. At stake are some large and important ethical, legal and social issues: the extent of our right to control our bodies, the distinction between killing and allowing to die, the potential consequences of legal and medical change, and how we understand life and death.

This collection of essays advances the discussion one step further. It could hardly come at a more opportune moment and it could hardly bring greater sophistication and sensitivity to the public argument. If ever there was a case of looking before we leap, then this is it. We have the chance to do so and this book is a good place to begin.

Daniel Callahan
President
The Hastings Center

Introduction

JOHN KEOWN

EUTHANASIA – the intentional killing of a patient, by act or omission, as part of his or her* medical care – is, without doubt, one of the most pressing and profound issues confronting the modern world. It is pressing in that there appears to have been, as Dan Callahan indicates in his Foreword, a sea change in the climate of opinion, which is now more receptive than before to euthanasia and assisted suicide, and profound in that it raises questions of fundamental importance not only for health care professionals and their patients, but for lawyers and legislators, philosophers and theologians, and indeed all members of society.

Questions raised include: Is it always wrong for a doctor intentionally to kill a patient, even if the patient is suffering and asks for death? Do beneficence and respect for autonomy not require that his or her request be carried out? Do patients enjoy a 'right to die' and, if so, what does it mean? Are only some lives 'worthwhile' and, if so, which and why? Is there a moral difference between intending to hasten death and foreseeing that life will be shortened, or between killing and letting die, or between euthanasia and assisted suicide? Can voluntary euthanasia be distinguished in principle from euthanasia without request? Can voluntary euthanasia be safely regulated or is the 'slippery slope' to euthanasia without request unavoidable? Is life a benefit for those in a 'persistent vegetative state' or should their treatment and feeding be stopped? Are 'living wills' a desirable mechanism for facilitating treatment decisions in relation to incompetent patients or are they a 'back door' to euthanasia?

* Throughout this volume, the use of the male pronoun shall be taken, unless the contrary is indicated, to include the female pronoun, and vice versa.

The debate about euthanasia and assisted suicide is both international and interdisciplinary, engaging experts and laypeople across the globe. In Washington State in 1991 and California the following year, proposals to legalise euthanasia narrowly failed to win majority support in public referenda. In 1994, in Oregon, a referendum proposal to decriminalise 'physician-assisted suicide' narrowly passed, though its implementation was then halted by a federal court pending the determination of its constitutionality. The passage of this proposal may well encourage similar proposals seeking to decriminalise physician-assisted suicide rather than euthanasia, not only in other states but also in other countries. In Michigan the activities of Dr Kevorkian with his 'suicide machine' have precipitated the enactment of legislation prohibiting assisted suicide, the constitutionality of which has already been challenged in the Michigan courts. It may not be long before the challenges to laws either prohibiting or allowing assisted suicide are all finally heard by the US Supreme Court. In Canada, Sue Rodriguez, a woman suffering from a paralysing terminal disease, almost succeeded in persuading the Supreme Court to strike down as unconstitutional the law against assisted suicide. In England, the conviction of Dr Nigel Cox, a respected consultant, for the attempted murder of a patient in severe pain, and the Law Lords' decision in the Tony Bland case that it can be lawful to stop tube-feeding a patient in a 'persistent vegetative state', even (according to a majority) with intent to kill, led to the establishment of a Select Committee of the House of Lords to consider the ethical, legal and clinical implications of life-shortening actions. In the Netherlands, where euthanasia has been officially condoned and widely practised for at least a decade, a wide-ranging empirical survey carried out on behalf of a government-appointed commission of inquiry has generated invaluable data about the practice of euthanasia by Dutch doctors but also fierce controversy over the proper interpretation of those data. Do they show that euthanasia can be controlled or that the Dutch are sliding down the 'slippery slope' to euthanasia without request?

As this book first went to press, a major development in Australia intensified the debate. In May 1995, the Legislative Assembly of the Northern Territory passed, by 13 votes to 12 the 'Rights of the Terminally Ill Bill', making Northern Territory the first place in the world to legalise physician-assisted suicide and euthanasia. When this legislation was subsequently brought into force, it permitted a patient with a 'terminal illness' (which it defines broadly to include an illness which would result in death because the patient refused treatment) who was experiencing pain, suffering and/or distress which he found 'unacceptable' to ask his doctor 'to assist the patient to terminate the patient's life', and it allowed the doctor, if satisfied that certain specified conditions had been met (including the examination of the patient by a second doctor holding a diploma in psychological medicine; the signing by the patient, no less than 7 days after he first indicated his decision to end his life to his doctor, of a certificate requesting assistance to end his life; and the passage of 48 hours since the patient's signature), to provide such assistance whether by prescribing, preparing or administering a substance. The scope and operation of this legislation clearly called for expert study, not least as similar Bills might well be introduced elsewhere in Australia and beyond.

The debate is not, however, only for the 'experts', the professionals and academics in the disciplines concerned. Everyone – doctor or patient, lawyer or legislator, ethicist or elderly – has a right to contribute to the debate, not least because how we as a society answer the questions raised above will ineluctably have a profound effect on the very nature of our society. But our contribution should be informed rather than ignorant, rational rather than emotional, and rest on argument rather than anecdote. To that end it is important to eschew prejudice, examine the evidence objectively, and dispassionately to evaluate the competing arguments.

How regrettable, then, that the debate is often characterised not by cool reason but by hot air, often fanned by a sensationalistic mass media which seeks, typically by way of an exclusive and manipulative focus on the 'human interest' angle, to generate emotion and disagreement rather than reflection and consensus.

This brings us to the purpose of this volume. This book seeks, by bringing together papers by some of the world's leading experts in ethics, medicine and law, to inform anyone interested in the debate. It is intended for the reader seeking rational debate rather than ranting polemic and is aimed at both experts and laypeople. It should be readily intelligible to the general reader: no expertise in ethics, law or medicine is either assumed or required.

The genesis of the idea for this book was a national conference on euthanasia held at the University of Leicester in October 1991. Five of the chapters are updated versions of papers delivered at the conference. The remaining papers have been specially commissioned for this volume.

The chapters cover ethics, law, medicine and theology. The first six chapters comprise a vigorous debate on the ethics of euthanasia (conducted within pre-arranged word limits) between two leading philosophers: John Harris, Professor of Applied Philosophy in the University of Manchester, and John Finnis, Professor of Law and Legal Philosophy in the University of Oxford. The former wrote a chapter setting out an ethical case for the legalisation of euthanasia and the latter a case against. Each was sent the other's chapter and wrote a reply. Finally, each wrote a concluding comment on the other's reply. This may well be the first time that two philosophers of such eminence have participated in a sustained debate on the issue, in a format which should help readers to follow the main lines of argument and grasp the main points of agreement and disagreement.

Lest it be thought that the Harris–Finnis debate exhausts the controversy, the next four chapters treat the reader to another complementary array of competing viewpoints. Chapters 7 and 8 consist of ethical arguments in favour of euthanasia by, respectively, Kenneth Boyd, a theologian with a special interest in medical ethics, and Jean Davies, a past-President of the World Federation of Right-to-Die Societies. Chapter 9 sets out the conclusions of the House of Lords Select Committee on Medical Ethics which in 1994 recommended against relaxing the law to permit active euthanasia. A critique of the Select Committee Report, and a reply to the arguments of Davies and Boyd, is then provided in Chapter 10 by Luke Gormally, Director of the Linacre Centre, one of the world's foremost Roman Catholic centres for medical ethics.

Perspectives on the debate by two eminent clinicians are provided by Dr Robert Twycross, who writes from his long experience as one of the world's leading hospice doctors, and Professor Bryan Jennett, an eminent authority on the 'persistent vegetative state', who describes this state and argues the case for withdrawing treatment and tube-feeding from such patients. In the following chapter, Professor Joseph Boyle, a philosopher, advances (without having seen Jennett's chapter) a contrasting view.

The remaining five chapters are all written by lawyers. In Chapter 14, Professor Dieter Giesen, a world authority on comparative medical law, presents a thorough overview of the law relating to euthanasia and assisted suicide from a comparative perspective. Professor Yale Kamisar, whose first seminal article on this subject was written almost forty years ago, contributes yet another in the form of a searching analysis of the arguments advanced by those who are advocating a constitutional right to assisted suicide and who are challenging the constitutionality of the law against assisted suicide under which Dr Kevorkian has been prosecuted. Professor Kamisar's critique of their alleged distinctions between physician-assisted suicide and euthanasia has assumed an especial significance in the light of the recent tactic of 'right to die' campaigners, which has proved so successful in Oregon, of proposing the decriminalisation of the former rather than the latter. In Chapter 16, the Editor examines the experience of the Netherlands, the only country in which euthanasia is officially condoned, and considers, in the light of recent empirical evidence, whether euthanasia is under effective control or whether the Dutch are sliding down the 'slippery slope'. In the following chapter,

Stuart Hornett, a practising barrister with a special interest in medical law, examines the legal status of 'advance directives' or 'living wills' and outlines a number of the main ethical questions to which they give rise. The final chapter is, fittingly, written by a legally trained theologian specialising in medical ethics, who considers euthanasia from a theological perspective.

This volume cannot attempt to cover all the issues raised by euthanasia and assisted suicide, nor does it attempt to do so. It aims rather to bring together leading experts from centrally relevant disciplines and a range of perspectives to set out their views clearly and readably in order to inform the general reader (whether professional or layperson) who wishes better to understand the cardinal questions involved and ways of answering them.

The aim has not been to produce a mathematical equality between contributors who argue the ethical case for and against, though there is indeed a very reasonable balance, but rather to ensure that some of the central arguments and some of the important data relevant to them are brought together in one volume and given a fair airing for the benefit of the general reader.

The contributions to this volume, written with clarity by experts at the forefront of their respective areas of expertise, will assist the reader to penetrate the fog of confusion which too often surrounds the euthanasia debate, much of it generated by some of the existing literature on the subject, which often presents a simplistic case for, ignores or caricatures the case against, and avoids any real engagement with the issues. The euthanasia question could hardly be more momentous; it demands the sort of close and informed consideration which this book seeks to provide.

Since the publication of the hardback edition of this book in 1995, the euthanasia debate has intensified. In 1996 two Federal Courts of Appeal in the US upheld a constitutional right to physician-assisted suicide, decisions which are criticised by Professor Kamisar in an updated Afterword to his chapter. In 1997, the US Supreme Court (citing his chapter and the Editor's) reversed both decisions. Moreover, the Australian Federal Parliament, after considering much evidence (including testimony from the Editor about the Dutch experience) repealed the Northern Territory's euthanasia legislation. In developments going the other way, however, voters in Oregon decided to retain its law permitting physician-assisted suicide, and it was reported that the Constitutional Court in Colombia, South America, has declared euthanasia lawful in certain circumstances. Clearly, the euthanasia debate worldwide is far from spent, and the essays in this book prove no less relevant and timely than when they first appeared.

1

Euthanasia and the value of life

JOHN HARRIS

THE MORAL SIGNIFICANCE of euthanasia is inevitably connected with the way that we understand the value of life and what it is to uphold and protect that value. As the argument unfolds I shall argue that on a particular understanding of the value of life, voluntary euthanasia as conventionally understood is morally and should be legally permissible. I shall end by suggesting that the real problem of euthanasia, its scale and also its real horror is not only misunderstood but largely ignored.

I shall concentrate on the moral arguments and I will largely ignore what I call practical questions. It is sometimes suggested that if voluntary euthanasia were to be legalised, this would inevitably lead to involuntary euthanasia. Similarly it has been said that the legal possibility of euthanasia will put pressure on those who are old or terminally ill to 'opt' for euthanasia and that the knowledge that doctors will perform euthanasia will undermine confidence in the medical profession. These questions are important but I have no space for them here. I believe, however, that if euthanasia is in principle morally acceptable, these practical questions are soluble with good will and care.[1]

To avoid possible misunderstanding I shall start by making clear how I shall be using the terms which define our subject. As I shall use the term, *euthanasia* is the implementation of a decision that a particular individual's life will come to an end before it need do so – a decision that a life will end when it could be prolonged. This decision may involve direct interventions (active euthanasia) or withholding of life-prolonging measures (passive euthanasia).[2] If that decision coincides with the individual's own wishes and he or she has consciously and expressly approved of the decision, I will call this *voluntary euthanasia*. Where the individual concerned does not know about the decision and has not consciously and expressly approved it in advance, I will call this *non-voluntary euthanasia* even where he or she is believed or presumed to be in accord. I shall not, for the most part, be concerned with involuntary euthanasia or murder where the individual is presumed or known to wish to go on living.

PRELUDE: TWO ENGLISH CASES

We should start in the real world with two recent cases which were resolved in the United Kingdom courts in 1993. They involved the fate of two individuals whose predicament shows one important reason why the issue of the ethics of euthanasia requires to be resolved.

Lillian Boyes

Lillian Boyes had been suffering acute pain from rheumatoid arthritis which her doctor of many years, Nigel Cox, found he could not control with analgesics. She repeatedly begged him to kill her and, in the face of her terrible anguish and his own inability to control the pain as he had promised her, Dr Cox gave Lillian Boyes a lethal injection of the poison potassium chloride. His action, which he had made no attempt to conceal, was reported by a nurse and he was charged with attempted murder.[3] Had Dr Cox administered a lethal dose of an opiate which also possessed analgesic properties he would probably never have been tried for attempted murder. In the event his honesty of purpose or lack of sophistication led to his eventual conviction for attempted murder and a suspended sentence of one year's imprisonment. The General Medical Council reprimanded him but permitted him to remain a practising doctor.[4]

Tony Bland

Tony Bland had gone to support his football team, Liverpool, who were playing at the Hillsborough stadium on 15 April 1989. In the course of the disaster which occurred on that day Tony Bland's brain was damaged so that he became permanently and irrevocably unconscious. His resulting condition has been termed a 'persistent vegetative state' – a state in which he was doomed to remain indefinitely without hope of recovery. Persistent vegetative state is not fatal and so long as feeding is maintained people like Tony Bland can remain alive for thirty or more years. His parents, who accepted that their son had ceased to exist in any real, biographical sense, although his body remained alive, were prevented from obtaining the solace of grief. In desperation they asked the English courts to declare that it would be lawful for medical staff to withdraw feeding and other life-sustaining measures so that he would die.[5]

Eventually the House of Lords ruled unanimously that such a course of action would be lawful, although it is not unfair to say that the reasoning of the five Law Lords was inconsistent and contradictory, as had been that of the three Lords Justices of Appeal before them.[6] The problem was of course that although Tony Bland had permanently ceased to have 'a life' in any meaningful sense of that term, he was not dead and would not die unless the courts permitted doctors to take steps to that end.[7]

We will return to one of these two cases after developing a theoretical framework within which to consider them.

I. THE LIBERAL ACCOUNT OF EUTHANASIA

I said at the start that what people believe about the ethics of euthanasia is likely to turn at crucial points on the account they give of the value of life. I had better start by trying to explain (though I will not have space to defend) the way in which I understand 'the value of life' and its intrinsic importance. I believe that there is a crucial distinction between the moral importance of the lives of *persons* and those of any other sorts of beings and that this importance derives from what it is that makes an individual a person. It is this difference (whatever explains and justifies it) that makes it permissible to sacrifice animals in the interest of humans or at least to rescue humans before animals in case of threats to their lives. Here of course the term 'person' is used to denote a particular sort of individual identified by its capacities or powers rather than by its species membership. On this account persons will constitute a large category of beings, including most humans from an early age, and perhaps also some animals. It also allows for the possibility of there being non-human persons on other worlds.

What sort of beings are persons?

I cannot attempt a complete account here of the point at which an individual becomes a person, but I can sketch the lines of such an account. Most current accounts of the criteria for personhood follow John Locke in identifying self-consciousness coupled with fairly rudimentary intelligence as the most important features. My own account[8] uses these, but argues that they are important *because* they permit the individual to value her own existence. The important feature of this account of what it takes to be a person, namely that *a person is a creature capable of valuing its own existence*, is that it also makes plausible an explanation of the nature of the wrong done to such a being when it is deprived of existence. Persons who want to live are wronged by being killed because they are thereby deprived of something they value. Persons who do not want to live are not on this account wronged by having their wish to die granted, through voluntary euthanasia for example. Non-persons or potential persons cannot be wronged in this way because death does not deprive them of anything they can value. If they cannot wish to live, they cannot have that wish frustrated by being killed. Creatures other than persons can, of course, be harmed in other ways, by being caused gratuitous suffering for example, but not by being painlessly killed. And the morality of ending their lives will have to take account of the wishes and interests of others as we shall shortly see.

The life-cycle of a given individual passes through a number of stages of different moral significance. The individual can be said to have come into existence when the egg is first differentiated or the sperm that will fertilise that egg is first formed.[9] This individual will gradually move from being a potential or a pre-person into an actual person when she becomes capable of valuing her own existence. And if, eventually, she permanently loses this capacity, she will have ceased to be a person.

The morality of killing persons

The harm you do in taking a life is the harm of depriving someone of something that they can value. But you may also wrong those who care about them and those who value life intrinsically or for what Ronald Dworkin, for example, has termed its 'investment' value.[10] The crucial issues are autonomy and integrity and we will be returning to these in a moment.

The distinction between persons and other sorts of creatures explains the difference between abortion, infanticide and murder and allows us to account for how we might have benefited persons by having saved the lives of the human potential persons they once were, but at the same time shows why we do not harm the potential person by ending that life, whether it be the life of an unfertilised egg or a newborn infant.[11]

This account, very starkly presented, yields a difference in the morality of ending the lives of persons and that of ending the lives of all other creatures including human non-persons.

The liberal view of euthanasia

If the harm of ending a life is principally a harm to the individual whose life it is and if this harm must in turn be understood principally as the harm of depriving that individual of something that they value and want, then voluntary euthanasia will not be wrong on this account. Such a view prioritising the individual's autonomy and her liberty to pursue it in her own way may be termed the liberal view of euthanasia. However, to understand both its force and its limitations we must see how and to what extent it needs to be understood in other terms.

II. EUTHANASIA AND RESPECT FOR PERSONS

Discussions of euthanasia and for that matter of other life and death issues such as abortion and experiments on embryos, are often cast in the terms of the value of life or of how the sanctity of life, its sacredness or its intrinsic importance are to be understood.[12] However, these accounts all assume a special importance attaching to human life or the life of some humans without trying to account for this special importance. In attempting to account for it, as I have done,[13] in terms of an answer to the question 'What is so special about the lives of persons?' a different perspective emerges. It is not so much *life* that is special, rather it is the individuals whose lives are in question that are special and special precisely because they are individuals of a certain kind. From this perspective it is not respect for *life* but respect for *persons* that is the moral imperative that has to be understood.

The idea of respect for persons

There are perhaps four distinct dimensions to the attitude to others that is encapsulated in the idea of 'respect for persons'. These are *concern for their welfare, respect for their wishes, respect for the intrinsic value of their lives* and *respect for their interests*. We will look at them briefly in turn.

Concern for welfare and respect for wishes

No one could, I believe, claim coherently to have genuine respect for persons unless at the very least they were prepared to show concern for their welfare and respect for their wishes. Normally these two ideas are complementary, but sometimes, where people have self-harming preferences, these two dimensions of respect for persons come into direct conflict and we have to decide which is to have priority. These self-harming preferences can of course range from the relatively mundane,[14] where people opt for an unhealthy diet or lifestyle, to the limiting case of suicide. Where we cannot show both concern for another's welfare *and* respect for their wishes, what should we do? To answer this question we need to remind ourselves of the point of valuing liberty – freedom of choice. The point of autonomy, the point of choosing and having the freedom to choose between competing conceptions of how, and indeed why, to live, is simply that it is only thus that our lives become in any real sense our own. The value of our lives is the value we give to our lives. And we do this, so far as this is possible at all, by shaping our lives for ourselves. Our own choices, decisions and preferences help to make us what we are, for each helps us to confirm and modify our own character and enables us to develop and to understand ourselves. So autonomy, as the ability and the freedom to make the choices that shape our lives, is quite crucial in giving to each life its own special and peculiar value.

Concern for welfare, and the paternalist control it is so often used to justify, ceases to be legitimate at the point at which, so far from being productive of autonomy, so far from enabling the individual to create her own life, it operates to frustrate the individual's own attempts to create her own life for herself. And of course this also applies in the limiting case of suicide or of course to voluntary euthanasia, where the individual's attempts to create her own life involve creating its ending also.

Welfare thus conceived has a point, as does concern for the welfare of others; it is not simply a good in itself. We need welfare, broadly conceived in terms of health, freedom from pain, mobility, shelter, nourishment and so on, precisely because welfare is liberating. It is what we need to be able to pursue our lives to best advantage. So that where concern for welfare and respect for wishes are incompatible one with another, concern for welfare must give way to respect for autonomy.[15]

Let us now turn to the remaining two dimensions that I mentioned: respect for the intrinsic value of life and respect for the interests of the people whose lives are in question.

These two ideas have recently been given powerful expression by Ronald Dworkin in an important new book which attempts to put euthanasia (and indeed abortion) in a new perspective.[16] I shall concentrate on his way of expressing and analysing these ideas.

Respect for the intrinsic value of life

Ronald Dworkin's book links discussions of abortion and euthanasia and he first introduces his account of the sanctity of life in the context of abortion.

> In discussing abortion, I defended a particular understanding of the sanctity of life: that once a human life has begun, it is a waste – an inherently bad event – when the investment in that life is wasted. I distinguished between two different dimensions of the investment in a human life that a decision for death might be thought to waste – what I called the natural and the human dimensions . . .[17]

Briefly, for Dworkin, 'natural investment' is simply the idea that nature itself makes an investment in terms of time, trouble and natural resources when life is created and that investment increases in a linear way as the life continues. Equally, distinguishing the human from the natural, there is human investment as well. There is both the investment of the human whose life it is (in terms of self-creation both conscious and unconscious); and the investment of the other people who invest time, effort and resources in creating and sustaining that life. On this view the wrong of euthanasia (and abortion) is the wrong of squandering this natural and human investment. A conservative view of the wrong of euthanasia prioritises natural investment; a more liberal view will prioritise a particular interpretation of the human contribution to a life.

There are a number of problems with such a view. Dworkin himself points out that even people who prioritise the natural contribution 'may plausibly believe that prolonging the life of a patient who is riddled with disease or no longer conscious does nothing to help realise the natural wonder of a human life, that nature's purposes are not served when plastic, suction, and chemistry keep a heart beating in a lifeless, mindless body, a heart that nature, on its own, would have stilled.'[18]

But such a moderation of the conservative view can scarcely be consistently defended. There are many hearts which beat today, with pacemakers for example, or with transplants either of the heart itself or of other vital organs (or perhaps even with the aid of antibiotics), which 'nature, on its own, would have stilled'. We must remember that nature is a profligate killer as well as a promiscuous and profligate generator.

However, Dworkin relies on denying 'that the natural contribution to life is dominant and insist[ing] that the human contribution is important as well, and that it, too, should not be frustrated or wasted.'[19]

Now there is an important difficulty with this idea of locating the value, the *sacredness*, of human life in the concept of waste of investment. In discussing abortion, Dworkin is rightly critical of the 'simple loss' view – the view that the waste of a life is the waste of what we might call its 'unelapsed time'.[20] He notes, plausibly enough, that:

> The death of an adolescent girl is worse than the death of an infant girl because the adolescent's death frustrates the investments she and others have already made in her life – the ambitions and expectations she constructed, the plans and projects she made, the love and interest and emotional involvement she formed for and with others, and they for and with her.[21]

Dworkin combines this with a form of what I have called 'the fair innings argument'.[22]

> We believe . . . that a successful human life has a certain natural course . . . It ends after a normal life span, in a natural death . . . But how bad this is – how great the frustration – depends on the stage of life in which it occurs, because the frustration is greater if it takes place after rather than before the person has made a significant personal investment in his own life, and less if it occurs after any investment has been substantially fulfilled, or as substantially fulfilled as is anyway likely.[23]

The problem with such a view of course is that it makes the value of a life vary with the degree of investment in it. Some of the ways in which this can happen are embarrassingly counter-intuitive. For example, the life of an infant which has had intensive investment is worth more than one which has not. So Jack, who resulted from massive emotional and material investment in his conception via *in vitro* fertilisation and surrogacy followed by a caesarian birth and post-natal intensive care, becomes more valuable in virtue of all this than Jill, who is exactly the same age but is trouble-free in every way. Jack's life must be more valuable, or sacred in these terms, because it has had immensely more investment in it. Equally, Dick and Harriet are the same age in the middle of their natural lives, but while Harriet's life is full, successful, rich in satisfying relationships and full of projects in mid course, Dick has a dull, lonely and mundane life. Harriet's death would represent the greater waste, so her life is more sacred, more worth saving.[24]

Dworkin largely ignores these difficulties because his account of the value of life mentions but does not really depend on the idea of investment at all. When the chips are down it is the notion of 'interests' that bears the full weight of his argument. However, as we shall see, it is doubtful whether this idea can bear single-handedly the weight put upon it. Having found both the conservative and the 'less conservative' accounts of the wrong of euthanasia problematic, Dworkin examines the denial that natural contribution to life is dominant and examines what follows from insisting on the importance of the human contribution. When this is unpacked, however, the contribution of humans, other than the individual whose life is in question, completely disappears. What remains as crucial is not that individual's own contribution to the richness of her life, but rather, simply her critical interests.

Respect for critical interests

We have come to the point where we must explain briefly Dworkin's distinction between what he calls *experiential* interests on the one hand and *critical* interests on the other.[25] This distinction is one that Dworkin develops with great subtlety over about fourteen pages and I can hope only to convey the gist, rather than the force, of the distinction as he draws it.

> First, everyone has what I shall call *experiential* interests. We all do things because we like the experience of doing them: playing softball perhaps or cooking or eating well . . . But most people think that they also have *critical* interests: interests that it does make their life genuinely better to satisfy . . . Most people enjoy and want close friendships because they believe such friendships are good, that people *should* want them . . . Having a close relationship with my children is not important because I happen to want the experience; on the contrary, I believe a life without wanting it would be a much worse one.[26]

In short, as Dworkin says, '[p]eople think it important not just that their life contain a variety of the right experiences, achievements and connections, but that it have a structure that expresses a coherent choice among these'[27] and he adds that this choice extends, sometimes crucially, to the moment and to the manner of life's end and beyond.

An important feature of critical, as opposed to experiential, interests is that they survive the permanent loss of the capacity to know whether or not these interests are being fulfilled. If, for example, I have a critical interest in the manner of my death, I have that interest even after I have fallen into a persistent vegetative state and will never know whether or not that interest is ever satisfied. And if I could be said to have such an interest in the manner of my burial or the disposition of my assets, then such an interest would also survive death.

What is it to respect persons?

> Anyone who believes in the sanctity of human life believes that once a human life has begun it matters, intrinsically, that that life go well, that the investment it represents be realized rather than frustrated. Someone's convictions about his own critical interests are opinions about what it means for his own human

> life to go well, and these convictions can therefore best be understood as a special application of his general commitment to the sanctity of life.[28]

So for Dworkin, not only has the natural contribution to someone's life been abandoned as an essential component of its sanctity, but so also has the human contribution of others. What we are left with is the individual's own convictions as to what is in his critical interests.

Now Dworkin has what I believe to be a genuinely noble, and at root, sustainable objective here. He wants to show that a person's beliefs about, and wishes concerning, his destiny, are an integral part of his conception of the value not only of his own life, but also of *the value of life*.[29] Dworkin's contention is that this conception can compete on an equal footing with other such conceptions, precisely because they are different conceptions of *the same concept*. And that where, in a decent and democratic society, such competing conceptions of the value of life exist, each person will respect the others' conception precisely because they will or should recognise it as just that: a principled, conscientious attempt to express and defend a shared value, albeit a value interpreted differently by different individuals or groups.

> Once again the critical question is whether a decent society will choose coercion or responsibility, whether it will seek to impose a collective judgement on matters of the most profound spiritual character on everyone, or whether it will allow and ask its citizens to make the most central, personality-defining judgements about their own lives for themselves.[30]

The answer is of course that society should choose responsibility, both in the case of euthanasia and in that of abortion. As Dworkin eloquently concludes of both abortion and euthanasia:

> Each involves decisions not just about the rights and interests of particular people, but about the intrinsic, cosmic importance of human life itself. In each case opinions divide, not because some people have contempt for values that others cherish, but, on the contrary, because the values in question are at the center of everyone's lives, and no one can treat them as trivial enough to accept other people's orders about what they mean. Making someone die in a way that others approve, but he believes a horrifying contradiction of his life, is a devastating, odious form of tyranny.[31]

It is difficult not to agree with the sentiment here, but it is important to be clear about the basis of the agreement. To be sure, making someone die in a way he finds horrifying is an odious form of tyranny. But is it significantly *more odious* because he also sees it as 'a contradiction of his life'? Dworkin adds this phrase because, in the attenuated conception of the sanctity of life with which he has left himself, it is all that marks the difference between *respect for a person's wishes about the shape and ending of his life* and *respect for their conception of the sanctity of life*. Of course, it also shows that the wish is a serious and important one (not all wishes are of equal importance to a person); but the individual can surely mark this importance in other ways. Does he have to admit that his horror of that method of dying is rooted in his belief that dying in *that way* somehow makes a nonsense of his life?

Of course, if people do see it in Dworkin's way, well and good, but do they *have to* see it that way?

If we take as our root idea the notion of *respect for persons* rather than that of *the sanctity of life*, and by root notion here I mean the same as Dworkin – an idea about what is of intrinsic, cosmic importance; we get the same answer (at the level of policy and legislation) to these issues as Dworkin does for a different, if related, reason. That reason is of course that whether what people take to be of cosmic importance they characterise as 'opinions about what it means for his *own* human life to go well' or as 'wishes to control their own destiny', what is at stake is a desire about a hugely important event in a person's history.[32] I deliberately do not say 'self-defining preference' because I wish to allow for the distinct possibility that while someone might have strong, and for them important, preferences about the manner and timing of their own death, these should be respected because they are just that, strong and important preferences; and not, if and only if, the individual also sees the manner and timing of their death as in some way self-defining.

So Dworkin's rich and interesting analysis of the sanctity of life, encompassing a combination of natural and personal investment in life and respect for an individual's critical interests, reduces, when the chips are down, to an individual's 'opinions about what it means for his own life to go well', and while I agree with Dworkin that these are, or can be, cosmically important, I do not believe it plausible to suppose that they are significantly more important than an individual's desire to control his or her own destiny, which will include preferences about the manner and timing of his or her own death.

Critical interests are objective

We should note for the record that Dworkin's idea of critical interests may conflict with respect for persons in another way. Respect for a person's critical interests may conflict with respect for the individual's wishes simply because the individual may misunderstand the meaning of her life and hence mislocate her critical interests. This would justify[33] a defence of paternalistic interference with an individual's desires 'in her own critical interests'. Thus the individual's desire to control her own destiny might, on a Dworkinesque view, be legitimately frustrated by another's plausible (and possibly true) claim the better to understand her critical interests and hence save her, at the last, from tragically misinterpreting her life and its meaning by implementing an inconsistent or self-defeating[34] desire at its end.

However, there are other important differences between accepting, as what is of intrinsic and cosmic importance, the idea of the *sanctity of life* on the one hand, and that of *respect for persons*, on the other. These have important consequences for our views about the value of life and in particular about the value of the lives of different sorts of human individuals. It is to these we must finally turn.

Euthanasia and respect for persons

To bring out the difference between Dworkin's position and my own and to show how the conception of respect for persons I have been using here[35] gives us importantly different answers to some of the crucial issues concerning euthanasia, we will look again at the issue of persistent vegetative state (PVS). This is the condition which was at issue in two crucial cases of highest jurisdiction in the United States and in the United Kingdom: those of Nancy Cruzan and Tony Bland.[36] For brevity we will concentrate on the details of the Bland case which we have already rehearsed. Both Nancy Cruzan and Tony Bland had been left in PVS following accidents. This, we noted, is an unconscious state which, after a year's duration, is accepted as permanent and irreversible. People in PVS do not require life support as this is usually understood,[37] although they do require tube-feeding and hydration. They are not, nor without assistance will they become, 'dead' according to any of the current criteria or accepted definitions of death.[38]

As we have seen, Tony Bland's parents asked the courts to rule that his death could be brought about by withdrawal of feeding and withholding of other life-sustaining measures including antibiotics.[39] In advance of the various hearings, it had been expected that the issue in court would turn on whether it was lawful to withdraw life-sustaining *medical* treatment, but no one considered feeding to be a 'treatment' and hence something that doctors could withdraw on the basis of their judgements as to whether the measure at issue was in the patient's best interests or could be afforded by the health care system. To their credit the courts did not attempt to stretch the meaning of 'medical treatment' to cover feeding, thus giving the doctors clinical discretion in the matter, but squarely faced the issue of whether or not Tony Bland should continue alive.

The decisions of the judges in both the Court of Appeal and the House of Lords were in the end given for a wide variety of different reasons, some of which contradicted others. For example, it was held both that death was appropriate because Tony Bland was no longer capable of possessing any interests at all, and that death was in his best interests. A third reason was that it was believed that, had he foreseen this contingency, Tony Bland would have wished to die in these circumstances.

Despite valiant attempts both by the three judges of the Court of Appeal and by the five judges in the House of Lords to pretend otherwise, their decision was in effect one permitting non-voluntary euthanasia. Since Tony Bland was not dead, and would not die unless the Law Lords permitted a definite course of action which would result in his death, their decision to the effect that it was permissible to end his life when it otherwise would have continued indefinitely,[40] effectively brought his life to an end. And indeed, such a decision was sought by Tony Bland's parents for precisely that reason.[41]

If we ask what justified the non-voluntary euthanasia of Tony Bland, I believe none of the reasons given by the various judges, nor those given by Dworkin and others, are satisfactory. If it is believed that the sanctity of life attaches to the lives of humans then as a live human Tony Bland does not relevantly differ from others whom it is wrong to kill. If, however, it is the lives of *persons* that are sacred in this sense and if the value of their lives is expressed in terms of the respect due to persons in virtue of their personhood, we get a different answer. For though a live human being, Tony Bland, at the time of the courts' deliberations, was no longer a person. Respect for persons no longer applied to him. However, he could and did still have critical interests – the interests persist even though the person is no more. These are due some weight. The critical question is: how much?

What weight is due to critical interests?

The answer to this question we can see most clearly if we imagine a variant of Tony Bland's predicament. Suppose John, who is also in PVS, had made an advance directive[42] (albeit not generally binding in English law)[43] which declared and explained a critical interest in staying alive indefinitely in PVS? What force should such a directive have? In particular how is such a post-conscious critical interest of John's to fare when set against the desires (and possibly the critical interests) of others to stay alive *and* remain self-conscious?

How important is it to respect critical interests of those who are capable of having interests of no other sort, as opposed to the wishes or interests of persons properly so called, those who have retained their capacity for self-consciousness?

How is my conscious critical interest in receiving a life-saving organ transplant to fare when in competition with your advance directive not to have your organs used after your death? Or where John's critical interest in staying alive indefinitely in PVS (at an estimated cost of some £150 per day)[44] involves not only the squandered resources but the lost opportunity costs of treating other patients in his bed, some of whose lives would certainly thereby be preserved?

The idea of respect for persons

Respect for persons requires that it is persons who will be respected and hence their interests, whether those interests are experiential or critical. Where, however, the person no longer exists, the critical interests of the former person, while still worthy of our respect, must of necessity give way to the significant[45] interests or preferences of actual people. Thus John's critical interest in a further thirty years of life in PVS would give way to the significant critical interests or preferences of any actual persons, persons to whom the satisfaction, or not, of their desires can continue to matter. And this would surely accord with our intuitions here. We would not, I imagine, think that someone who could no longer benefit from, or appreciate, the life he was leading should have that life sustained when to do so would cost the lives of others who could appreciate, and benefit from, their existences.[46]

Tyranny and tolerance

'Making someone die in a way that others approve, but he believes a horrifying contradiction of his life, is a devastating, odious form of tyranny'. I have tried to show that if this is so, it is not because it involves the frustration of a particular class of belief, namely one that involves 'a contradiction of his life', or of his conception of its sanctity, but because it is simply a form of tyranny; an attempt to control the life of a person who has her own autonomous views about how that life should go. The evil of tyranny does not require explication in terms of the nature of the sanctity of life, but rather in terms of respect for persons and of their autonomy.

Euthanasia should be permitted, not because everyone should accept that it is right, nor because to fail to do so violates a defensible conception of the sanctity of life, but simply because to deny a person control of what, on any analysis, must be one of the most important decisions of life, is a form of tyranny, which like all acts of tyranny is an ultimate denial of respect for persons. And because it is not only the dead who are beyond the reach of tyrants but also those who have permanently lost personhood, respect for persons demands that the values and critical interests of persons be given priority over those of former persons or potential persons,[47] even though both of these sorts of beings can have interests. Former persons can have persisting critical interests and potential persons experiential ones.

The real problem of euthanasia

This brings us to the final and I believe the real problem of euthanasia, which is simply and briefly stated. The real problem of euthanasia is the tragedy of the premature and unwanted deaths of the thousands of people in every society who die for want of medical and other resources or who are allowed to die or are killed because others believe their lives are not worth sustaining. It is, I believe, an idle and perverse arrogance to frustrate the wishes of those who want to die or to preserve indefinitely the lives of those who have irrevocably lost personhood when the wishes of people who do not want to die are consistently and callously disregarded.[48]

NOTES

I would like to thank Margaret Brazier, Inez de Beaufort, Charles Erin and Søren Holm for helpful comments on an earlier draft of this chapter.

1 See for example James Rachels, *The End of Life*, Oxford University Press, Oxford, 1986, Chapter 10. And a number of the contributions to A. B. Downing & Barbara Smoker (eds.) *Voluntary Euthanasia*, Peter Owen, London, 1986.

2 I do not believe that there is any useful moral distinction to be drawn between active and passive euthanasia. See my *Violence and Responsibility*, Routledge & Kegan Paul, London, 1980. And my *The Value of Life*, Routledge, London, 1985, Chapter 2.

3 Lillian Boyes' body had by this time been cremated and there was no evidence that the injection had been the operative cause of death – hence the charge of attempted murder.

4 Subject to a registration conditional upon him working under supervision.

5 It is not clear why there was any necessity to take the *Bland* case to the courts since it was already well established that there was no obligation to sustain a baby by feeding. See *Re C* [1989] 2 All England Law Reports 782 and *Re J* [1990] 3 All England Law Reports 930.

6 *Airedale NHS Trust* v. *Bland* [1993] Appeal Cases 789.

7 A more recent case was concluded in the Court of Appeal in January 1994. The Master of the Rolls Sir Thomas Bingham held, in a bizarre judgement with which the other two Lords Justices of Appeal concurred, that it was permissible for doctors to end the life of a patient by

refusing life-prolonging treatment when the consultant and 'a number of other doctors' agreed that such a course was in the patient's best interests and 'no medical opinion contradicted it'. See *Frenchay Healthcare NHS Trust* v. *S* [1994] 2 All England Law Reports 403 (C.A.).

8 See *The Value of Life*, Routledge, London, 1985 and 1992, Chapter 1.

9 See my *Wonderwoman and Superman*, Oxford University Press, Oxford, 1992, Chapter 3.

10 Ronald Dworkin, *Life's Dominion*, Harper Collins, London 1993. See for example Chapter 3.

11 See my *The Value of Life*, Routledge, London, 1985 and 1992.

12 See Helga Kuhse, *The Sanctity of Life Doctrine in Medicine*, Oxford University Press, Oxford, 1987.

13 See my *The Value of Life*, Routledge, London, 1985 and 1992, Chapter 1.

14 Though not trivial.

15 Of course I am aware that I have not said enough to be persuasive let alone conclusive on a point of such complexity and importance. I have here space simply to indicate the way my argument is constructed rather than to attempt to produce the complete structure.

16 Ronald Dworkin, *Life's Dominion*, Harper Collins, London, 1993.

17 Ibid., pp. 213–214.

18 Ibid., p. 215.

19 Ibid.

20 Ibid., p. 87. See also my own discussion of these problems in my *The Value of Life*, Routledge, London, 1985, Chapter 5.

21 Dworkin, op. cit., p. 88.

22 Harris, op. cit.

23 Dworkin, op. cit., p. 88.

24 See my discussion of some of these problems in my 'Justice, Age and Ageism' in *Bioethics*, Vol. 8 No. 1, January 1994.

25 Dworkin's own account of this occurs in a number of places but the account I shall be drawing upon here occurs between pages 201 and 217 of *Life's Dominion*.

26 Dworkin, op. cit., pp. 201–202.

27 Ibid., p. 205.

28 Ibid., p. 215.

29 *Life* here of course meaning that life which is, or those lives which are, intrinsically valuable.

30 Ibid., p. 216.

31 Ibid., p. 217.

32 I do not say 'even in one's life' because of problems that would in this context be tedious as to whether or not death is strictly speaking an event *in* someone's life or rather an event that limits that life.

33 Uncharacteristically for Dworkin.

34 Literally as well as logically.

35 And which I have defended at some length in my *The Value of Life*, Routledge, London, 1985.

36 *Cruzan* v. *Director, Missouri Department of Health*, 497 U.S. 261 (1990); *Airedale NHS Trust* v. *Bland* [1993] Appeal Cases 789.

37 They are not on ventilators for example.

38 They are not brain stem dead for example and because they have spontaneous heartbeat and respiration are not dead by any normal conceptions of death either.

39 After withdrawal of feeding he was expected to succumb to infections from which he would die without antibiotics.

40 Some patients survive in PVS as long as thirty years or more.

41 Since the Law Lords knew his parents and doctors fully intended to halt tube-feeding if they permitted it, they knew Tony Bland's life or death hung on their decision.

42 See Charles A. Erin and John Harris, '"Living wills", anticipatory decisions and advance directives', *Reviews in Clinical Gerontology*, Vol. 4 No. 3, 1994, pp. 269–275.

43 While a refusal to accept treatment expressed in an advance directive may be upheld in English courts, a general directive as to positive measures to be taken is unlikely to be upheld.

44 Based on estimates of the costs to the National Health Service of sustaining Tony Bland in PVS. Dr Jim Howe pointed out to me that the lost opportunity costs of treating others in cases like this, taking an average figure of one patient per bed per five days,

would mean 70 patients a year who might be treated in that bed.

45 The interests will have to be sufficiently important to justify denial of the critical interests of former people.

46 This discussion has been, of necessity, abbreviated. For a more detailed discussion see my *The Value of Life*, Chapters 1, 5 and 12.

47 This suggestion differs from the conventions of respecting testamentary dispositions in that such dispositions determine the fate of the former agent's own resources and cannot bind the use of those of third parties or of the public. We must also remember that even the private resources of the deceased are liable to tax in the public interest.

48 There is a more extended discussion of this idea in my *The Value of Life*, Routledge, London, 1985, Chapter 4.

2

A philosophical case against euthanasia

JOHN FINNIS

I. 'EUTHANASIA'

Devised for service in a rhetoric of persuasion, the term 'euthanasia' has no generally accepted and philosophically warranted core of meaning.

The Dutch medical profession and civil authorities define euthanasia as: killing at the request of the person killed. But I shall call that *voluntary euthanasia*, and distinguish it from non-voluntary euthanasia (where the person killed is not capable of either making or refusing to make such a request) and involuntary euthanasia (where the person killed is capable of making such a request but has not done so).[1] It is certain that deliberate killing of patients by Dutch medical personnel, with the more or less explicit permission of civil authority, extends well beyond cases where death has been requested by the person killed; the Dutch practice of euthanasia includes non-voluntary and perhaps some involuntary euthanasia. Rightly (as we shall see) the Dutch commonly reject as morally irrelevant the distinction sometimes drawn between 'active' and 'passive' euthanasia, i.e. between killing by use of techniques or instrumentalities for hastening death, and killing by omitting to supply sustenance and/or treatment which, but for the decision and intent to terminate life, would been have supplied.

In Nazi discourse, euthanasia was any killing carried out by medical means or medically qualified personnel, whether intended for the termination of suffering and/or of the burden or indignity of a life not worth living (*Lebensunwertes Leben*), or for some more evidently public benefit such as eugenics (racial purity *and hygiene*), *Lebensraum* (living space for

Germans), and/or minimising the waste of resources on 'useless mouths'.

In pluralist democracies today, there is understandable reluctance to be associated with Nazi ideas and practices. Racist eugenics are condemned, though one comes across discreet allusions to the burden and futility of sustaining the severely mentally handicapped. Much more popular is the conception that some sorts of life are not worth living; life in such a state demeans the patient's dignity, and maintaining it (otherwise than at the patient's express request) insults that dignity; proper respect for the patient and the patient's best interests requires that that life be brought to an end.

Since this paper is to present a philosophical case against euthanasia, my working definition of euthanasia should satisfy two requirements. It should ensure that the type of proposal to be argued against is identified under its most attractive or tempting true description. And it should also identify the full range or set of proposals which, for the purposes of applying the relevant moral principles and norms, fall within the same morally significant type and are the subject matter of a single moral conclusion.

So I define the *central case* of *euthanasia* as the adopting and carrying out of a proposal that, as part of the medical care being given someone, his or her life be terminated on the ground that it would be better for him or her (or at least no harm) if that were done. But this definition should be taken with two related and inter-related points. The moral norms which, I shall argue, rule out the central case will rule out *every* proposal to terminate people's lives on the ground that doing so would be beneficial by alleviating human suffering or burdens, whether the proposal arises within or outside the context of medical care. And, conversely, if the central case of euthanasia is not morally ruled out, neither are proposals to terminate people's lives outside the context of medical care and/or on the ground that doing so would benefit *other people* at least by alleviating their proportionately greater burdens.

To make this last point is not to insinuate some crude 'slippery slope' argument from the anticipated bad consequences of allowing euthanasia of the paradigm sort. It is merely to indicate at the outset, proleptically, that neither the true moral principles at stake in the discussion, nor any plausible (though untrue) principles which if true would justify euthanasia of the paradigmatic type, give warrant for thinking that the conclusion of the moral argument might depend upon the medical (or non-medical) character or context of lethal conduct, or upon the identity of the person(s) for whose benefit a proposal precisely to terminate life might be adopted as a means. It is, in other words, to indicate that hereabouts one will find 'slippery slope' arguments of a valid[2] and sophisticated type, adverting not so much to predictions and attempted evaluative assessments of future consequences and states of affairs, but rather to the implications of consistency in judgment.

One of those valid arguments from consistency will conclude that there is no morally relevant distinction between employing deliberate omissions (or forbearances or abstentions) *in order to* terminate life ('passive euthanasia') and employing 'a deliberate intervention' for the same purpose ('active euthanasia'). So my definition even of the narrow central case of euthanasia is wider than the definition offered by those who, like the Walton Committee,[3] wish (for good reason) to oppose euthanasia but (for no detectable reason of principle) are unwilling to challenge the line between 'positive actions intended to terminate life' and 'omissions intended to terminate life' – the line drawn, for example, in *Airedale NHS Trust* v. *Bland*,[4] by Law Lords who admitted its legal misshapenness and moral irrelevance.[5]

II. HOW INTENTION COUNTS

The Select Committee on Medical Ethics (Walton Committee), which was set up by the House of Lords in the wake of the *Bland* case and reported in early 1994, unanimously rejected any proposal to 'cross the line which prohibits any *intentional* killing, a line which we think it essential to preserve'.[6] The Committee described the 'prohibition of intentional killing' as 'the cornerstone of law and of social relationships'.[7] They then showed their understanding of the nature and importance of *intention* by rejecting outright the view[8] that the rightness or wrongness of administering analgesics or sedatives, in the knowledge that the dose will both relieve pain and shorten life, depends not upon the intention with which the medication is administered and only upon the comparative value of the respective outcomes. The Committee's view was this:

> [W]e are satisfied that the professional judgment of the health-care team can be exercised to enable increasing doses of medication (whether of analgesics or sedatives) to be given *in order to* provide relief, even if this shortens life. In some cases patients may in consequence die sooner than they would otherwise have done but this is not in our view a reason for withholding treatment that would give relief, *as long as* the doctor acts in accordance with responsible medical practice *with the objective of* relieving pain or distress, and *with no intention to kill* . . . the doctor's intention, and evaluation of the pain and distress suffered by the patient, are of crucial significance in judging double effect. If this *intention* is the relief of pain or severe distress, and the treatment given is appropriate to that *end*, then the possible double effect should be no obstacle to such treatment being given. Some may suggest that intention is not

> readily ascertainable. But juries are asked every day to assess intention in all sorts of cases.[9]

In this passage, the Committee rightly deploy some of the various synonyms which common speech deploys as alternative ways of expressing what is signified by their key general term 'intentional': 'with the intention to', 'in order to', 'with the objective of' and 'to that end'.[10]

I mention the Walton Committee's conclusions not as an appeal to authority, but as convenient evidence of a fact confirmed in many recent philosophical studies. Intention is a tough, sophisticated and serviceable concept, well worthy of its central role in moral deliberation, analysis and judgment, because it picks out the central realities of deliberation and choice: the linking of means and ends in a plan or *proposal*-for-action *adopted* by *choice* in preference to alternative proposals (including: to do nothing). What one intends is what one chooses, whether as end or as means. Included in one's intention is everything which is part of one's plan (proposal), whether as purpose or as way of effecting one's purpose(s). The parts of the plan are often picked out by phrases such as 'trying to', 'in order to', 'with the objective of', 'so as to' or, often enough, plain 'to'.

In recent years, the English courts have firmly set their face against a view widely and for many years propounded by legal academics, but most clearly put by Henry Sidgwick:

> for purposes of exact moral or jural discussion, it is best to include under the term 'intention' all the consequences of an act that are foreseen as certain or probable.[11]

It was settled by the Law Lords in *R.* v. *Moloney* (1985) and *R.* v. *Hancock* (1986) that it is a fatal misdirection to instruct a jury on Sidgwick's lines. Foresight of consequences is evidentially relevant to the question what the accused intended, but a jury can rightly hold that what one foresees as probable or even certain to result from one's action is nevertheless no part of what one intends.[12] (And 'jural discussion' about the law of murder is intended by the judges to track sound 'moral discussion'.) The 'oblique intention' of Bentham, Sidgwick, Holmes and Glanville Williams is not intention at all; it is a state of foresight and acceptance that one will cause such and such as a side-effect. These thinkers claim one *should* have the same moral responsibility for foreseen (or foreseeable?) side-effects as one has for what one intentionally brings about. But that claim depends not on a clear and realistic analysis of action but on a (highly contestable) theory about the content of true moral norms. In a sound theory of human action, the utilitarian construct 'oblique intention' is a mere deeming, a fiction, but the *intention* known to common sense, law and exact philosophy alike is action's central reality. It is what one forms in choosing to act on *this* proposal/plan rather than that or those. In carrying out one's intention, one *does* precisely what one intends. The primary and proper description of one's act, and thus its primary identity as a human act, morally assessable by reference to relevant moral norms, is settled by what one intends, what one means to do.

So, in common sense and law alike, there is a straightforward, non-artificial, substantive distinction between choosing to kill someone with drugs (administered over, say, three days in order not to arouse suspicion) in order to relieve them of their pain and suffering, and choosing to relieve someone of their pain by giving drugs, in a dosage determined by the drugs' capacity for pain-relief, foreseeing that the drugs in that dosage will cause death in say three days. The former choice is legally and morally murder (in mitigating circumstances); the latter is not. The latter *may* still be morally and legally culpable, not by virtue of the moral and legal norm which excludes intentionally terminating life, but by virtue of other legal and moral norms, those which apply to the causing and accepting of side-effects unfairly or in some other way unreasonably. So if the pain were in any case likely to abate, and the patient was not in any case dying, the imposition of death even as an unintended consequence (side-effect) of pain-relief would normally be grossly unfair and unreasonable, and in law a case of manslaughter though not murder.

The distinctions between what is intended as means or end and what is accepted as a side-effect do not depend upon whether the side-effect is desired or undesired, welcomed or accepted with reluctance. Provided that one in no way adjusts one's plan so as to make them more likely, side-effects may be welcomed as a 'bonus' without being intended. It can be reasonable for someone to welcome death precisely insofar as it involves an end to misery or is envisaged as the gate of heaven. Of course, such a desire for death can be or become a temptation to form an intention to terminate or secure the termination of one's life, even if only a conditional ('If things get worse, I'll . . .') or hypothetical intention ('If I had the nerve to do it, I'd . . .'). But a desire for death need not result in the forming of such an understandable but always fundamentally different (and immoral) intention.

So the moral argument which condemns euthanasia as a kind of intentional killing does not condemn the use of drugs which cause death as a side-effect, and does not condemn the longing that some people have for death. Nor does it condemn the decision of those who decline to undergo some life-saving or life-sustaining form of treatment because they choose to avoid the burdens (e.g. pain, disfigurement or expense) imposed by such treatment, and accept the earlier onset of their death as a side-effect of that choice. Such decisions may be more or less immoral because lacking in fortitude and/or perseverance in reasonable commitment, or because unfair to dependents or colleagues, and so forth. But provided that they in no way involve the choice (intention) to terminate life by omission, they are not suicidal, and a similar decision made on someone's behalf is not euthanasiast.

Turn the coin over. Intentionally terminating life by omission – starving someone to death, or withholding their insulin, etc., etc. – is just as much murder as doing so by 'deliberate intervention' ('commission', 'active euthanasia'). Without squarely confronting the issue, at least a majority of the Law Lords in *Bland* slid, via a confused analysis of 'duty of care', into a position tantamount to denying this implication of the significance of intention. And the Walton Committee unfortunately so arranged their definitions and discussions that they managed to avoid even confronting the need to identify euthanasia by deliberate omission for what it is, and to distinguish it from the refusal or withholding of burdensome or futile treatment.

III. WHY INTENTION COUNTS

The distinction between what one intends (and does) and what one accepts as foreseen side-effect(s) is significant because free choice matters. There is a free choice (in the sense that matters morally) only when one is rationally motivated towards incompatible alternative possible purposes (X and Y, or X and not-X) which one considers desirable by reason of the intelligible goods (instrumental and basic) which they offer – and when nothing but one's choosing itself settles which alternative is chosen. In choosing one adopts a proposal to bring about certain states of affairs – one's instrumental and basic purposes – which are precisely those identified under the description which made them seem rationally appealing and choosable. And what one thus adopts is, so to speak, synthesised with one's will, i.e. with oneself as an acting person. Rationally motivated choice, being for reasons, is never of a sheer particular. So one *becomes* a doer of the *sort* of thing that one saw reason to do and chose and set oneself to do and accomplish – in short, one becomes the sort of person who has *such* an intention. Nothing but contrary free choice(s) can reverse this self-constitution.

Forming an intention, in choosing freely, is not a matter of having an internal feeling or impression; it is a matter of *setting oneself* to do something. (Here and hereabouts 'do' and 'act' include deliberate omissions such as starving one's children to death.) No form of voluntariness other than intention – e.g. the voluntariness involved in knowingly causing the side-effects one could have avoided causing by not choosing what one chose – can have the self-constituting significance of really forming an intention.

The distinction between the intended and the side-effect is *morally* significant. One who chooses (intends) to destroy, damage or impede some instantiation of a basic human good chooses and acts contrary to the practical reason constituted by that basic human good. It can never be reasonable – and hence it can never be morally acceptable – to choose contrary to a reason, unless one has reason to do so which is rationally preferable to the reason not to do so. But where the reason *not* to act is a *basic* human good, there cannot be a rationally preferable reason to choose so to act. (For the basic goods are aspects of the human persons who can participate in them, and their instantiations in particular persons cannot, as reasons for action, be rationally commensurated with one another. Indeed, if they could be, the reason which measured lower on the scale would, by that very fact, cease to be a *reason* and the higher-ranked reason, having *all* the value of the lower *and some additional value*, would be rationally unopposed; so the situation would cease to be one of morally significant choice, choice between rationally appealing alternatives. But, to repeat, because of many factors including the self-constitutive significance of free choices, reasons for action (goods and bads) involved in alternative proposals for action are not commensurable *prior* to *moral* judgment and choice. Immoral proposals, though not fully reasonable, can and often do have rational appeal and morally significant choice between right and wrong remains eminently possible.) So, one who *intends* to destroy, damage or impede some instantiation of a basic human good necessarily acts contrary not merely to a reason but to reason, i.e. immorally.

Such, in very abstract terms, is the rationale of the more concrete and traditional moral wisdom: there are means which cannot be justified by any end; do not do evil that good may come; it is better to suffer wrong than to do it – not to mention the restatement made by Kant in opposition to early utilitarianism: treat humanity in oneself and others always as an end and never as a mere means.

The exceptionless moral norms which give specificity to these principles are – and, if morality is to give coherent direction to conscientious deliberation, must be – negative norms about what is chosen and intended, not about what is caused and accepted as a side-effect. But while one can always refrain from *choosing to harm* an instance of a basic human good (i.e. from resorting to unjustifiable means, doing evil, doing wrong, treating someone's humanity as a mere means), one *cannot* avoid *causing harm* to some instances of human goods. For every choice and action has some more or less immediate or remote negative impact on – in some way facilitates the damaging or impeding of – some instantiation(s) of basic human good(s). And since such harm is inevitable, it cannot be excluded by reason's norms of action. For moral norms exclude irrationality over which we have some control; they do not exclude accepting the inevitable limits we face as rational agents. Accepting – knowingly causing – harm to basic human goods as side-effects will be contrary to reason only if doing so is contrary to a reason of another sort, viz., a reason which bears not on choosing/intending precisely as such but rather on acceptance, awareness and causation. As I indicated in relation to choices to administer pain-relieving drugs, or to refuse or withhold life-saving treatment, there certainly are reasons of this other sort – particularly reasons of impartiality and fairness (the Golden Rule), and reasons arising from role-responsibilities and prior commitments. Still, one can be certain that harmful side-effects are *not* such as to give reason to reject an option, if the feasible alternative option(s) involve *intending* to destroy or damage some instantiation of a basic human good such as someone's life.

IV. WHY IT IS ALWAYS WRONG TO CHOOSE TO TERMINATE THE LIFE OF THE VERY YOUNG, THE VERY ILL AND/OR THE VERY OLD

The Walton Committee, having expressed its judgment that the prohibition of intentional killing is the cornerstone of social relationships, immediately adds: 'It protects each one of us impartially, embodying the belief that *all are equal*.'[13] All who/what? The answer is evident enough: people, including the vulnerable and disadvantaged.[14]

In virtue of what (if anything) are people, with all their manifold differences, equal and so entitled to be valued and treated as – not merely *as if*! – equals? To answer that question is also to answer the question of whether and why human life is a basic good which one may never rightly choose to destroy in any of its instantiations (living human beings).

What do all human beings have in common? Their humanity. This is not a mere abstraction or nominal category; nor is it Kant's thin, rationalistic reduction of one's humanity (*Menschlichkeit*) to that aspect of one's nature which one does not share with other terrestrial creatures: one's reason and rational will. Rather, one's humanity is one's capacity to live the life, not of a carrot or a cat, but a human being. And one's having this radical capacity is, again, no mere abstraction; it is, indeed, one's very life, one's being a living human being. Carrots and cats, too, are alive. But human life is not partly carrot-life and partly cat-life. It is human through and through, a capacity – more or less actualised in various states of existence such as waking, sleeping, infancy, traumatic unconsciousness, decrepitude, etc. – for human metabolism, human awareness, feelings, imagination, memory, responsiveness and sexuality, and human wondering, relating and communicating, deliberating, choosing and acting. To lose one's life is to lose all these capacities, these specific forms and manifestations of one's humanness; it is to lose one's very reality as a human being.

That reality is through and through the reality of a person, a being with the radical capacity to deliberate and choose. Free choice, as I have already said, is wonderful in its freedom from inner and outer determination and its world-shaping and self-determining creativity for participating in intelligible goods. Personal life accordingly has the dignity which the tradition sought to capture with the phrase 'image of God' – a phrase which serious philosophers such as Socrates, Plato and Aristotle would not have dismissed as a mere theological flourish foreign to philosophy's reflection on the ultimate principles of everything.[15] That dignity is most fully manifested in the dispositions and activities of people and communities who think wisely, and choose and act with the integrity and justice of full reasonableness. But, once again, thinking (and thinking straight) and choosing (with the freedom of full reasonableness unfettered by deflecting emotions) are *vital* activities, life-functions, actualisations of that *one* radical, dynamic capacity which is actuated in all one's activities, metabolic, sensitive, imaginative, intellectual and volitional.

Every living human being has this radical capacity for participating in the manner of a person – intelligently and freely – in human goods. That is, every living being which results from human conception and has the epigenetic primordia (which hydatidiform moles and, even more obviously, human sperm and ova lack) of a human body normal enough to be the bodily basis of some intellectual act is truly a human being, a human person. But, to repeat again, the human being's life is not a vegetable life supplemented by an animal life supplemented by an intellectual life; it is the one life of a unitary being. So a being that once has human (and thus personal) life will remain a human person while that life (the dynamic principle for that being's integrated organic functioning) remains – i.e. until death. Where one's brain has not yet developed, or has been so damaged as to impair or even destroy one's capacity for intellectual acts, one is an immature or damaged human person.

The alternative is some sort of dualism according to which a human person inhabits and uses a living, organically human body while that body is in a certain state of development and health, but at other times (earlier and in many cases also later) is absent from it because the body, though living, cannot yet or can no longer support personal existence. But dualism – every such attempt to distance human bodily life from person or selfhood – has been subjected to devastating philosophical criticism. For a dualistic account of personal existence undertakes to be a theory of something but ends up unable to pick out any unified something of which to be the theory. More specifically, it sets out to be a theory of one's personal identity as a unitary and subsisting self – a self always organically living but only discontinuously conscious, and now and then inquiring and judging, deliberating and choosing, communicating, etc. – but every dualistic theory renders inexplicable the unity in complexity which one experiences in every act one consciously does. We experience this (complex) unity more intimately and thoroughly than any other unity in the world; indeed, it is for us the very paradigm of substantial unity and identity. As I write this, I am one and the same subject of my fingers hitting the keys, the sensations I feel in them, the thinking I am articulating, my commitment to write this paper, my use of the computer to express myself. Dualistic accounts, then, fail to explain *me*; they tell me about two things, other and other, one a nonbodily person and the other a nonpersonal body, neither of which I can recognise as myself, and neither of which can be recognised as me by the people with whom I communicate my perceptions, feelings, thoughts, desires and intentions by speaking, smiling, etc. Careful philosophical reflection on human existence rejects the casual, opportunistic dualism of the many bio-ethicists who want to justify the non-voluntary killing of small, weak, or otherwise impaired people but, for some ill-explained reason, are reluctant to accept that such killing puts to death persons. It also exposes the arbitrariness with which these bio-ethicists attempt to draw a line between living human beings deemed to be persons and living human beings deemed to be not yet or no longer or never persons.

In short, human bodily life is the life of a person and has the dignity of the person. Every human being is equal precisely in having that human life which is also humanity and personhood, and thus that dignity and intrinsic value. Human bodily life is not mere habitation, platform or instrument for the human person or spirit. It is therefore not a merely instrumental good, but is an intrinsic and basic human good. Human life is indeed the concrete reality of the human person. In sustaining human bodily life, in however impaired a condition, one is sustaining the person whose life it is. In refusing to choose to violate it, one respects the person in the most fundamental and indispensable way.

In the life of the person in an irreversible coma or irreversibly persistent vegetative state, the good of human life is really but very inadequately instantiated. Respect for persons and the goods intrinsic to their well-being requires that one make no choice to violate that good by terminating their life. On the other hand, fair-minded persons may well be unwilling to impose on themselves or their families or communities the burden of expense involved in medical treatment and non-domestic care for the purpose of sustaining them in such a deprived and unhealthy state. To preserve human solidarity with such people, and to respect rather than violate the one good in which they still participate – bodily life bereft of participation in other human goods such as knowledge and friendship – the care to be provided to them need not, I think, be more than is provided (save in times of most desperate emergency) to anyone and everyone for whom one has any respect and responsibility: the food, water and cleaning that one can provide at home. To do less than that (save in desperate emergency when one must attend to more urgent responsibilities) would scarcely be intelligible save as manifesting a choice – perhaps even a choice once made by the patient and set down in some advance directive – to proceed *on the basis that* such patients and/or anyone who is responsible for caring for them would be better off if they were dead. But such a choice involves the intent to terminate life and thus violates a basic and intrinsic good of human persons, and denies such people's still subsisting equality of value and worth, and their equal right to life.

Is this to say that the autonomy of the patient or prospective patient counts for nothing? By no means. Where one does not know that the requests are suicidal in intent, one can rightly, as a health-care professional or as someone responsible for the care of people, give full effect to requests to withhold specified treatments or indeed any and all treatments, even when one considers the requests misguided and regrettable. For one is entitled and indeed ought to honour these people's autonomy, and can reasonably accept their death as a side-effect of doing so.

But suicide and requests which one understands to be requests for assistance in suicide are a very different matter. It is mere self-deception to regard the choice to kill oneself as a 'self-regarding' decision with no impact on the well-being of people to whom one has duties in justice. The point is not merely that 'the death of a person affects the lives of others, often in ways and to an extent which cannot be foreseen'.[16] More importantly, it is this. If one is really exercising autonomy in choosing to kill oneself, or in inviting or demanding that others assist one to do so or themselves take steps to terminate one's life, one will be proceeding on one or both of two philosophically and morally erroneous judgments: (i) that human life in certain conditions or circumstances retains no intrinsic value and dignity; and/or (ii) that the world would be a better place if one's life were intentionally terminated. And each of these erroneous judgments has very grave implications for people who are in poor shape and/or whose existence creates serious burdens for others.

For: If one claims a right to suicide, assistance in suicide and/or euthanasia, one is making a claim which is not and rationally cannot be limited by reference to one's own particular identity and circumstances. Nor can it plausibly be restricted to cases where the person to be killed has autonomously chosen to act on one or both of the two (erroneous) judgments. For the first judgment claims that death – and thus being killed – is *no harm* (indeed may be a benefit). So it renders unintelligible any principled moral exclusion of non-voluntary and even of involuntary euthanasia. And the second judgment, too, cannot be plausibly defended by reasons such that its range of application would be limited to suicide, assisted suicide and voluntary euthanasia; its sense and its grounds alike extend to include non-voluntary euthanasia.

The moral errors underlying claims to a right to assistance in suicide or to voluntary euthanasia are errors which do the most vulnerable members of our communities the great injustice of denying, in action, the true judgments on which depend both the acknowledgment of their dignity and their right to life (and so too all their other rights).

NOTES

1 These definitions of 'voluntary', 'non-voluntary' and 'involuntary' euthanasia correspond to those employed by the House of Lords Select Committee on Medical Ethics (Walton Committee) (see House of Lords Paper 21-I of 1993–94, para. 23), and seem more serviceable than the different definitions offered in Harris, *The Value of Life* (Routledge, London, 1985), 82–83.

2 See Douglas Walton, *Slippery Slope Arguments* (Clarendon Press, Oxford, 1992).

3 Report of the Select Committee on Medical Ethics [Chairman Lord Walton], 31 January 1994 (House of Lords Paper 21-I of 1993–94), paras. 20–21.

4 [1993] Appeal Cases 789.

5 See John Finnis, '*Bland*: Crossing the Rubicon?' (1993) 109 Law Quarterly Review 329–337.

6 House of Lords Paper 21-I of 1993–94, para. 260. Here as elsewhere emphases are by me unless otherwise indicated.

7 Ibid., para. 237.

8 Expressed to the Committee by the British Humanist Association, thus: 'The doctrine of double effect seems to us a sophistry which is morally particularly damaging. When there are two outcomes of a given action, one good and one bad, the action is justified only if the good outweighs the bad in moral significance; and the moral weights of the two outcomes depend on the outcomes and the overall context, and are quite independent of the doctor's self-

described intentions.' Ibid., para. 76.

9 Ibid., paras. 242, 243.

10 Thus the Committee make it clear that they use 'intentional' as equivalent to 'intended' or 'with intent to', and not in the weaker sense (equivalent to 'not unintentional(ly)', i.e. not accidentally or mistakenly or unexpectedly) found in some common idiom and some philosophical treatments of these issues.

11 *The Methods of Ethics* ([1874], 7th edn., London, 1907), 202.

12 See Finnis, 'Intention and side-effects' in R. G. Frey and Christopher Morris (eds.), *Liability and Responsibility* (Cambridge University Press, Cambridge, 1991) 32 at 33–35, 45–46; Lord Goff of Chieveley, 'The Mental Element in the Crime of Murder' (1988) 104 Law Quarterly Review 30 at 42–43.

13 House of Lords Paper 21-I of 1993–94, para. 237.

14 See ibid., para. 239.

15 See e.g. Aristotle, *Metaphysics* XII.7: 1072b14–30.

16 Walton Committee, House of Lords Paper 21-I of 1993–94, para. 237.

3

The philosophical case against the philosophical case against euthanasia

JOHN HARRIS

JOHN FINNIS has produced an elegant and closely argued case against euthanasia. The argument is complex and I would like to take issue with almost all of it, although I think that very often the differences between us are not so great as may at first appear. Of necessity I will have to confine myself to one or two key points.

The case against euthanasia, as Finnis presents it, rests upon three foundations. They are his account of the moral importance of intention, his account of personhood and the distinction he makes between two types of killing. We will accordingly look at these in turn, taking note of some tangential issues along the way.

Before doing so, however, it is good to be able to start with a point of agreement. We both agree that 'there is no morally relevant distinction between employing deliberate omissions . . . *in order to* terminate life ("passive euthanasia") and employing "a deliberate intervention" for the same purpose ("active euthanasia")'.[1] We disagree, however, as will be obvious, as to what precisely counts as 'employing' either acts or omissions to a particular end.

I. THE MORAL IMPORTANCE OF INTENTION

Few would deny that we are morally responsible for the acts that we intend. The crucial issue is whether we are also and equally responsible for things we, voluntarily, bring about, for the things that are the consequences of our free choices. Finnis claims we are principally morally responsible only for what we intend in a narrow sense. We are, on his account, less responsible for things that we voluntarily bring about but do not positively desire, or which are not our primary objective in acting or refraining.

This seemingly clear distinction is complicated to unravel. After drawing this distinction in characteristically robust style Finnis notes that:

> In recent years the English courts have firmly set their face against a view widely and for many years propounded by legal academics, but most clearly put by Henry Sidgwick: 'for purposes of exact moral or jural discussion, it is best to include under the term "intention" all the consequences of an act that are foreseen as certain or probable'.[2]

Finnis rightly suggests that we do not necessarily intend all the foreseeable consequences of our acts, and that Sidgwick and others are wrong to claim otherwise; but goes on to conclude something rather different. Namely that:

> These thinkers claim one *should* have the same moral responsibility for foreseen (or foreseeable?) side-effects as one has for what one intentionally brings about. But that claim depends not on a clear and realistic analysis of action but on a (highly contestable) theory about the content of true moral norms. In a sound theory of human action, the utilitarian construct 'oblique intention' is a mere deeming, a fiction, but the *intention* known to commonsense, law and exact philosophy alike is action's central reality . . . The primary and proper description of one's act . . . morally assessable by reference to relevant moral norms, is settled by what one intends, what one means to do.[3]

I have quoted this key passage of Finnis at length because of a number of issues between us that it raises. Finnis conflates the false claim of Sidgwick and others that oblique intention is somehow intention properly so-called, with the far less vulnerable and quite distinct claim (which it is true they *also* make) that one should have the same moral responsibility for foreseen consequences as for what one intentionally brings about.[4]

Anthony Kenny produced a knockdown argument against the claims of Sidgwick and others that we necessarily intend the foreseen or foreseeable consequences of our actions.[5] However, his example also shows that those consequences are part of what we choose and of that for which we are properly and fully morally responsible. 'If I get drunk tonight', said Kenny, 'I may well foresee that I will have a hangover tomorrow, but it would be false to claim that I intend to have a hangover tomorrow'. True enough, but I am clearly responsible for my hangover; it is something I have done to myself, as is the liver disease which was consequent upon my getting drunk every night.

No sound theory of action could surely ignore things like this that we deliberately do to ourselves.

It is true that the law has been preoccupied with intention as a marker of moral responsibility, hence Sidgwick's concern to bring his conception of moral responsibility within its scope. However, as I have argued at length elsewhere[6] and will suggest again now, it is more plausible to think of our moral responsibility as covering what we knowingly and voluntarily bring about. The differences between, and the rival merits of, these different accounts can be highlighted by discussion of the distinction as Finnis explores it in this example:

> So, in commonsense and law alike, there is a . . . distinction between choosing to kill someone with drugs (administered over, say, three days in order not to arouse suspicion) in order to relieve them of their pain and suffering, and choosing to relieve someone of their pain by giving drugs, in a dosage determined by the drugs' capacity for pain-relief, foreseeing that the drugs in that dosage will cause death in say three days.[7]

Now I must say that I fail to see any moral distinction at all here. If we delete the question-begging and tendentious parentheses about the guilty desire to avoid suspicion, and substitute a more impartial qualification – perhaps '(administered over, say, three days in order to avoid unpleasant side-effects)' – then in each case the drugs have been administered to control pain *and* to bring about the death which will permanently end irremediable suffering. That is what has been done in each case. If the death was not an acceptable part of the act of administering the drugs, then it would not be defensible to administer them for any reason, knowing that death would result.

Finnis sees part of this for he says:

> So if the pain were in any case likely to abate, and the patient was not in any case dying, the imposition of death even as an unintended consequence (side-effect) of pain-relief would normally be grossly unfair and unreasonable, and in law a case of manslaughter though not murder.[8]

The crucial issue is: Who is responsible for what and why? Finnis wants to claim that only where death is intended is full moral responsibility for that death attributable. Where it is an unintended, though voluntarily caused consequence, it is 'morally and legally culpable, not by virtue of the moral and legal norm which excludes intentionally terminating life, but by virtue of other legal and moral norms, those which apply to the causing and accepting of side-effects unfairly or in some other way unreasonably.'[9] The question we must press is: Why would the causing of these side-effects in these circumstances be unfair and unreasonable? Why would bringing about someone's death in this way be an unfair and an unreasonable thing to do?

First, of course, because these 'side-effects' are someone's death. The victim, if she is a victim, is surely less concerned about whether her untimely death is an intended consequence or a side-effect, than in whether or not it occurs at all. And if she is not a victim, but seeks death, then the same is still true. The reason why these effects are unfair and unreasonable cannot be explained without reference to their consequences. They are not free-standing norms that apply whatever the consequences. Her death is unfair if she does not want to die, and unreasonable if her death is too big a price to pay for pain relief. So what makes causing the death morally permissible either intentionally or knowingly, is whether or not the person should die, not whether or not their death should be intended or merely foreseen as a consequence. We can determine neither the morality of the intention, nor that of the voluntary action, nor even the nature of these mysterious 'other legal and moral norms', without *first* determining whether or not *this death is morally permissible in these circumstances howsoever caused*.

If someone should not die in these circumstances then their death should neither be intended nor brought about voluntarily though not intentionally. If they should not die, if causing their death would be unfair and unreasonable or even downright wicked, then it would be equally wrong to bring it about intentionally or voluntarily. Their death should neither be an object nor a 'side-effect' of any free action. And the converse is surely also true, namely that if it is right that they should die in these circumstances (because death is the only reliable and sure way to relieve their suffering and they want to die) then it is morally right to bring their death about for these reasons either intentionally or voluntarily or both.

In section III of his paper Finnis offers a gloss on his account of why intention counts. His answer is simply that 'free choice matters'. I agree. We differ as to what counts as choice, we have different theories of action.

Why what matters is what we voluntarily bring about

If free choice matters, as Finnis and I agree, it matters because of the effects of choosing, whether those effects are defined as 'side' or not. It is important to choose, because choosing makes a difference. Now choosing makes a difference to the person who chooses and it makes a difference to the world. The chooser is a world maker and a character builder at the same time. The chooser is the sort of character who creates this sort of world rather than that. So far I think Finnis and I would agree. The disagreement is over what counts as world building. For Finnis, an agent only builds, and is hence only responsible for, the worlds he intends. For me the agent chooses the world which she voluntarily creates, the world she could have chosen not to create or to create differently, the world which results from her actions (or conscious omissions).

I believe that we are responsible for the whole package of consequences which we know will result from the choices we make. We cannot, I believe, evade responsibility by only narrowly intending some of the consequences of our choices. We are responsible for the consequences of our choices because we know the sorts of world those consequences will help to shape.

With Finnis, I agree that we are the sorts of people who make particular sorts of worlds. Finnis is more interested in moral character – in the state of a person's soul – than what happens in the world. I put more emphasis on the worlds we create than on the sorts of people who create them, although we both agree that *both these dimensions are inseparable parts of a theory of action*. It is the scope of the theory about which we differ.

Intention matters because we are interested in what people do and have done, what is rightly 'down to them'. But for the same reasons, what people voluntarily create also matters, is also down to them and hence is also something for which they are morally responsible; and responsible because it is part of what they have done in choosing freely.

I believe Finnis is marking a distinction without a significant moral difference – not enough of a moral difference to make death defensible when it is a 'side-effect' and not when it is directly intended. The relevant question for the ethics of euthanasia is: Is the distinction sufficiently weighty to justify condemning those whose deaths cannot occur as what Finnis calls 'side-effects', to suffering and a denial of what they believe to be an important and appropriate end to their lives, while those fortunate enough to be vulnerable to death as a side-effect of the administration of analgesics are permitted the death they seek? What matters, I believe, is whether this person should die, not whether their death will be a side-effect.

II. WHAT IS A PERSON?

'In virtue of what (if anything) are people, with all their manifold differences, equal and so entitled to be valued and treated as – not merely *as if*! – equals?' This is the question as Finnis poses it and it is also one that I posed and attempted to answer in my book *The Value of Life*. Finnis's answer to this question is simple and correct. It amounts to defining personhood in terms of certain personhood-enabling capacities. In *The Value of Life*, I argued that the relevant capacity is the capacity to value existence. Finnis identifies two basic capacities, which in combination enable the individuals who possess them to value existence. 'To lose one's life', suggests Finnis, ' . . . is to lose one's very reality as a human being . . . [and] That reality is through and through the reality of a person, a being with the radical capacity to deliberate and choose'.

Finnis claims that every 'living human being has this radical capacity for participating in the manner of a person – intelligently and freely – in human goods'. As stated this is simply false. It was false of Tony Bland after he came to be in a persistent vegetative state. Bland had then permanently lost that radical capacity. On my account he had, at that point, ceased to be a person because he had ceased permanently to possess the radical capacity which Finnis and I agree is required for personhood.

Finnis's problem, as I see it, is that he wants both to hold that the radical capacity to deliberate and choose is definitive and constitutive of personhood and to hold that where 'one's brain has not yet developed, or has been so damaged as to impair or even destroy one's capacity for intellectual acts, one is an immature or damaged person'. He needs persons to have this radical capacity to deliberate and choose, for without it they are not morally distinguishable from cats and canaries. However, he also wants to hold that when human beings lack these capacities, they are still persons, although they then possess no capacities that relevantly distinguish them from cats and canaries. He believes the alternative to his position is a philosophically discredited dualism which divides the person into the body and mind and fails to account for unity in complexity. But his account of the way in which unity in complexity functions, simply fails to make this obscure charge stick.

> As I write this, I am one and the same subject of my fingers hitting the keys, the sensations I feel in them, the thinking I am articulating, my commitment to write this paper . . . Dualistic accounts, then, fail to explain *me*; they tell me about two things, other and other, one a nonbodily person and the other a nonpersonal body.[10]

The account of personhood that I (and others) have developed is not dualistic in this sense. We hold that a person is a unified complex being, but that complexity is part of what it is to possess the radical capacities of intelligence and autonomy – in short, the capacity to value existence. When these are lacking the person has ceased to exist (or has not yet come into being). All the things Finnis mentions as examples of experiencing unity in complexity are dimensions of what it is to have intelligence and autonomy.

They are, as he rightly demonstrates, manifestations of that intelligence and autonomy which has no separate existence. When intelligence and autonomy are permanently lost or have not yet developed, all those complex unified phenomena are also necessarily absent. They come into being together, non-dualistically, and they vanish together – just as they do at death, but not only as they do at death. For example, in persistent vegetative state it is not that the person is absent from the body, it is that, as in death, the body has ceased to be the body of a person. It is a living human body (as in a sense it often is when brain death is diagnosed on a life-support system – it is warm, the blood circulates and so on) but it is not the living human body of a person.

I do not know whom Finnis has in mind when he comments:

> Careful philosophical reflection on human existence rejects the casual, opportunistic dualism of the many bio-ethicists who want to justify the non-voluntary killing of small, weak, or otherwise impaired people but, for some ill-explained reason, are reluctant to accept that such killing puts to death persons.[11]

The position I have outlined in these papers and elsewhere is shared by many bio-ethicists to some degree. It is neither casual, nor opportunistic, nor dualism. If it remains ill-explained it is not for want of trying. Nor does it, as Finnis suggests, pick on the weak. It does not justify the *non*-voluntary euthanasia of any persons however weak or strong. Those persons whose deaths are permitted must autonomously choose to die. It is in disagreement with Finnis to be sure, but it is at least as careful and well motivated as his own philosophy.

III. THERE IS KILLING AND KILLING

Finnis ends by re-emphasising the distinction he believes exists between two types of killing:

> Respect for persons and the goods intrinsic to their well-being requires that one make no choice to violate that good by terminating their life. On the other hand, fair-minded persons may well be unwilling to impose on themselves or their families or communities the burden of expense involved in medical treatment and non-domestic care for the purpose of sustaining them in such a deprived and unhealthy state. To preserve human solidarity with such people . . . the care provided to them need not, I think, be more than . . . the food, water and cleaning that one can provide at home.[12]

If it is known, as it will so often be clearly known, that people this ill cannot long survive with home care alone, or indeed in hospitals with what is sometimes described as 'nursing care only', then by declining to impose on themselves or the community the expense and the burden of care which will effectively preserve such patients' lives, 'fair-minded people' will be effectively condemning them to death.

What else can it be when such fair-minded people are faced with alternative courses of action like these? In one, hospital care, with a full nursing team to turn the patient etc., tube-feeding and perhaps antibiotics, will preserve life indefinitely (in the case of persistent vegetative state for perhaps thirty years or more). In the other, the patient will soon die for want of 24-hour nursing care (three nurses plus expensive machinery), untreated infection or lack of food. To choose home care or its hospital equivalent is to choose death precisely because there is an alternative choice available which will preserve the patient's life.

Again the test is similar to the one proposed by Finnis himself. Would it be legitimate to give such home 'care' to someone with a condition in which he would die at home but make a full recovery to normal functioning (my personhood) in 'hospital'? Certainly to choose the home care is not to treat that individual as the equal of someone treated in hospital. Finnis would admit that such a choice would be unfair and unreasonable. I say it would be unfair and unreasonable *because* it would be to choose to kill the patient.

Finnis is prepared to allow patients to refuse treatment, even by advance directive, so long as they do not refuse treatment in order to commit suicide, or so long as the patients keep their motives secret and the health professionals do not know for sure that 'the requests are suicidal in intent'. Finnis insists that 'requests for assistance in suicide are a very different matter. It is self-deception to regard the choice to kill oneself as a "self-regarding" decision with no impact on the well-being of people to whom one has duties in justice'. Of course, but it is equally self-deception to take a decision, the consequence of which is your premature death, and think that this has no impact on others. It is also surely self-deception if 'fair-minded people' think they are not killing someone when they deliberately choose a regime of treatment which they know will result in the patient's death, when there is an alternative which will keep the patient alive.

Finnis ends by asserting that voluntary euthanasia involves:

> proceeding on one or both of two philosophically and morally erroneous judgments: (i) that human life in certain conditions or circumstances retains no intrinsic value and dignity; and/or (ii) that the world would be a better place if one's life were intentionally terminated . . . the first judgment claims

> that death – and thus being killed – is *no harm* . . . So it renders unintelligible any principled moral exclusion of non-voluntary and even of involuntary euthanasia. And the second judgment['s] . . . sense and its grounds alike extend to include non-voluntary euthanasia.[13]

Both of Finnis's claims here are false. There is no entailment of the sort he describes, because one can sensibly hold that such intrinsic value as life retains is not so important as to deny people the right autonomously to terminate their own life along with its remaining intrinsic value. It is rational to believe that life without autonomy, or where autonomy is denied, is not worthless but simply not worth enough. That is perhaps why so many people will fight, and sometimes die willingly, for freedom as they perceive it.

Finnis's second claim is doubly false; it is false that someone who would end their own life must believe the world would be a better place without them. Why should they necessarily believe that? It is also false to claim that the second judgment necessarily 'extend[s] to include non-voluntary euthanasia'. One can rationally hold that even if the world would undoubtedly be a better place without some people (I can think of many living people of whom this is true) one is not entitled to end the life of a person against their will. And if an individual regards their own life as diminished in value *to them*, it does not follow that they are any the less a full person and hence fully entitled to have their life respected by others. Persons are valuable because they have the capacity to value their own lives, not because they *do* value them. Someone who wants to die, even if they have this wish because they have ceased to value their own life, is still a person. We respect the value of the lives of persons *by respecting their autonomy*. It is thus an affirmation of the value of life to respect the wishes of the person whose life it is about the appropriate way for that life to end.

Non-persons, even if human, are as we have seen, a different matter.

NOTES

1 John Finnis, 'A Philosophical Case against Euthanasia' (Chapter 2 in this volume, hereafter 'Chapter 2') p. 25. See my *Violence and Responsibility*, Routledge and Kegan Paul, London, 1980, for a detailed account of why this is so.

2 Chapter 2, p. 26.

3 Ibid., pp. 26–27.

4 It will be noted that I have substituted for the question-begging term 'side-effects', the term 'consequences' in this paraphrase.

5 In a conversation with the author about intention.

6 In my *Violence and Responsibility*, Routledge and Kegan Paul, London, 1980.

7 Finnis holds that it is possible to withdraw treatment from people who will die without it, without any intention of ending their

life. Despite Finnis's identification of his own position with the common tradition, this view is not a common one to take. Even the Law Lords (not noted consequentialist bio-ethicists or opportunists) seem to accept my interpretation here and fail to see a moral distinction precisely where I fail to see one. Lord Mustill, for example, in his judgment in the *Bland* case (detailed in my first essay: Chapter 1 in this volume), concluding that Bland's tube-feeding could lawfully be stopped, said: 'The conclusion . . . depends crucially on a distinction drawn by the criminal law between acts and omissions, and carries with it inescapably a distinction between, on the one hand what is often called "mercy killing", where active steps are taken in a medical context to terminate the life of a suffering patient, *and a situation such as the present where the proposed conduct has the aim for equally humane reasons of terminating the life of Anthony Bland by withholding from him the basic necessities of life*. The acute unease which I feel about adopting this way through the legal and ethical maze is I believe due in an important part to the sensation that however much the terminologies may differ *the ethical status of the two courses of action is for all relevant purposes indistinguishable*.' My emphasis added. [1993] Appeal Cases 789 at 887.

8 Chapter 2, p. 27.

9 Ibid.

10 Ibid., p. 32.

11 Ibid.

12 Ibid., p. 33.

13 Ibid., pp. 33—34.

4

The fragile case for euthanasia: a reply to John Harris

JOHN FINNIS

THE NOTABLE DIFFERENCES between John Harris's essay (chapter 1) and his earlier writings suggest the fragility of the grounds he offers for abandoning our deeply meditated traditions and embracing euthanasia. The ground he marks out is indeed shifting.

I. 'INDIVIDUAL'

Harris's definition of euthanasia, and much of his discussion, employs the term 'individual'. The theme of our exchange, of course, is not abortion. But it would be wrong to overlook his essay's striking assertion that 'the individual can be said to have come into existence when the egg is first differentiated or the sperm that will fertilise that egg is first formed'. Contrast this with chapter 1 of *The Value of Life* (often cited in the essay), where Harris maintained that 'fertilisation does not result in an individual even of any kind' and that 'the emergence of the individual occurs gradually', *after* conception.[1]

In 1985, Harris had two arguments for denying that a human individual begins at conception: that the 'fertilised egg' (i.e. the early embryo) will divide into two elements (the embryo proper, as distinct from the placenta and related tissues), and that some early embryos split to form twins. Both those arguments are quite inadequate bases for denying what the definite article in the otherwise tendentious phrase '*the* fertilised egg' bears witness to: that from conception there is at all stages an individual organic entity. The specification of embryonic tissues into embryoblast and trophoblast, and the development of the latter into the placenta and related tissues, is neither more nor less than the development of an organ *of the embryo*, an organ which it will discard at birth. The division of an embryo into twins or triplets is simply a change from one individual into two; whether or not the original individual was predetermined to become two, we find at all stages of this remarkable biological process nothing other than an individual or two or more individual human beings.

Before conception, on the other hand, it is not possible to say with confidence that 'the egg' will be fertilised. Still less is it possible to say which of many millions of sperm will fertilise it, if it is fertilised. Only the most unreconstructed Laplacean determinist could deny that the identity of the fertilising sperm – i.e. the question which one among the many millions of sperm which are formed at about the same time will in fact fertilise an egg – is a matter partly of chance and other non-determined factors (such as the free choice of the parents to have intercourse at such and such a precise time and in such and such a precise way). The first time at which the egg and sperm referred to by Harris become even in principle identifiable is the time of conception. Only by making an extravagant extrapolation backwards in time from that point can Harris suggest that the individual which emerges in the union of that egg and sperm already constituted an individual – indeed, already constituted *that* individual – from the earlier time when the fertilising sperm was first formed. Harris's willingness to affirm that there is an individual from that earlier time is dependent upon his projecting forward the futures of two individuals (only hypothetically identifiable at that moment).

This willingness to project or extrapolate *individuals* backwards and forwards, in a manner quite foreign to a biologist's understanding of what is and is not an organism, not only stands in uneasy contrast to Harris's 1985 discussion. It also contrasts dramatically (and, I think, inexplicably) with his *un*willingness to project backwards or forwards those *capacities* which characterise the being of *persons*. His arbitrarily constrained conception of *having a capacity* is the basis of his artificial and fragile concept of being a person. It is thus the basis of his claims that a person does not exist until such and such a (very vaguely described) stage in the life of an individual human being, and that a person has ceased to exist before, perhaps long before, the death of the (so to speak) corresponding human individual.

II. 'PERSON'

Like Harris, the tradition has an understanding of persons which 'allows for the possibility of there being non-human persons on other worlds'. That understanding is not anthropocentric; it respects and promotes the human, and recognises inviolable human rights, not because humanity is *our* species and we just do favour our own, but because to be human is to have some share in the dignity of persons. Unlike Harris, however, the common tradition holds that where a product of human conception has the epigenetic primordia of a human body normal enough to be the organic basis of some intellectual act,[2] it is not only a human being or individual but is indeed a person. And such a bodily individual is a bodily person not only from the outset but also, until death, irrevocably, whether or not he or she happens ever to engage in an intellectual act or is prevented temporarily or permanently from doing so by sleep, disease, injury, immaturity or senility. Though there may be bodily persons who are not human, there are no human individuals who are not persons.

Like Harris, the tradition considers that self-consciousness and intelligence are 'criteria for personhood' in one sense of that very elusive phrase. To be a person is to belong to a kind of being which is characterised by rational (self-conscious, intelligent) nature.[3] To have a particular nature is to be so constituted, dynamically integrated, as to have certain *capacities* (e.g. for self-awareness and reasoning). But if being a person ('personhood') were not as radical and fundamental to one's dynamic constitution as being a human being is, but were rather an acquired trait – something as extrinsic and therefore potentially transient as, say, the magnetism of a piece of iron – then one's being a person would not have the significant depth, the dignity, which even Harris acknowledges.

What is distinctive about Harris's position, both in his essay and his book, is his attempt to link *being a person* with *being capable of valuing one's own existence*. Once again, the tradition accepts this link or criterion, provided that 'capable of' is understood as signifying having a nature of the kind whose flourishing involves such valuing, whether or not an individual or such a nature happens to be in a position to exercise those capacities. But if 'capable of' is understood as Harris does, then people's personhood will come and go.[4] If, furthermore, the term 'valuing' is taken to signify a self-conscious intellectual act (such as mice and dogs, though wanting things, presumably cannot perform),[5] then personhood will be so much the more transient and the class of human persons so much the more restricted.

And since the presence or absence of this more than merely animal 'valuing' is so elusive, indeterminate and non-determinable, the class of persons, of *people with equal rights*, becomes, even in principle, a matter of sheer decision, of selecting some point along a spectrum. Then the 'we' in Harris's 'What we have in common is our *capacity* to value our own lives and those of others'[6] takes on the somewhat sinister connotation of a self-defined discrimination between 'us' and 'you' or 'them' (the immature, the mentally defective, the senile . . .).

Harris preserves a discreet silence about Ronald Dworkin's recognition that a person who becomes demented remains a person.[7] But whether or not he in fact agrees with that judgment, the fact is that Harris's criterion of personhood allows him no rational basis for a judgment on the matter. All depends on how strongly and narrowly one understands 'able to value his own life', given that 'to value its own life, a being would have to be aware of itself as an independent centre of consciousness with a future that it was capable of envisaging and wishing to experience.'[8] And why not pick out other features which characterise human nature in its flourishing – say, linguistic articulacy,[9] sense of humour, and/or friendship more deep, transparent and supple than friendship between man and dog? Why not then call one or other or some set of these the capacity which, while it is enjoyed, makes us people and 'entitles an individual to be considered a person'?[10]

It is the fragility of Harris's method that impresses, its character as a process of *selecting grounds* on which to *adopt* a conception of personhood. It is a conception narrower and wider[11] than *humanity*, and it is selected, constructed or interpreted, from a range of conceptions or interpretations, for its apparent congruence with current views about 'the peculiar *status that we give* to creatures possessing such features'.[12]

As the discussion in section I above suggested, Harris fails to understand organic identity, and the *substantial* change – change of organic identity – which occurs at conception and death.[13] His notion of *capacity* is as narrow and shifting as it is because, misconceiving organic identity, he misconceives what he calls 'the potentiality argument' and mistakenly thinks he has refuted 'it'. He misconceives the relevant point as a claim that 'since the fertilised egg is potentially a human being we must invest [!] it with all the same rights and protections that are possessed by actual human beings'.[14] But the relevant argument instead claims that the embryo is actually a human being because it already possesses, albeit in undeveloped or immature form, all the capacities or potential that any other human being has. Harris's counter-arguments fail. They are worth considering here, not because our theme is abortion, but because failure to grasp what is involved in organic integration, unity and identity makes it impossible to give a true account of the changes which an organism undergoes in illness, decay, injury and the process of dying.

Harris's first argument about 'potentiality' is that 'the bare fact that something will become X . . . is not a good reason for treating it now as if it were in fact X. We will all inevitably die, but that is . . . an inadequate reason for treating us now as if we were dead.'[15] This argument fails to grasp the difference between an active capacity and a vulnerability or susceptibility. An organic capacity for developing eye-sight is not 'the bare fact that something will become' sighted; it is an existing reality, a thoroughly unitary ensemble of dynamically inter-related primordia of, bases and structures for, development.

Harris's second counter-argument equally disregards the real distinction between what pertains to one organism and what does not. 'The unfertilised egg and the sperm' [which sperm?] 'are equally potentially new human beings'.[16] But this claim flies in the face of the biological understanding of reality to which it appeals. Even if 'the sperm' could be identified in advance of fertilisation (as even in principle it cannot), there is no sense whatever in which the unfertilised ovum and that sperm constitute one organism, a dynamic unity, identity, whole. The zygote is precisely that: a new human being. It will remain one and the same (unless it twins) until its death, whether days or decades later. The same organising principle which integrates a human individual and directs his or her development continues to do so until death. So this individual remains the same organic individual even if gravely impaired by immaturity, senility or illness.

Someone may say that to speak of organisms is one thing but to speak of persons quite another. And it is true that just as physics as such knows nothing of chemical compounding, and chemistry as such knows nothing of the living cell, so biology as such knows nothing of persons. But a philosophical anthropology attentive to all the relevant data, including biological and zoological realities, can make a well-grounded affirmation of the personal nature of the human organism. An organism of human genetic constitution normal enough to provide, or develop sufficiently to provide, at least the organic basis of some intellectual act is a personal entity, even when too impaired to perform such an act. To deny this is either to ignore the personal characteristics of normal adult human existence (characteristics most perfectly represented by the bodily-intellectual reality of language), or else to embrace a kind of dualism according to which a person temporarily *inhabits*[17] an organism. That kind of dualism is unsustainable for reasons some of which I sketched in my first essay (Chapter 2).[18]

III. 'CRITICAL INTERESTS'

We now reach the most interesting aspect of Harris's essay – interesting not least for its divergence from the position advanced in his book *The Value of Life*. It is the theory, which he adopts or perhaps adapts from Dworkin, of *critical interests*. The link between this new theme and the matters just discussed can be seen in Harris's remarkable thesis: a human being who – or rather, which, or that – has ceased to be a person may nonetheless retain critical interests. One can have a critical interest, he says, even when one can no longer want or value anything; Tony Bland, when 'no longer a person', 'could and did still have critical interests'.[19] This whole thesis dramatises the artificiality of Harris's conception of personhood. The idea of critical interests also, as I shall argue, undermines his case for voluntary euthanasia and his 'liberal' objections to the 'tyranny' or 'paternalism' allegedly involved in proscribing it.

Harris makes some acute observations on Ronald Dworkin's case for euthanasia. But, so it seems, he now accepts the idea which Dworkin names *critical interests*.

Dworkin distinguishes between experiential and critical interests. One's experiential interests, he says, are one's interests merely because one likes the experiences involved in satisfying them; and 'the value of these experiences . . . depends precisely on the fact that we do find them pleasurable or exciting *as experiences*.'[20] But critical interests are 'interests that it does make [one's] life genuinely better to satisfy, interests [one] would be mistaken, and genuinely worse off, if one did not recognise.'[21] So these are not just interests which one happens to have and happens to want satisfied. Rather they are 'critical' precisely because they are interests which one judges one '*should* want' (Dworkin's italics).[22]

> [W]e not only have, in common with all sensate creatures, experiential interests in the quality of our future experiences but also critical interests in the character and value of our lives as a whole. These critical interests are connected . . . to our convictions about the intrinsic value . . . of our own lives. A person worries about his critical interests because he believes it important what kind of a life he has led, important for its own sake and not merely for the experiential pleasure that leading a valuable life (or believing it valuable) might or might not have given him . . . he is the kind of creature, and has the moral standing, such that it is intrinsically, objectively important how his life goes.[23]

Harris notes, indeed headlines, that 'critical interests are objective'. He notes how this objectivity entails that one can misunderstand what is important about life and mislocate one's critical interests, and how this possibility provides the basis for a 'defence of paternalistic interference with an individual's desires "in her own critical interests"'. He seems unhappy with this implication of the notion of critical interests, yet rejects neither the soundness of the implication nor the notion of critical interests itself. Indeed his essay concludes by accepting and deploying the notion, if not the implication, with some enthusiasm. He seems not to see what havoc it plays with his fundamental conclusion that forbidding voluntary euthanasia is 'a form of tyranny which like all acts of tyranny is an ultimate denial of respect for persons'.

Harris's allegation about the tyrannical character of laws found in all civilized states cannot be sustained. The argument of section IV of my first essay (Chapter 2) is here reinforced by the conception of critical interests. For if it is the case, as I argued, that those who choose to ask to be killed are (in Harris's paraphrase of Dworkin) 'tragically misinterpreting' their own life and its meaning – not to mention the meaning and value of the life of any bodily person and thus any human being – it must also be the case that action to prevent persons from acting on such a misinterpretation need involve no 'ultimate denial of respect for persons' but rather can manifest the most profound respect for persons, including even the persons so prevented.

I suspect that Harris hopes to escape this implication of the idea of critical interests by 'reinterpreting' the idea. On Dworkin's understanding of it, what is objectively important is how one's life goes, and one can rightly speak of the 'intrinsic, cosmic importance of human life itself'.[24]

Harris hopes, I think, to replace this understanding of *critical interests* with a more subjective understanding of it: what is 'of intrinsic, cosmic importance' (as Harris puts it) is the individual's *opinions about* what it means for his or her own life to go well. But this subjectivising of Dworkin's conception cannot be carried through without abandoning the very notion of critical interests. Dworkin could of course accept, and may well in fact accept, that amongst the items of cosmic importance are the strong and genuine preferences and self-referential opinions of persons – right or wrong. But there is no plausibility whatever in the notion – which seems to be what Harris is hinting at – that the *only* items of cosmic importance are the preferences or self-referential opinions themselves, regardless of their rightness. If nothing else about human existence and its forms and conditions be of objective importance, there are no grounds for thinking that the sheer fact of having an opinion or preference *is* of such importance and does call for such respect.

As Dworkin says, in a passage quoted by Harris with qualified approval, opinions about the importance of human life concern values which 'no one can treat . . . as trivial enough to accept other people's orders about what they mean'.[25] Swept along by his prejudicial rhetoric about 'orders' and his imminent declamation about 'devastating, odious tyranny', Dworkin fails to see that his thesis in this passage cuts both ways. Since the 'values' are indeed as important as he says, one can hardly treat them as trivial enough to stand idly by when someone within one's care makes a mistake about them which threatens to have irreversible consequences, directly for that person and indirectly for others. Harris in turn fails to see that if the values themselves lack 'cosmic importance', so too must people's opinions about them. For if a human person's very being, self and flourishing or ruin are of no cosmic importance, it is mere baseless conceit to attribute that kind of importance (as Harris does) to people's self-assessments or self-disposition.

IV. NON-VOLUNTARY AND INVOLUNTARY EUTHANASIA

Harris says 'the real problem of euthanasia is the tragedy of the premature and unwanted deaths of the thousands of people in every society who die for want of medical or other resources'. By thus deliberately treating *intention to kill* as irrelevant, Harris wilfully obfuscates the debate about euthanasia. According to him 'whenever life-saving resources are "spent" on things other than saving lives',[26] those who decide to spend these resources on something other than saving life have (or treat themselves as having) 'moral reasons for killing' the person whom they could have saved, and are indeed killing that person.[27] Since money can almost always buy life-saving resources, almost everyone who spends money on anything other than such resources is deciding to kill, and killing. This debauching of our language by Harris is most readily explicable as intended to soften up his readers to support wide programmes of deliberate, intentional killing.

The definitions of voluntary and non-voluntary euthanasia offered in his first essay (Chapter 1) are significantly different from those offered in his book, *The Value of Life*. But all are syntactically misleading. The phrase common to all of them, 'decision that a particular individual's life will come to an end', would be taken in good faith by most readers as meaning the same as 'decision *to* bring an individual's life to an end', i.e. a decision executing a choice or *intention to* terminate life (whether by 'act' or omission). But Harris intends the phrase to include decisions by Parliament not to increase the health budget by the sums that would be required to save every life that could be saved – i.e. all decisions to spend money on something other than life-saving. On this basis, he can freely and quite misleadingly denounce 'the government's euthanasia programme'.[28] His definition's allusion to 'a *particular* person's life' is thus a red herring, and it is hard to think of any appropriate reason for his including it.

Harris is fully entitled, of course, to argue that more should be spent on life-saving, and that failure to do so is very culpable. He is fully entitled to argue (though he will be mistaken in doing so) that the distinction between what is intended and what is merely accepted as a side-effect has no moral significance. But it is, I suggest, profoundly misleading of him simply to ignore the distinction, without fair notice, and to hijack the term 'murder' – which centrally connotes *intention to kill*, both in law and common morality – by claiming, as he in substance does, that any governmental or private limiting of life-saving is 'involuntary euthanasia or murder'. This sleight of hand even does duty to relieve him of his obligation to *argue* that such limiting is unjustified.

Meanwhile, everyone should notice what the moral principles, the conception of value and the conception of responsibility employed by Harris entail. On his view of things, there is no barrier of principle which excludes either non-voluntary euthanasia (whether on his definition or Walton's and mine) or involuntary euthanasia (again, on his or my definition). Even his 'liberal' conception of respect for people's 'autonomy' is subject to a tacit qualification that autonomy, being one value among many, can be outweighed.[29] Since the weights and measures for this 'balancing' of values are not supplied by reason, our right not to be deliberately killed could scarcely – if Harris were correct – be a right, so radically subject would it be, even in principle, to the sentiments of those who subscribe to arguments like his. Shifting, unsteady ground.

NOTES

1 Harris, *The Value of Life* (Routledge and Kegan Paul, London, 1985 and 1992), p. 11.

2 Thus a hydatidiform mole, though an organic individual with human origins and a human genetic structure, is not a human person.

3 See e.g. David Wiggins, 'Locke, Butler and the Stream of Consciousness: and Men as a Natural Kind', *Philosophy* 51 (1976) 131–158 and the works cited in his note 33. Wiggins integrates Locke's conception of personhood into his own more adequate account.

4 Sometimes the capacity is understood by Harris in such a narrow and stringent way that it becomes equivalent to exercising the capacity. Thus he says (*The Value of Life*, p. 18): 'To value its own life, a being would have to be aware of itself as an independent centre of consciousness, existing over time with a future that it was capable of envisaging and wishing to experience. Only if it could envisage the future could a being want life to go on, and so value its continued existence . . . On this concept of the person, the moral difference between persons and non-persons lies in the value that people *give to their lives*. The reasons it is wrong to kill a person is [*sic*] that to do so robs that individual of something they value and of the very thing that makes possible valuing

anything at all' (emphasis added).

5 'For valuing is a conscious process and to value something is both to know what we value and to be conscious of our attitude towards it': ibid., p. 15. But apes and perhaps some other creatures satisfy Harris's own understanding of his criteria for being a valuer: ibid., pp. 19–21.

6 Ibid., p. 16.

7 Ronald Dworkin, *Life's Dominion* (Harper Collins, London, 1993), p. 237.

8 Harris, *The Value of Life*, p. 18.

9 'If there are, as there may well be, as many accounts of what it is that makes life valuable as there are valuable lives these accounts in a sense cancel each other out. What matters is not the *content* of each account but rather *that the individual in question has the capacity to give such an account*': ibid., p. 16 (emphasis added to last 13 words).

10 Ibid., p. 14. Some individual human beings, then, are not 'entitled' to be 'considered' persons.

11 'I think that she [Washoe, a chimpanzee] clearly can [speak] and is therefore equally clearly a person': ibid., p. 20.

12 Ibid., p. 15 (emphasis added).

13 And, it seems, in the relatively rare case of twinning.

14 Ibid., p. 11.

15 Ibid., p. 11.

16 Ibid., p. 11; see also p. 12.

17 See e.g. Ronald Dworkin, 'The Right to Death', *New York Review of Books*, 31 January 1991, 14 at 17.

18 See also David Braine, *The Human Person: Animal and Spirit* (Duckworth, London; University of Notre Dame Press, 1993). (This is a book which itself is in more ways than one a triumph of the human as described in its sub-title.)

19 'An important feature of critical, as opposed to experiential, interests is that they survive the permanent loss of the capacity to know whether or not these interests are being fulfilled': Harris, 'Euthanasia and the Value of Life' (Chapter 1 in this volume). Why this should be so Harris never, I think, even vaguely indicates.

20 Dworkin, *Life's Dominion*, p. 201.

21 Ibid., p. 201.

22 Ibid., p. 202. Dworkin illustrates his point: 'Having a close relationship with my children is not important just because I happen to want the experience; on the contrary, I believe a life without wanting it would be a much worse one.'

23 Ibid., pp. 235–236.

24 Ibid., p. 217.

25 Ibid., p. 217.

26 Harris, *The Value of Life*, p. 260.

27 Ibid., pp. 65–66.

28 Ibid., pp. 84–85.

29 See ibid., p. 66.

5

Final thoughts on final acts

JOHN HARRIS

THE TONE of Finnis's contribution to these exchanges about the ethics of euthanasia has two noteworthy features. The first is his penchant for attesting to the truth of his own assertions. His response to my first essay does this in the very title and repeatedly thereafter; his own first contribution, perhaps following Sidgwick, also repeatedly purports to confirm the truth of its own claims. In one orgy of self-endorsement, within the space of fourteen lines, he describes his own claims, directly or obliquely, as 'sound' (twice), 'common sense' (twice) and once each as 'true', 'exact philosophy', 'proper description', 'clear and realistic analysis', 'primary and proper description', 'straightforward, non-artificial' and 'substantive'. If only saying so could make it so!

The second is his apparent willingness to attribute the most discreditable of motives to those with whom he disagrees. When he concludes his second essay (Chapter 4) by asserting: 'This debauching of our language by Harris is most readily explicable as intended to soften up his readers to support wide programmes of deliberate, intentional killing', he is using the language of the holocaust. To invoke such an image to suggest that I am attempting to incite the commission of mass murder is, to put it as mildly as I can, unworthy. The passage to which Finnis refers explicitly argues against the killing of people who have not consented to die.

In this brief final fling in our exchanges about euthanasia I will take up some points made by Finnis in his second essay (Chapter 4) and re-emphasise what I take to be the crucial issue between us. I will start with his discussion of critical interests and then move to individuality and personhood.

I. CRITICAL INTERESTS

Finnis makes great play with the thought that I now accept 'this idea which Dworkin names *critical interests*'. Well, I do accept it and have done for a long time, in the sense that I think there are such things as critical interests or, as I called them some time ago, 'persisting interests'.[1] However, Finnis misconceives the whole argument about such interests as deployed in my first essay (Chapter 1). I do not attempt to replace Dworkin's conception of critical interests 'with a more subjective understanding' of such interests. I do not rely on it in any sense. Rather I attempt to show that Dworkin's use of such interests and the role they play in his argument effectively reduces such interests to claims about autonomy. I then argue that critical interests ultimately play no role at all in the argument, either because they reduce to claims about autonomy or because they are subordinate to such claims. I am glad Finnis found so much to interest him in this part of the discussion, but his criticisms all miss the point. Let me repeat what I said in the first essay (Chapter 1):

> So Dworkin's rich and interesting analysis of the sanctity of life, encompassing a combination of natural and personal investment in life and respect for an individual's critical interests, reduces, when the chips are down, to an individual's 'opinions about what it means for his own life to go well', and . . . I do not believe it plausible to suppose that they are significantly more important than an individual's desire to control his or her own destiny, which will include preferences about the manner and timing of his or her own death.[2]

I end the first essay (Chapter 1) by repeating my explanation of the wrong done when we deny people the right to euthanasia. Denial of euthanasia is wrong, not because it involves the frustration of critical interests, but because:

> it is simply a form of tyranny; an attempt to control the life of a person who has her own autonomous views about how that life should go. The evil of tyranny does not require explication in terms of the nature of the sanctity of life, but rather in terms of respect for persons and of their autonomy.[3]

II. INDIVIDUALITY AND PERSONHOOD

Finnis has a lot of trouble with the notion of individuality. It is perhaps my fault because I did not quote the full argument behind my assertion that 'the individual can be said to have come into existence when the egg is first differentiated or the sperm that will fertilise that egg is first formed'.[4] I was indeed extrapolating back from adulthood in order to explain why it might be reasonable to say that material changes (in the genetic constitution for example) that are made to the gametes, are part of the life history of an individual.[5] It does not follow that the egg, say, is necessarily the same individual as the adult it eventually becomes, any more than the zygote could logically be the same individual as each of the twins it becomes, if it twins (although Finnis seems to think that it could).

While it is possible to talk of the origins of an adult person in the gametes from which she developed, you cannot extrapolate capacities back and forth. This is because an individual either possesses a capacity or she does not. Misunderstanding of this point leads Finnis to make a fairly basic mistake about the nature of capacities.

> What is distinctive about Harris's position, both in his essay and his book, is his attempt to link *being a person* with *being capable of valuing one's own existence*. Once again, the tradition accepts this link or criterion, provided that 'capable of' is understood as signifying having a nature of the kind whose flourishing involves such valuing, whether or not an individual of such a nature happens to be in a position to exercise those capacities. But if 'capable of' is understood as Harris does, then people's personhood will come and go.[6]

Finnis, it will be noted, constantly contrasts what I say with what he calls 'the common tradition', with which he aligns his own views. I am not averse to being in a minority of one, but while Catholic theology certainly constitutes *a* tradition it could hardly be fairly described as *the common* tradition. However, the main difficulty is how he understands what it is to possess a capacity. Finnis's understanding of capacities allows him to say that an individual *possesses* a capacity which she never *acquires* nor ever has the *power to exercise*. On the Finnis understanding, a zygote *actually has* the capacity for self-awareness and reasoning, even if it dies before ever developing either of these capacities. This, I am afraid, is just nonsense. The ability to speak French and ride a bicycle are capacities possessed by an individual if and only if they are things the individual in question is capable of. They develop with practice and the acquisition of knowledge and could not sensibly be said to be possessed by anyone who has not a word of French and always falls off his bicycle.

My conception of personhood does not permit capacities to come and go (at least not more than once, which even in Finnis's conception they sometimes do). What Finnis has in mind, I guess, is the familiar problem of whether or not people possess the capacity for self-consciousness, or for speaking French, while asleep or unconscious. The answer is simple, though not always simple to ascertain. I have retained while unconscious the capacity to speak French, or while my leg is broken to ride a bicycle, if, when I regain consciousness or my leg mends, I can once again speak French and ride a bicycle without having to acquire these capacities again *de novo*. It is true of me that I speak French and can ride a bicycle and these remain true facts about me even when I am asleep or unconscious. In those states I possess capacities which I am temporarily unable to exercise. I have not lost those capacities, for if I had I would have to re-acquire them each morning on waking. The zygote, of course, has yet to acquire any of these capacities.[7]

In the centre of Finnis's discussion of capacities comes more of what he himself (when talking of others) characterises as 'prejudicial rhetoric':

> Then the 'we' in Harris's 'What we have in common is our *capacity* to value our own lives and those of others' takes on the somewhat sinister connotation of a self-defined discrimination between 'us' and 'you' or 'them' (the immature, the mentally defective, the senile . . .).
>
> Harris preserves a discreet silence about Ronald Dworkin's recognition that a person who becomes demented remains a person.[8]

I may preserve a silence, but I find it difficult to keep a straight face when presented with such inept innuendo. The reason I preserve a silence is not, as Finnis tendentiously implies, discreetly, in the hope that no one will notice that my position denies the demented personhood, for the simple and sufficient reason that it does not. Almost no people suffering from dementia or 'senility' will have lost the capacity to value existence and hence personhood. Perhaps one to five percent of those diagnosed with dementia will have lost all capacity for self-consciousness. This small percentage will be in a condition akin to persistent vegetative state, a condition which, even Finnis allows, renders them vulnerable to death-dealing treatment.[9] To imply that my position denies personhood to 'the immature, the mentally defective, the senile . . . ' *en bloc*, is a travesty.

Finnis repeatedly asks: 'which sperm?' will fertilise the egg and insists that the sperm is not, 'even in principle', identifiable before conception. For someone who often talks of his own position in laudatory terms as being 'attentive to all the relevant data, including biological and zoological realities' this is singularly inattentive.[10] There are now frequently used *in vitro* techniques which allow an individual sperm to be inserted into the egg via a pipette, thus identifying it in advance, on some occasions, *both in principle and in practice*. For the record, two slightly different techniques to achieve this are known, by their acronyms, as ICSI (Intra-Cytoplasmic Sperm Injection) and SUSI (Subzonal Sperm Injection).

Finnis ends by claiming that on my view 'there is no barrier of principle which excludes non-voluntary euthanasia'. Since he quotes the very passage in a footnote, Finnis has no excuse for having failed to notice that I explicitly articulate the relevant principle: 'the reason it is wrong to kill a person is that to do so robs that individual of something that they value, and of the very thing that makes possible valuing anything at all.'[11] The wrong of killing is therefore located in the *principle* that it is wrong to take autonomously valued life. Non-voluntary and involuntary euthanasia of persons is always wrong.

Finnis concludes his section on individuality by asserting that the 'individual remains the same organic individual even if gravely impaired by immaturity, senility or illness'. He concedes, however, that 'someone may say that to speak of organisms is one thing but to speak of persons quite another'. He responds by asserting, again, that one can make 'a well-grounded affirmation of the personal nature of the human organism':

> An organism of human genetic constitution normal enough to provide, or develop sufficiently to provide, at least the organic basis of some intellectual act is a personal entity, even when too impaired to perform such an act.[12]

Finnis's position involves the claim that the moral importance of the human individual derives solely from it possessing 'the organic basis of some intellectual act', even if it is so impaired as never actually to develop the capacity to perform such an act.

Finnis insists that the organic basis of the intellectual act is enough. I am unsure what this organic basis could amount to in a one-cell zygote, nor how, if it is possessed by the one-cell zygote, it could be totally absent from the elements, sperm and egg, which, without remainder, form the zygote. However, if it is the intellectual capacity that is important, we are entitled to ask how a creature that has never possessed, and will never possess, the ability, the power (dare I say the capacity) to perform such an act, can be valuable solely in virtue of such a remote (unrealisable and forever unrealised) connection with such an act. Finnis believes that 'if being a person . . . were not as . . . fundamental . . . as being a human being is, but were rather an acquired trait . . . transient . . . then one's being a person would not have the significant depth, the dignity, which even Harris acknowledges'. It should be noted that this is just an unsupported assertion – a claim about how we should *feel*. But if, as Finnis and I both accept, *the dignity comes from the trait, the dignity resides in an individual being a creature which can value existence*, then it is *possession* of the trait that is crucial. Its transience is no more significant than the transience of life itself.

This is why I believe that, despite all the prejudicial rhetoric, we are not so far apart. We both recognise that it is only in virtue of the possession of a capacity to perform some intellectual act that the human individual is morally important. We differ only as to when its plausible to *attribute* such a capacity. We both believe, I do not doubt in good faith, that we have solid grounds for attributing such a capacity to different individuals at different times. We are surely sufficiently close for Dworkin to be right to claim that neither side has the moral right to force someone, through legislation, 'to die in a way that others approve' but which he himself finds unacceptable. I can only repeat that in view of this, it seems to me that opposition to voluntary euthanasia constitutes 'a devastating, odious form of tyranny'.

NOTES

1 *Wonderwoman and Superman*, Oxford University Press, Oxford, 1992, p. 100. I follow Dworkin's usage in these essays for simplicity.
2 'Euthanasia and the Value of Life' (Chapter 1 in this volume), p. 16.
3 Ibid., p. 19.
4 But note the conditional nature of the claim. It is conditional on the coming into being of the person who develops from that individual gamete. See my *Wonderwoman and Superman*, Oxford University Press, Oxford, 1992, Chapter 3, for the full story.
5 Ibid.
6 Finnis, 'The Fragile Case for Euthanasia: A Reply to John Harris' (Chapter 4 in this volume, hereafter 'Chapter 4') p. 48.
7 I grant it is difficult to say precisely when the human infant does acquire them.
8 Chapter 4, pp. 48–49.
9 Although this characterisation of their vulnerability is of course a point at issue between Finnis and me.
10 And perhaps indicates he is not a completely reliable witness as to what 'true' science or 'exact philosophy' demonstrates.
11 *The Value of Life*, Routledge and Kegan Paul, London, 1985, p. 19. In his footnote Finnis erroneously suggests that I conflate *having* a capacity with *exercising* it. This is because, with characteristic attention to all the relevant data, he fails to notice that I explicitly talk of what it takes to value life and not what it takes to possess the capacity for valuing life.
12 Chapter 4, p. 50.

6

Misunderstanding the case against euthanasia: response to Harris's first reply

JOHN FINNIS

JOHN HARRIS's second essay (Chapter 3) depends upon some striking misunderstandings of the positions central to my 'A philosophical case against euthanasia' (Chapter 2). These misunderstandings or misstatements are of more than local or personal interest. They are characteristic of euthanasiast attempts to rationalise the sentiments which are the movement's real guide.

Chapter 3 is notable also for its open reliance upon the thought that there are persons who simply 'should die'. To the notion that there are people who lack the status of 'persons', the thought that some innocent people who concededly do have that status nevertheless *should* die, and so should be killed, adds something equally sinister.

I have not, of course, seen Harris's third essay (Chapter 5). But at the end of the debate readers will, I think, wish to ask: Has Harris offered any clear and settled reason for doubting that all living human beings are people (persons), however disabled? Or for doubting that intention matters to the content of our fundamental rights, and duties of respect? Or that allowing sentiment to preside in these matters will propel us down a slippery slope into fearful oppression of the aged and infirm?

I. RESPONSIBILITY FOR SIDE-EFFECTS

Although he even quotes one of the passages in which I speak about our serious moral and legal responsibility for side-effects of our choices, Harris insinuates that on my 'theory of action' one can 'ignore' all side-effects, such as the hangovers or liver disease one incurs through over-drinking. 'For Finnis, an agent . . . is . . . only responsible for the world he intends'. Battling against this straw man, Harris contends that 'our moral responsibility [covers] what we knowingly and voluntarily bring about'. On other occasions, however, he tacitly acknowledges that my theory indeed affirms moral (and legal) responsibility for side-effects. But his acknowledgments are misshapen.

For he claims that, on my view, we are '*less* responsible for things we . . . do not *positively desire*, or which are not our *primary objective*'; we do not 'have *the same* responsibility', or '*full* moral responsibility' for side-effects. I have italicised the misstatements. Intention, on my account, is not a matter of desire, still less of positively desiring; rather, it is a matter of choosing ends and means, often against the tug of contrary desires. Intention extends not only to primary objectives, but also to secondary objectives and chosen means (however reluctantly they may be chosen). The difference between our responsibility for what we intend and our responsibility for what we choose is not that the latter cannot be 'full', or is necessarily 'less' than (and in that quantitative sense not the 'same' as) the former. It is rather, as the very passage Harris quoted makes clear, a real and often very grave moral responsibility, but one governed, measured and identifiable by moral norms *different* from those applicable to our intending and choosing of ends and means.

Harris's misunderstanding is not merely of my text and my theory of action and account of morality. It is a thoroughgoing misunderstanding of the whole common tradition recently manifested in passages of the Walton Report noted in my first essay (Chapter 2). Where Walton, the law, the common tradition and I all distinguish between giving drugs *to kill* and giving the same drugs *to suppress pain*, Harris 'fail[s] to see any moral distinction at all'. (His changing my hypothetical euthanasiast doctor's motives for taking three days to do the job is quite beside the point.) Each of these two administrations of drugs, says Harris, is '*to* bring about the death'. This claim is false, for the very reasons which Harris acknowledges when he admits, against Sidgwick, that the average drunkard does not drink *to* get a hangover or *to* get liver disease.

Nor does the point depend upon whether the side-effects are altogether unwanted (as hangovers and liver disease usually are) or unwanted in one respect but welcome in another. Suppose a commander orders the bombing of a factory, regretting as a human person the civilian deaths (unwanted side-effect) from inevitable misses but also welcoming as a combatant the impact ('bonus' side-effect) of these civilian deaths on enemy morale. He can truthfully say that (unlike many immorally ruthless commanders) he is not bombing *to* undermine civilian morale at all, but only *to* destroy the factory. This claim will be true if he has in no way calibrated or adjusted his plans so as to achieve civilian deaths – not even as a secondary objective – and if he stops the bombing as soon as the factory is destroyed.

Harris thinks this sort of distinction is of interest only to people who, like me (he says), are 'more interested in moral character – in the state of a person's soul – than what happens in the world'. This contrast is misconceived. The moral principles and norms which rely on the distinction between the intended and the unintended (side-effect) are vastly important for 'what happens in the world'. The effects, 'in the world', of abandoning those principles, so as to treat ends (consequences) as potentially justifying any and every type of means, are and will be enormous. To the extent that we accept Harris's (or Machiavelli's or Bentham's) invitation to set aside moral norms which pivot on intention, and to make moral judgments by looking only to ends or expected or actual results, we become persons and societies of a different sort, we change character in a way that must (*if and to the extent that we are self-consistent*) involve extensive changes in the ways we act and thus in 'the worlds we create'.

Recognition of the absolute human (personal) rights and exceptionless duties of respect, so central to the morality Harris rejects, has had incalculably beneficial effects on these worlds, i.e. on the real people who would otherwise be the victims of acts intended to suppress their life. The beneficial effects on character, on the souls of those who unconditionally respect personal dignity, have been and are side-effects (albeit inbuilt and welcome), not the primary motivation of that respect. It is, as Elizabeth Anscombe has observed, 'quite characteristic of very bad degenerations of thought on such questions that they sound edifying'.[1] She was speaking precisely of the thesis which Harris articulates thus in his second essay (Chapter 3); 'the agent chooses . . . the world which results from her actions (or conscious omissions) . . . we are responsible for the whole package of consequences which we know will result from the choices we make.' This sounds edifying. So too does Harris's later claim that those who choose a regime of treatment which results in earlier death are choosing to kill because there is an alternative which (at whatever cost) will delay the patient's death. But such claims are manifestations of a thought which is manifested also by one of Harris's claims on which I commented in my second essay (Chapter 4): when Parliament chooses to spend funds on education which might have been spent on life-saving surgery it is choosing and running a programme of euthanasia. The same thought entails also the conclusion that when one chooses to take one's children for a walk, thus passing up the opportunity to take a plane to Calcutta to save street children, one is responsible for the deaths of – indeed, is choosing to kill (by omission) – those far-away street children.

Taken with the refusal to acknowledge that there are moral norms which relate precisely to what one intends as distinct from what one foresees and causes as a side-effect, this thought yields the conclusion that intentional killing – indeed as much intentional killing as seems likely to promote overall human welfare – is not merely justified but actually required. The degeneration involved in reaching such a conclusion is not only of personal and social character, with grave consequences for everybody (the world). It is, in Anscombe's words, a degeneration *of thought*, a refusal or failure to attend steadily and openly to reality, to real distinctions between trying to get and accepting, and to real and insuperable limitations on our knowledge and capacities and thus on our responsibility.

II. PEOPLE 'WHO SHOULD DIE'

Harris misunderstands that common tradition of moral thought, and thus too my first essay, when he offers to explain why, as I said, it could well be grossly wrong to administer pain-killing drugs for the purpose exclusively of relieving pain (and in no way intending to kill) but knowing that the dosage is liable to kill someone who might otherwise recover from their illness. He thinks that what makes such a knowingly though not intentionally lethal administration immoral is that, independently of any moral assessment of the choice to administer drugs, the person in question 'should not die'. Correspondingly, there are people who (he says) 'should die', and to whom drugs can therefore rightly be administered precisely with the intent to kill them.

Harris's willingness thus to categorise *people as people who should live* and *people who should die* is a vivid illustration of the change of character, heart – and thus of conduct and world – which is introduced by the shift from the common tradition to his consequentialist ethic. In the common tradition, the question whether a lethal but not intentionally lethal act or omission[2] is culpable is answered not by making such a categorisation. Rather it is answered by considering the interrelationships of the various competing responsibilities of the person whose acts or omissions are under consideration (who could also be the person whose life is at stake).

It can be perfectly reasonable to *feel* that death would be a welcome relief for someone suffering from hopeless debility or illness, or from intense and intractable pain, and to *wish for* that relief from suffering which death promises to bring. It cannot be reasonable to form the *judgment* that all things considered this person would be better off dead, or the world would be better off if this person were dead, or this person is someone who *should die*. Nor can it be reasonable to rely upon that judgment to 'outweigh' the reason which every basic and intrinsic good of a person gives one not to choose to destroy that basic good (see section III of Chapter 2). Making and relying thus upon such a judgment irrationally ignores the incommensurability of the personal goods and bads, and the incalculable perils and opportunities, involved in the life and death of anyone. It unreasonably treats the dignity of the person (whose life is his or her very existence as a person) as if it were a factor which like money or other instrumental goods can be weighed in a balance and found wanting.

The morality of choices which involve no intent to kill or harm but foreseeably will result in death is to be assessed by reference to moral standards of which the most important and pervasive is the standard of fairness, the Golden Rule. This is a *rational* standard, identifying and critiquing the unreasonableness of discriminating between persons (other than for reasons e.g. of commitment or vocation). But in determining what counts as discrimination, the Golden Rule relies primarily upon the measure of *feelings*. Do to others as you *would be* (i.e. feel willing to be) done by. Do not do to others what you would not feel willing to do to those for whom you feel affection. And so on. (To play this proper and necessary role in giving content to a rational standard (fairness), such feelings must be coherent with the other requirements of practical reason – acknowledgment of the worth and pursuitworthiness of all the basic personal goods, fidelity to reasonable commitments, and so forth; but within the forms and limits established by those rational considerations, *feelings* (which themselves are not rational) *about the consequences of one's options* can be one's measure and guide in deliberation.) By such a discernment of feelings one can measure the extent of one's responsibility to undergo burdensome treatments to preserve or restore one's own health; or of one's responsibility to impose on one's family or heirs or society the costs of expensive treatment (whether of oneself or of others) which promises rather little improvement.

In this way (here only sketched) one can justifiably make decisions and choices which one knows will or may well have the death of oneself or another person as their side-effect. And one can reasonably reach such decisions without ever making a judgment of the form: this person is a *person who should die*. Such judgments are not only irrational, hubristic, and in their practical implications deeply sinister. They also are not necessary to the identification and justified rejection of treatment which is burdensome or futile, and thus excessive, inhumane or unfair.

Each of Harris's attempts to explain how causing death as a side-effect can be unfair and unreasonable is, in fact, absurd. First he suggests that it is unfair 'because these "side-effects" are someone's death'. But this ignores the many cases where such a consequence is the inevitable outcome of a 'triage' situation, or where death could be averted only by heroic efforts and expenditures far out of line with people's normal willingness to accept *lethal* risks avertable only at great expense. Then he suggests that it 'is unfair if she does not want to die'. But this ignores those cases where a person's wish could be satisfied only by imposing on others burdens which she would not accept if she were in their shoes. Finally he proposes that the fairness or unfairness of causing death depends on the judgment whether or not 'the person should die' – a judgment for which no criteria are offered except the implicit appeal to an imagined assessment of how killings of innocent persons would, overall, sufficiently (!) diminish 'the level of suffering in the world' or perhaps sufficiently enhance some other 'very weighty cause'.[3] But this, as I have argued, absurdly exaggerates the power of human reasoning to commensurate the consequences of choices, and overlooks the dignity of the persons whose intrinsic goods make rational claims to our untradable respect.

For good measure, this paragraph in Harris's second essay (Chapter 3) ends by openly asserting that the morality of causing death (whether intentionally or by side-effect) cannot be determined without 'first determining whether or not this death is morally permissible in these circumstances howsoever caused'. That is a hopelessly vicious circle. It also involves a category mistake about permissibility, which is predicable only of actions and their consequences precisely as such, and not of events or occurrences considered prior to any consideration of a human action.

In this same essay, Harris more than once suggests that 'the persons whose deaths are permitted must autonomously choose to die'. This purported restriction of permissible euthanasia to voluntary euthanasia must be taken cautiously and with a large pinch of salt. Cautiously, because as he says in the essay's chilling final words, 'non-persons, even if human, are . . . a different matter'. And with a large pinch of salt, because in his book *The Value of Life* (1985, 1992) Harris unambiguously affirms that the persons who may rightly (indeed should) be killed include not only those who autonomously choose to die but also 'those who are living in circumstances to which death is preferable or who face a future in which this will be true, but who are unable to express a preference for death',[4] and also those other innocents whose death, although not desired by them, is expected to 'promote [ ] other values' of sufficient weight.[5] Are Harris's present essays really recanting his book's promotion of both non-voluntary euthanasia and the deliberate and intentional killing of innocent and unwilling persons? It would be rash to think so.

III. RADICAL CAPACITY, CAPACITY AND DUALISM

The discussion of capacity, personhood and dualism in Harris's second essay (Chapter 3) is another tissue of muddles.

Ignoring, even while quoting, my distinction between 'capacity' and 'radical capacity', Harris claims that I 'want [ ] to hold that when human beings lack these capacities, they are still persons'. But 'these capacities' refers back to his own immediately preceding sentence, in which he says that I 'need [ ] persons to have this *radical* capacity to deliberate and choose'. Thus his exposition severely mangles my claim, which was this. Every living human being has the *radical capacity* to deliberate and choose, even when a given individual human person's capacity to do so – ability to exercise the radical capacity – has been destroyed. And why is this is so? Because, as I said, 'thinking . . . and choosing . . . are *vital* activities, life-functions, actualisations of that *one* radical, dynamic capacity which is actuated in all one's activities, metabolic, sensitive, imaginative, intellectual and volitional.'

The alternative, as I showed, is some kind of dualism which overlooks the *unity* of the bodily and mental in the life of the human being. I recalled the experience we have of this unity – say, the experience (as one composes on a word-processor) of being the single subject of one's fingers hitting the keys, the sensations in those fingers, the thinking one is articulating, and so forth. Harris quotes this passage, and then declares that:

> all the things Finnis mentions as examples of experiencing unity in complexity are dimensions of what it is to have intelligence and autonomy. They are, as he rightly demonstrates, manifestations of that intelligence and autonomy which has no separate existence.

Harris is quite mistaken. I 'rightly demonstrate' no such thing. For some of the things I mention are not 'manifestations' or 'dimensions' of 'what it is to have intelligence and autonomy'. Sensing one's fingers hitting keys, for example, is rather a 'dimension' or 'manifestation' of what it is to be a living body, intelligent or not. Of course, in the human subject bodily life in all its manifestations is a dimension of the *one human life* by which a person composing onto a word-processor *also* exercises and experiences intelligence and autonomy, and by which a sleeping person breathes, metabolises air and food, dreams, and responds to stimuli.

Having thus yet again mutilated my argument, Harris provides a fairly clear affirmation of his dualism. A living human being in persistent vegetative state is 'a living human body' but no longer the body of a person. But this affirmation entails that one and the same living human body at one time was the body of a person and at another time was not. The person comes (at some ill-defined stage in fetal or infant development) and goes (at some ill-defined stage in illness or decay), while the bodily life of the being that can move and perhaps also sense its fingers subsists throughout, until death. This division between person and body is the very dualism to which my arguments were directed, and they remain unanswered.

I called such dualism casual and opportunistic because the grounds for it, e.g. in Harris's *The Value of Life*, seem to me just that. In his case, they are little more than a definition of 'person' resting uncritically on the authority of an under-interpreted and rationally most vulnerable proposal by Locke.[6]

The living principle (dynamic and constitutive inner source) which actively animates, organises and informs every aspect of one's existence from one's conception to one's death establishes, constitutes, one's radical capacity to metabolise, feel, move, notice, understand, respond, want, choose and carry out choices all in a human way. That radical capacity remains even when the breakdown of one or more of one's organs deprives one of the capacity (ability) to exercise that radical capacity in one or more of its dimensions. A Tony Bland in deep and irreversible persistent vegetative state is in a profoundly disabled state. He has lost the capacity (ability) to think and feel – but not the humanity, the *human* life, which until his death goes on shaping, informing, and organising his existence *towards* the feeling and thinking which are natural to human life (i.e. which human life is radically capable of and orientated towards).

The 24-year-old patient 'S.', who died in southern England in January 1994 after the judicially authorised discontinuance of nutrition and hydration and all other life-sustaining measures, was judged by his nurses and at least one of the neurologists attending him to be suffering pain from time to time, making non-verbal noises and moving about in his bed.[7] He was less disabled than Bland, occupying a somewhat different place on the great spectrum of human beings in different states of flourishing and impairment of capacity. That is the spectrum which Harris divides somewhere into two: those states of human life which qualify one as a person and those which qualify one as now a mere living human body without rights or intrinsic value. His division, as I argued in my second essay (Chapter 4), is a matter of sheer decision, so indeterminate and indeed shifting are his criteria.

IV. AUTONOMY, VALUE, AND UNFAIR GROUNDS OF CHOICE

At the end of my first essay (Chapter 2) I argued that if one is really exercising autonomy (not merely yielding to impulse or compulsion) in choosing to kill oneself or to be deliberately killed, one will be proceeding on one or both of two philosophically and morally erroneous judgments: (i) that human life in certain conditions or circumstances retains no intrinsic value or dignity; and/or (ii) that the world would be a better place if one's life were intentionally terminated; and that these erroneous judgments, being inherently universal, have grave implications for the weak and disabled.

Despite Harris's free and not too carefully posited assertions that I was mistaken, my argument stands. But it could be made more precise. The first of the two types of erroneous judgment which I identified could be stated more exactly: (i) that one's human life in certain conditions or circumstances retains no intrinsic value or dignity, or on balance no net value, so that one's life is not worth living and one would be better-off dead.

Against this, Harris asserts that 'one can rationally hold' that even people whose life has no net value have a right not to be killed against their will or without the exercise of their autonomous choice. Harris's use of the indefinite passive phrases 'one can sensibly hold' and 'one can rationally hold' is significant. Whatever others might rationally hold, no one with a theory of value and morality such as Harris's can rationally, i.e. consistently and for reasons, hold that there are human rights (or entitlements and corresponding disentitlements) not grounded in assessments of the overall balance of values and disvalues in the situation. As I indicated at the end of section III above, Harris's book *The Value of Life* contends that many people (persons) can rightly be killed without having made a choice to be killed, and that at least some persons can be killed against their will. Autonomy, in his scheme of things, is a value and can be outweighed by other values, by 'very weighty causes'.[8]

In the common tradition which I have been defending and Harris wishes to replace, autonomy is indeed a great good. But its exercise should be consistent with the rights of others and with all the other requirements of humane and decent behaviour. No man is an island. That is why it is important to try to understand the premises on which autonomous choices are made, to reflect on the implications of those premises. Exercises of autonomy which proceed from premises which are both false and, in their implications, injurious to other members of society, can rightly be overridden by law.

NOTES

1 Anscombe, 'Modern Moral Philosophy', *Philosophy* 33 (1958), reprinted in *The Collected Philosophical Papers of G. E. M. Anscombe*, vol. 3, *Ethics, Religion and Politics* (Blackwell, Oxford, 1981), p. 35.

2 As Lord Mustill (quoted in note 7 of Harris's 'The Philosophical Case against the Philosophical Case against Euthanasia', Chapter 3 in this volume) rightly noted in *Bland*, and as I noted at the end of part I of my first essay (Chapter 2), there is no morally relevant distinction between a positive act intended to achieve an effect and an omission intended to achieve the same effect. The unargued assumption by some of the Law Lords in *Bland*, that the withdrawal of life-sustaining measures was being chosen by the plaintiffs in that case with the intention (aim, purpose) of terminating Bland's life, may well have been a justified assumption on the record of the proceedings in that litigation. But it in no way amounts to a ruling, nor does it in any way entail, nor does judicial or other common sense suggest, that all withdrawals of 'treatment from people who will die without it' must be intended to end their life.

3 See Harris, *The Value of Life* (Routledge and Kegan Paul, London, 1985 and 1992), p. 81.

4 Ibid., p. 78. See also p. 83: 'Non-voluntary euthanasia . . . will be wrong unless it seems certain that the individual concerned would prefer to die rather than go on living under the circumstances which confront her *and* it is impossible to find out whether the individual concerned shares this view' (Harris's emphasis). On Harris's peculiar use of 'wrong', which will allow other cases of fully justifiable non-voluntary (and involuntary) euthanasia, see note 5 below.

5 Ibid., p. 81. Harris sometimes uses the word 'wrong' in a confined, technical and highly idiosyncratic way, according to which an action can be 'wrong' but fully justifiable and precisely the caring thing to do. Thus at p. 83 of *The Value of Life* he sums up his position: 'So that involuntary euthanasia [killing an individual against that individual's express wishes: p. 82] will always be wrong, although it may be *justifiable* for any of the reasons considered earlier' (Harris's emphasis)!

6 Ibid., p. 15. On the incoherences in Locke's account of persons and the arbitrariness in contemporary quasi-Lockean definitions such as Harris's, see B. A. O. Williams, 'Memory and Identity', in his *Problems of the Self* (Cambridge University Press, Cambridge, 1973); Jenny Teichman, 'The definition of a person', *Philosophy* 60 (1973).

7 *Frenchay NHS Trust* v. *S.* [1994] 2 All England Law Reports 403 at 407, 410.

8 See Harris, *The Value of Life*, p. 81.

7

Euthanasia: back to the future

KENNETH BOYD

The Fixed Period (Trollope 1990), Anthony Trollope's science-fiction novel, was published in 1881 but set a century later, on the imaginary island of Britannula, somewhere off New Zealand. The constitution of Britannula, originally a British colony but now a prosperous little republic, provides compulsory euthanasia for all of its citizens on reaching the age of $67\frac{1}{2}$ – Trollope's own age when he wrote the novel. The euthanasia measure, together with the abolition of capital punishment, was freely voted in by the island's first republican parliament. Two arguments carried the day: euthanasia would relieve those who had lived out their 'fixed period' of active life from having to suffer the miseries and indignities of old age; and it would relieve their families and the republic of the cost of maintaining them.

The euthanasia measure was passed, however, at a time when none of Britannula's citizens, all settlers, was aged much above 30. Thirty years later, the first of them to reach his allotted span is about to be 'deposited' at the 'College' where he will enjoy 12 months' preparation for euthanasia. But he is as fit as a fiddle and most unwilling to go – as are the next few citizens in line. The President of the republic, Mr Neverbend, is all his name suggests and insists that the law, which they all agreed to, must be upheld.

In the end, the impasse is broken when the British government sends a gunboat to depose the President, reannex Britannula and repeal the euthanasia law. Mr Neverbend goes into exile to write his memoirs, convinced that while he may have got some of the details wrong, the 'Fixed Period' is an idea whose hour will come. Trollope himself seems to have been ambivalent about this, and the novel is not perhaps one of his best. But his view of late twentieth century euthanasia is not entirely irrelevant to what has actually transpired. I want to use the novel, therefore, to frame some comments related to theology, philosophy and the law, and then to say something about what Trollope failed to foresee, before ending with a practical suggestion.

RELIGION, PHILOSOPHY AND THE LAW

Part of the current debate on euthanasia is a much older debate about suicide, on which religion has traditionally held strong views. In *The Fixed Period*, the British Governor, who is sent out to replace Mr Neverbend, tells the Britannulans that they should 'leave the question of life and death in the hands of the Almighty'. To support this he quotes not Scripture, but Hamlet's remark about 'the Everlasting' having 'fixed his cannon 'gainst self-slaughter'. In Trollope's manuscript, although not in the published version of the novel, a contrary view is expressed by Mr Neverbend. Recalling the original parliamentary debate on the euthanasia measure, he observes that 'we were told that it was against God's ordinance' and he comments (Trollope 1990:175)

> What ordinance? How? When? Where? Quote the words. Show us even by deduction that the Lord has intended that we should keep old men alive in these miseries.

Trollope here, clearly if not consciously, is echoing David Hume's footnote at the end of his *Essay on Suicide* (Hume 1963: 262): 'There is not a single text in scripture which prohibits it'. Hume is not usually cited, of course, as a religious authority. But this and other arguments of the kind he used have greatly undermined the traditional theological and deontological view that suicide is always a grave sin or morally wrong. Hume's rebuttal of the claim that suicide usurps God's role is well-known (Hume 1963: 256f):

> Were the disposal of human life so much reserved as the peculiar province of the Almighty, that it were an encroachment on his right for men to dispose of their own lives, it would be equally criminal to ask for the preservation of life as for its destruction. If I turn aside a stone which is falling upon my head, I disturb the course of nature; and I invade the peculiar province of the Almighty, by lengthening out my life beyond the period which, by the general laws of matter and motion, he has assigned it.

Hume was not the first to question the traditional Christian condemnation and consequent criminalisation of suicide. This was done in earlier centuries by two of the greatest glories of the English Church: St Thomas More by implication in a not unfavourable account of euthanasia in his *Utopia* (More 1951), and John Donne, much more directly and using some arguments similar to Hume's, in his *Biathanatos* (Donne 1982). More recently, while most Jewish, Christian and Islamic authorities have continued to prohibit suicide and euthanasia, awareness has grown that this is not the only religious view of the matter. Some strands of Eastern religion and the Western Stoic tradition, for example, hold that suicide may be justified in some circumstances. Historical examination of the origins of Christian and to some extent Jewish opposition to suicide, moreover, suggests that the strength of this opposition might be proportionately related to the inducement to martyrdom felt by Christians and some Jews in the early centuries (Battin 1982). Later, after the great era of martyrs passed, Christianity continued to commend self-sacrifice, for example in ministering to the sick. By this point it had developed a clearer definition of what distinguished suicide from self-sacrifice – namely suicide's self-regarding as opposed to other-regarding motives. But the trouble with this, of course, is that in a post-Freudian era, this distinction has become harder to discern.

Some of the firmest foundations on which to mount a theological or deontological 'cannon 'gainst self-slaughter', in other words, now seem to have been deconstructed. The discernment of motives is still a crucial part of any moral judgement about a particular case of suicide. But it is now increasingly realised that such judgements are for the conscience of the individual concerned rather than for third parties. Donne sums it up (Donne 1982: 40):

> Thou knowest this man's fall, but not his wrestling, which perchance was such that almost his very fall is justified and accepted of God.

This view of suicide clearly has significant implications for the debate on euthanasia. Their sociological aspect is perhaps sufficiently illustrated by the fact that only a minority in the Dutch Reformed Churches now reject euthanasia absolutely (de Wachter 1992).

Trollope's 'rather grim little jeu d'esprit', as a contemporary reviewer called it (Trollope 1990: xii), may have done more to reflect than urge forward this process of deconstruction – it was not often reprinted. But Trollope had another philosophical movement in his sights, also of relevance today. For all his sympathy for Mr Neverbend, Trollope's portrayal of him also betrays the author's own ambivalence about the antipodean President's utilitarianism. Under the euthanasia law, Neverbend enthusiastically calculated (Trollope 1990: 3f):

> we should save on an average £50 for each man and woman who had departed. When our population should have become a million, presuming that only one in fifty would have reached the desired age, the sum actually saved to the colony would amount to £1 000 000 a year. It would keep us out of debt, make for us our railways, render our rivers navigable, construct our bridges, and leave us shortly the richest people on God's earth! And this would be effected by a measure doing more good to the aged than to any other class of the community!

Trollope's critique of utilitarianism, of course, derived from his civil-service experience of its crasser political and bureaucratic, as opposed to philosophical aspects. But it would be naive to forget that such utilitarian considerations, no doubt expressed in much more plausible and sophisticated terms, may still arise in many people's minds when considering the advantages of euthanasia. So it is not at all unrealistic to fear that legalising euthanasia might put many vulnerable individuals, especially the frail elderly, at risk. Whether this is the greatest fear of many elderly people themselves, and what precisely 'legalising euthanasia' might mean, I shall come back to later. But if the ethics of suicide is to be a matter for individual conscience, the exercise of that conscience clearly should be protected as much from undue utilitarian, as from undue religious external pressures.

The Fixed Period reflects the deconstruction of deontological arguments condemning and criminalising suicide. It also reminds us that, human nature being what it is, we may need a law against euthanasia – or at least one which declines to distinguish between murder and euthanasia. But what is the ultimate justification, not for protecting vulnerable individuals from being pressurised into asking for euthanasia, nor for protecting them against non-voluntary or involuntary euthanasia, but for using the law to achieve this? Trollope deftly raises this question when he makes the British Governor advise the Britannulans to 'leave the question of life and death in the hands of the Almighty'. The Governor says this with his ship's '250-ton steam-swiveller' gun trained on the republic's capital, and as the representative of an imperial power which, unlike Britannula, has not abolished capital punishment.

Trollope's point, of course, might have been more telling for us had he chosen to set *The Fixed Period* a couple of decades or so earlier in the twentieth century – at the time of Suez, well before Britain actually pensioned off the public hangman. Even so, his wry observation does more than simply expose the flank of religious positions which prohibit suicide while being prepared to defend just wars and capital punishment. It also recalls the interesting question posed (since I have mentioned deconstruction) by Jacques Derrida (Derrida 1992: 6):

> How are we to distinguish between the force of law of a legitimate power and the supposedly originary violence that must have established this authority and that could not in itself have been authorized by any anterior legitimacy . . . ?

Applying this question to euthanasia, one might ask: 'Is a social mechanism ultimately based on violence the most appropriate means of protecting old ladies from going to heaven or hell in their own way?' The obvious answer, which all civil servants know, is 'What is the alternative?' To try to answer that, I want now to turn to what Trollope failed to foresee.

MODERN MEDICINE

Noticeably absent from *The Fixed Period* is any role for medicine in euthanasia. President Neverbend has a vague idea that he might do it himself, in Abrahamic fashion, at least for the first few candidates. It is not that doctors do not appear in the novel – in fact they play a crucial part in Trollope's twentieth-century Test Match, by patching up cricketers who sustain near-fatal injuries from their opponents' deadly bowling machines. But more to the point, perhaps, were the injuries of a different kind, which one of the nineteenth-century's most famous physicians sustained as a result of having read Trollope's novel.

Sir William Osler, in his farewell address to Johns Hopkins University before moving on, at the age of 55, to Oxford, referred light-heartedly to 'that charming novel, *The Fixed Period*', with its 'admirable scheme of a college into which at sixty men retired for a year of contemplation before a peaceful departure by chloroform' (Trollope 1990: xii). But Osler's joke misfired – so badly that he had to insert an apology when his address was eventually published. It was ironical that 'Oslerisation' became for a time a synonym for euthanasia. Three years earlier, in an article entitled 'Our attitude toward incurable disease', Osler had written (Cowley *et al.* 1992):

> If a life is worth living at all, it is certainly worth living to the very end, a position from which the conscientious physician has no possible escape in the care of cases which he is called upon to treat.

What Trollope and perhaps Osler could not have foreseen, in other words, was the public reaction to an Oslerian 'attitude towards incurable disease', once that attitude was armed with the technological means and setting of late twentieth century medicine. What many people, including many elderly people, now most fear, and what creates most of the demand to 'legalise euthanasia', is not living beyond 'the fixed period' of active life – which few now regard as ending at $67\frac{1}{2}$ – but of being kept alive in a mentally or physically debilitated or painful state, either by medical technology or in long-term care. This fear is compounded by an awareness that for most people there is no longer any nice, well-known-to-the-family Sir William, who will do the right thing by you when your time comes.

Now most of this, as anyone familiar with health care knows, is no argument for euthanasia – or to be precise, as the Dutch are, for 'the purposeful acting to terminate life by someone other than the person concerned upon request of the latter' (van der Maas *et al.* 1992: 5). The great majority of the lay public's suitable candidates for euthanasia are either (1) elderly people with dementia but without insight into their condition or a living will – in whose case 'purposeful acting to terminate life' may be impossible to justify; or (2) people in whose case there is no justification for euthanasia because their needs and wishes can be met within the agreed terms of 'not prolonging life by disproportionate or extraordinary means' or 'relieving terminal pain by appropriate and necessary means'.

In addition to these people, however, there are at least three groups for whom voluntary euthanasia *may* be justified. They are (1) those, not necessarily near death, but who are totally paralysed and respirator dependent; (2) others, within weeks or months of death, who have either extreme difficulty in breathing or other very distressing symptoms, not necessarily painful, which cannot be relieved; and (3), more controversial, people with dementia, some insight, and who have explicitly requested euthanasia if these circumstances should arise. No less disturbing, to complicate this picture, are all the people whose needs and wishes *could* be met without euthanasia but *are* not, because of a lack of resources, time or skill.

Euthanasia, I am suggesting, should not be needed in the case of this last group, and may or may not be justified in the case of the three other groups whose predicament it may be difficult to relieve in any other way. This still may not be a good argument for 'legalising euthanasia'. But it does seem to reflect a situation which the law finds difficult to handle. The law's problem, I think, in turn reflects a feature of literate as opposed to pre-literate societies which has been well-observed by the anthropologist Jack Goody. This is that 'written formulations encourage the decontextualization . . . of norms' (Goody 1986: 12). For example, as Goody goes on to note (Goody 1986: 167):

> In real life the assessment of a killing depends upon the context and the category. This is true even in literate societies, the reaction depending upon whether the victim is inside or outside the group, whether the act is defined as war, feud, manslaughter or straight murder. But the written code tends to present the complex set of practices in the form of more simplified rules.

Having these general features, then, the present law appears not only to make no distinction between murder and euthanasia, but also so to decontextualise medical treatment as to view it as assault by consent. But a law which shows doctors that this is what it thinks of them, in practice tends to encourage defensive medical practice, and to discourage doctors from empowering patients to make their own sensitively informed choices. Lord Mustill's remarks in the recent House of Lords judgement on the *Bland* case, thus seem applicable to a much wider range of issues. Describing the present legal structure as 'both morally and intellectually misshapen', he called for (*Airedale NHS Trust* v. *Bland* (1993): 891)

> the establishment by legislation not only of a new set of ethically and intellectually consistent rules, distinct from the general criminal law, but also of a sound procedural framework within which the rules can be applied to individual cases.

A PRACTICAL SUGGESTION?

Now this, of course, is easier said than done, and as a theologian I should perhaps now confine myself to cheering the lawyers on from the sidelines. But at the risk of making an unholy fool of myself, let me add a few further points on the way to my eventual suggestion.

I have argued that deconstruction of deontological arguments condemning and criminalising suicide means that the proper place for debating the ethics of suicide is in the individual conscience of the person concerned. I would of course want to hedge that around by saying that the internal debate should be informed and that there are many suicide attempts which others may have a duty to try to prevent, and indeed will be thanked for so doing. But I accept that there are some rational suicides, and by extension that some requests for euthanasia are also rational. What I find more difficult to specify, however, beyond the very general categories I mentioned a few moments ago, are any more precise criteria for determining whether or not a particular request can be justified. The relevant judgement, I think, can only be made as the agreed outcome of a conversation, in some depth, between the person making the request and another individual – a conversation of the kind once described by Simone Weil as one in which 'each one of them, without ceasing to think in the first person, really understands what the other also thinks in the first person'. In these circumstances, Simone Weil argued, justice 'occurs as a natural phenomenon' (Weil 1957).

This argument probably can be traced back to Kant, although his application of it to suicide is too close to the traditional view for it to be fair to cite him for the present case (Paton 1948: 91–93). And of course Simone Weil's own self-sacrifice, a hair's-breadth from suicide, may make her too a problematic counsellor. But a similar point is also made by Derrida, when he writes (Derrida 1992: 17):

> To address oneself to the other in the language of the other is, it seems, the condition of all possible justice . . .

Derrida goes on, however, to point out that this may be impossible to do; and with particular reference to the law, he asks:

> How are we to reconcile the act of justice that must always concern singularity, individuals, irreplaceable groups and lives, the other or myself as other, in a unique situation, with rule, norm, value or the imperative of justice which necessarily have a general form, even if this generality prescribes a singular application in each case?

Derrida's argument, needless to say, is more complicated than this. But the point I want to extract from it is a fairly simple one. At those times when a request for euthanasia *may* be morally justified, the closest we can get to determining whether it *is* morally justified is in the kind of conversation where, in Derrida's terms, one addresses 'oneself to the other in the language of the other', or when, to repeat Simone Weil's words, 'each of one of them, without ceasing to think in the first person, really understands what the other also thinks in the first person'.

This, clearly, is a counsel of perfection. But given the obvious need for anyone requesting euthanasia to understand all their options, I suggest that the closest we can get to this kind of conversation, and hence the closest we can get to determining by its agreed conclusion whether a request for euthanasia is morally justified, is in a conversation between a doctor and a patient. To say this is not to claim that doctor–patient conversations are always or even often of this kind – clearly they are not, and an important aspect of Simone Weil's argument is the immense difficulty of having this conversation when one party is stronger and the other weaker, as is often the case between doctor and patient. Nor is it to deny that for 'doctor' you can sometimes read 'other health worker', or even 'informed friend', or that these others need be excluded from the doctor–patient conversation, even when that may make it more difficult. The point is simply that a doctor–patient conversation, insofar as it approximates to Derrida and Weil's ideal, is the best we can do if we want to determine whether the request is morally justified.

A further point I want to draw from this also is fairly simple. Lord Mustill's desire for 'a new set of ethically and intellectually consistent rules' is, I think, probably asking too much from human nature. In this connection I am reminded, to go back again to the nineteenth century, of Maine's remark about 'the exaggerated respect which is ordinarily paid to the doubtful virtue of consistency' (Maine 1986: 58). But at the same time I am also reminded of two further observations by Maine. The first reflects Goody's point and gets to the root of why the present law still declines to distinguish euthanasia from murder and regards medical treatment as assault by consent. In *Ancient Law*, Maine wrote (Maine 1986: 16):

> Prohibitions and ordinances, originally confined, for good reasons, to a single description of acts, are made to apply to all acts of the same class, because a man menaced with the anger of the gods for doing one thing, feels a natural terror in doing any other thing which is remotely like it.

As a theologian, for whatever that is worth nowadays, I would like to beseech the law to think it possible that it may be mistaken about the gods in this respect.

The second of Maine's observations, from the same book, is what he has to say about his 'three agencies by which Law is brought into harmony with society . . . Legal Fictions, Equity, and Legislation'. The Legal Fiction, an 'assumption which conceals or affects to conceal, the fact that a rule of law has undergone alteration, its letter remaining unchanged, its operation being modified' (Maine 1986: 21f), may be what the Netherlands has opted for and might be seen as an option for England also. But what, speaking as a total legal ignoramus, I find more intriguing is Maine's concept of Equity (Maine 1986: 23):

> any body of rules existing by the side of the original civil law, founded on distinct principles and claiming incidentally to supersede the civil law in virtue of a superior sanctity inherent in these principles.

In terms recognisable by the law, no doubt, the concept of Equity has little or nothing to do with the doctor–patient conversations I have been talking about. But I cannot help feeling that the notion of principles with a 'superior sanctity' must in some way be applicable to the principles inherent in those conversations, and that legislation ought to recognise this, even if at the end of the day the law must reserve a right to preserve patients from assault by maleficent doctors.

My suggestion for the future is very modest. There are, I believe, some people whose request for euthanasia is morally justified; and the best way of determining this is in these conversations. But the law as it stands inhibits many doctors from being open to what the patient really thinks in the first person, because to take this on board in some cases means risking the wrath of the law. This is unjust to any patient whose request for euthanasia is morally justified. We need, therefore, to find some way of creating a buffer between these conversations and the criminal law. How exactly we should do this, I am not qualified to say. But there are precedents: the system of confidential review of perinatal or surgical deaths suggests one way of investigating and supervising the occasions when euthanasia may be necessary. That precedent alone, no doubt, will seem too like an insider enquiry, and a strong public voice will be required. If so, there is the precedent of the growing confidence of lay members on ethics of research committees and on statutory bodies such as the Animals (Scientific Procedures) Committee and other national committees. The development, in the United States, of hospital as opposed to research ethics committees is another important precedent, since one of the main functions of these committees is educational, and continuing education of doctors and nurses in alternatives to euthanasia acceptable to both patients and professionals is crucial.

But no less crucial is the thought, for patients who have come to the end of their tether, that the possibility of euthanasia is always there as a last resort. The reassuring existence of that possibility, paradoxically, may be the best assurance that fewer people will, in the end, require euthanasia. Finally, no procedural framework is likely to provide public reassurance that justice is being done in this difficult area unless far more patients than at present experience conversations which begin to approximate to the ideal I have suggested. The most pressing aspect of the problem of euthanasia, therefore, is how to improve the quality of medical education in ethics and communication.

REFERENCES

Airedale NHS Trust v. *Bland* [1993] Appeal Cases 789.

Battin, M. P. 1982. *Ethical Issues in Suicide*. Englewood Cliffs: Prentice Hall.

Cowley, L. T., Young, E. and Raffin, T. A. 1992. Care of the dying: an ethical and historical perspective. *Critical Care Medicine* 20,10: 1473–1482.

Derrida, J. 1992. Force of law: the 'mystical foundation of authority'. In *Deconstruction and the Possibility of Justice*, ed. D. Cornell, M. Rosenfield & D. G. Carlson, pp. 3–67. London: Routledge.

de Wachter, M. A. M. 1992. Euthanasia in the Netherlands. *Hastings Center Report* 22,2: 23–30.

Donne, J. 1982 (1647). *Biathanatos*. New York: Garland Publishing.

Goody, J. 1986. *The Logic of Writing and the Organization of Society*. Cambridge: Cambridge University Press.

Hume, D. 1963 (1777). *On Suicide*. In *Hume on Religion*. London: Collins.

Maine, H. S. 1986 (1861). *Ancient Law*. USA: Dorset Press.
More, T. 1951 (1516). *Utopia*. London: Dent.
Paton, H. J. 1948. *The Moral Law*. London: Hutchinson.
Trollope, A. 1990 (1881). *The Fixed Period*, ed. R. H. Super. Ann Arbor: University of Michigan Press.
van der Maas, P. J., van Delden, J. J. M. and Pijnenborg, L. 1992. *Euthanasia and Other Medical Decisions Concerning the End of Life*. Amsterdam: Elsevier.
Weil, S. 1957. *Intimations of Christianity among the Ancient Greeks*. London: Routledge.

8

The case for legalising voluntary euthanasia

JEAN DAVIES

> The law is in effect the codification of the will of the people, and when there is such tension between a legal verdict and the people's thinking then it is time to reconsider the law.[1]

The verdict referred to in this *British Medical Journal* editorial is Dr Nigel Cox's conviction for attempted murder.[2] His patient of long standing, Lillian Boyes, who had made her wish for a tranquil death very plain to him, was dying in extreme agony when he gave her a lethal injection. Similar comments were made in the *Lancet*, and most of the quality newspapers; it amounted, in Professor Ronald Dworkin's view,[3] to the launching of a campaign to legalise euthanasia in such cases.

The general expectation was that a Royal Commission would be the appropriate body to examine the issue, but in the event it was a House of Lords Select Committee on Medical Ethics which was set up for this purpose. It reported in February 1994. Its terms of reference were:

> to consider the ethical, legal and clinical implications of a person's right to withhold consent to life-prolonging treatment, and the position of persons who are no longer able to give or withhold consent;
>
> and to consider whether and in what circumstances actions that have as their intention or a likely consequence the shortening of another person's life may be justified on the grounds that they accord with that person's wishes or that person's best interests;
>
> and in all the foregoing considerations to pay regard to the likely effect of changes in law or medical practice on society as a whole.

TERMINOLOGY

It was interesting that the word 'euthanasia' was not used, though the first paragraph would until recently have been generally regarded as a description of passive euthanasia, i.e. allowing an incurably ill patient to die even though medical intervention could postpone the death.

The second paragraph describes voluntary euthanasia, when deliberate action is taken to shorten an incurably ill patient's life at that patient's steadfast request. It also includes involuntary euthanasia where the justification of the act is not the patient's wish but what is judged by others to be the patient's best interests.

As its name implies, the voluntary euthanasia movement is not concerned with involuntary euthanasia. The arguments supporting the former are very different from those that would justify the latter. Legislation proposed by those who want the choice of voluntary euthanasia to be available would sharply distinguish between them and confine itself entirely to medical help to die given at the patient's considered and enduring request.

It is the Nazi misuse of the word euthanasia to mean the destruction of handicapped people regardless of their wishes that has led to the widespread avoidance of the word. The late John Dawson said that 'the word euthanasia is hopelessly overloaded with emotional connotations'.[4] His comment was startlingly brought to mind at the British Medical Association's annual conference in 1993 when the Chairman of the Ethics Committee used the Nazi meaning in his response to a resolution on voluntary euthanasia. Nevertheless the British Voluntary Euthanasia Society, which was founded in 1935, has continued to use the word in its original Greek-derived sense of a gentle death and the means of bringing this about, and to rely on the distinction between voluntary and involuntary being clear. Judging by the Society's rapidly growing membership – it has more than doubled from about 7000 to well over 14 000 between 1988 and 1994 – this has been well understood by the general public. In this chapter it will be assumed that the reader shares that understanding.

The British Society was the first in the world. The only other to be founded before World War II is in New York and that abandoned the word euthanasia in favour of Choice in Dying. The Australians and New Zealanders call their analogous organisations Voluntary Euthanasia Societies. Most of the other societies which make up the World Federation of Right-to-Die Societies – over thirty in number, and constantly being augmented – acknowledge the contamination of the word 'euthanasia' by choosing synonyms in their titles.

ADVANCE DIRECTIVES

Returning, then, to the first concern of the House of Lords Select Committee, the refusal of life-prolonging medical treatment, it is well established in English law that the consent of the patient is required to any proposed medical treatment. Doubt has arisen in the past about whether an incompetent patient's previously known wish to refuse treatment may be ignored by the doctor. A number of the appeal judges[5] who declared it lawful to discontinue the maintenance of the life of Tony Bland (a victim of the disastrous crush at the Hillsborough soccer stadium) in his persistent vegetative state, were agreed that if he had left any instruction forbidding artificial feeding such instruction would have been legally binding. Since that case there has been another which specifically addressed the issue of the patient's power to limit future treatment at a time of incompetence. The judgment was that the patient's refusal to have his gangrenous leg amputated was to be respected even if he became incompetent before he died.[6]

The Select Committee accepted the binding nature of the latter judgment and the evidence to the same effect given by the Crown Prosecution Service. One might expect the latter body's pronouncement to weigh particularly heavily with any doctor tempted to ignore such prospective decisions by a now incompetent patient.

The All-Party Parliamentary Voluntary Euthanasia Group has yet to decide whether it is now necessary to proceed with their Bill to give statutory authority to these judgments. This Bill would also make it possible to appoint a proxy to make health care decisions in the case of future incapacity. The nomination of such a proxy can often be of great help to the doctor when rival relatives have different views and each claims the right to speak on behalf of the patient. The Select Committee Report is uncharacteristically confused on the value of proxies. On the one hand it says of proxy decision-making 'we do not favour the more widespread development of such a system' and in the next sentence 'there is however no reason why an advance directive should not contain a request to doctors to consult if practicable with a third party'. This is precisely what members of the voluntary euthanasia movement have in mind when they ask to be able to nominate their preferred health spokesperson, or proxy. Perhaps the explanation lies in the fact that the Select Committee had examined the system, often used in the United States, of the court appointing a proxy after the patient becomes incompetent. This proxy will usually be a stranger to both patient and doctor, and when used in this sense the voluntary euthanasia movement is also against such a system. As it is, the suggestion of including the name of the person they hope will be speaking on their behalf (whether or not the House of Lords regards this person as a 'proxy') will be gladly accepted.

The British Medical Association has recently recommended the completion of a signed and witnessed document (known in this country as an advance directive and in the United States as a living will) in order to make one's treatment preferences known in case of future incompetence.

Internationally Britain is lagging in this respect. All of the states making up the United States and several Australian states have already passed Acts establishing the legal validity of advance directives. In Denmark a central register is kept of such recorded decisions and the number of people completing the widely available documents far exceeds the level expected when the law was recently passed. In the United States matters have gone further and Federal Law[7] requires that all medical facilities in receipt of public funds must on admission of patients discuss the limits of treatment they are prepared to accept. These decisions must be recorded and acted upon when the time comes.

So even in the field of refusing unwanted treatment further measures could be taken to ensure that the patient's wishes are respected. Nevertheless the House of Lords Report represents a major step forward in agreeing with the Crown Prosecution Service, the Centre of Medical Law and Ethics and the Law Commission that the legal validity and binding force of advance directives is now beyond question.

ACTIVE VOLUNTARY EUTHANASIA

The legalisation of positive medical help to die for the incurably ill and intolerably suffering, the major aim of the voluntary euthanasia movement in Britain, is a different matter.

As we have seen, the recent reconsideration of the law in relation to voluntary euthanasia was precipitated by the general agreement that it was wrong to convict a conscientious doctor of attempted murder when he ended the life of his intolerably suffering and dying patient. Few people would wish to have law-making by referendum but it is true that for the law to be respected and effective it must, in a democracy, embody what is generally regarded as right. In this case there is evidence from a series of properly conducted opinion polls that such a change in the law was wanted by a majority of the population (69%) when the first poll was held (1969) and that that percentage has steadily increased to 79% in 1993.[8] The Select Committee's response to this body of evidence was that the result produced is much influenced by the way the question is worded. This seems to imply an insultingly low estimate of the ordinary citizen's ability to comprehend the substance of the matter. And, given the immense numbers of such polls in so many countries, all worded slightly differently and all giving at least two-thirds majorities in favour, details of wording seem unlikely to be the determining factor.

Actually bringing about a change in the law that the majority of citizens want is not easy, especially when it is not a party political topic. The usual method in Britain is by a Private Member's Bill and the Parliamentary time such Bills are allotted is very small. In the United States the constitutions of many of the states include an initiative process by which a majority of citizens can propose and pass a law without using the usual parliamentary means. In Washington and California Bills to legalise medical aid-in-dying have recently been narrowly defeated following massively funded publicity campaigns in the weeks before the voting. The public relations firm employed to conduct the campaign opposing the Bill in California found that 68% of voters were in favour at the outset. By presenting vivid portrayals of what they alleged to be the likely abuse of this new power by doctors they managed, by voting day, to reduce this figure to 49%. The money for the campaign came mainly from Catholic sources. In these states citizens are preparing to try again and in Oregon in 1994 a Bill passed. Bills to similar effect have been introduced by the ordinary parliamentary process in New Hampshire, Iowa, Maine and Michigan. The Canadian Parliament also has a Bill on its agenda. Northern Territory, Australia, has passed one.

SOME ARGUMENTS AGAINST LEGALISING VOLUNTARY EUTHANASIA

The opponents of decriminalising voluntary euthanasia in Britain do not depend entirely on the inertia of our Parliamentary process, of course. They argue that personal autonomy should not be given the moral weight that it undoubtedly has in modern society. Today most people do aspire to make their own choices about education, career, marriage and lifestyle. They see no reason why they should not at the end of life choose a quicker death with less suffering if that blessing seems likely to be denied them. Telling them they should not want this choice cuts little ice. Moreover the English legal system gives priority to personal autonomy when other guiding principles come into conflict with it, as the appeal judges in the *Bland* case pointed out very clearly.[9]

The sanctity of human life is no longer advanced as an overriding principle by most of those who want voluntary euthanasia to remain a crime. Presumably this is because sanctity is a religious concept and they recognise that few people in contemporary Britain think in those terms.[10] The alternative wording is now 'respect for human life'. Of course everyone agrees that this is a fundamentally important principle, but most people define being humanly alive in broader terms than, for example, being in a persistent vegetative state. They distinguish between being alive and having a life;[11] as Lord Justice Hoffmann put it, 'the stark reality is that Anthony Bland is not living a life at all'.[12]

The persistent vegetative state is an extreme consequence of continuing advances in medical knowledge and technology. These have made it possible to extend the span of full life and, paradoxically, to extend the dying process beyond what most people think is sensible. The new capabilities require changes in our attitudes to the medical profession and the laws that define its proper practices. The doctors cannot be left to make crucial decisions within a framework of laws that were appropriate to a simpler medical world.

Research achievements of the hospice movement are sometimes claimed to have removed the need for voluntary euthanasia by increasing skill in coping with many of the distresses of dying. But even if it were possible to alleviate all of these – and the hospice doctors do not claim that it is – there are still many people who do not want to go on to the bitter end and do not see why that should be required of them.

ASSISTED SUICIDE

It is sometimes suggested that the comparatively recent decriminalisation of suicide offers an escape for the patient without doctor involvement. It is true that the 1961 Suicide Act at least removed the shadow of a possible criminal prosecution for those recovering from a failed suicide attempt. Some of those suffering from incurable illness succeed in ending their own lives, though the records do not separate these from the suicides who suffer predominantly from mental illness, so the numbers are not known. Doctors, dentists and retired army officers continue to be the occupational categories having the highest rates of suicides. They, unlike the rest of the population, have access to the necessary drugs or to guns. A book of advice on how to end one's own life successfully, and with the least distress for those who have to deal with the aftermath, has recently been a best-seller in the United States and is selling well in the rest of the world, translated into many languages. But society shows little sympathy with those who choose this escape route, no matter how rationally, as can be seen when it happens to an eminent person. The obituaries of Bruno Bettelheim,[13] for example, tended to relate his death by suicide to his experience of Buchenwald and Dachau fifty years earlier, rather than to his circumstances at the time of his death. These were that he had an oesophageal condition that meant he could not eat solid food, his wife of long-standing had died several years earlier, he was 86 years old and in a nursing home, dreading a third stroke.

Many people flinch at the stigma attaching to death by suicide and the extra grief this will cause their family. Since it is a criminal offence to aid, abet, counsel or procure a suicide the death must be accomplished alone and unaided, and for many this is no longer physically possible. Early in 1994 a group of doctors successfully filed suit in Washington State[14] declaring that the denial of physician-assisted suicide was unconstitutional since it discriminated against those unable to act for themselves. In some countries, notably Germany, Switzerland and recently Sweden, aiding a suicide is not a crime and a doctor can provide appropriate drugs to an incurably ill patient though not administer them. In the Australian state of Victoria a Bill has been prepared which would allow doctors similar powers. In New Zealand[15] and Britain[16] recently the courts have treated leniently friends who provided assistance to incurably ill and suicidal patients. Legalising the assistance of suicide in Britain might be more acceptable to the medical profession than making it legally possible for them to participate directly in the action that brings about the death. In spite of the drawbacks for some patients this would certainly help a large number and would be welcomed by those who would nevertheless prefer properly practised voluntary euthanasia.

ALLOWING TO DIE AND HELPING TO DIE

Most philosophers agree that allowing to die and helping to die are morally equivalent behaviour for the doctor, in that both recognise that a gentle death is the only remaining good thing that can happen to this patient. Whether the doctor then expedites the death by action or inaction does not affect the moral quality of responding to that recognition. This opinion is reflected in a Working Party Report of the Institute of Medical Ethics (1992) which said 'A doctor, acting in good conscience, is ethically justified in assisting death if the need to relieve intense and unceasing pain or distress caused by an incurable illness greatly outweighs the benefit to the patient of further prolonging his life. This conclusion applies to patients whose sustained wishes on this matter are known to the doctor and should thus be respected as outweighing any contrary opinions expressed by others.'[17]

Even so, many doctors share the view expressed in the British Medical Association (1988) Report of the Working Party to review guidance on euthanasia,[18] that the practice is intuitively wrong. Presumably this means that they could find no rational argument against it but had feelings of reluctance to do it. It is worth stressing, therefore, that no proposed legislation requires a doctor to act against his or her conscience.

The doctors who prefer the present system to a change in the law that would bring carefully controlled voluntary euthanasia within the scope of good medical practice give many reasons for their preference. Some of these used to be raised against their profession being involved in birth control: 'Only God can give or take life. We cannot play God', for example or 'Nature must take its course'. The emptiness of these assertions in relation to actual medical practice can be seen in the determined (and laudable) attempts that are made to restore to health those hovering on the brink of death by reason of accident or treatable infection. In fact the whole practice of medicine could be defined as one long struggle to prevent 'Nature taking its course'.

One fact that doctors do not openly state as an objection is that in voluntary euthanasia the patient is the decision-maker. In theory patient autonomy prevails for all medical treatment, but in Britain the tradition has been for the doctor to decide. The common parlance is of 'doctor's orders' rather than 'doctor's advice'. This makes it difficult for doctors, even those who thoroughly approve of patient autonomy, to step back from their traditional role of making the choice of treatment and having their decision accepted without question. It must be this that gives rise to the frequent assertion that voluntary euthanasia will inevitably lead to involuntary euthanasia. The doctor (suddenly transformed from a caring and, if possible, curing professional) will only pay lip-service to the patient's wishes and take the opportunity to clear the wards of anyone without strength or relatives to object! It is sad to record that the same British Medical Association Report[19] quotes such a disgraceful scenario. 'We shall start by putting patients away [*sic*] because they are in intolerable pain and haven't long to live anyway; and we shall end up by putting them away because it's Friday night and we want to get away for the weekend.' The much-revered founder of the hospice movement, Dame Cicely Saunders, frequently voices similar sentiments. Needless to say, action of this kind, without the patient's explicit request, would continue to be outside the law.

Another reason advanced for not seriously considering and possibly responding to the terminally ill patient's request for help to die is that no patient must be deprived of hope.[20] Hope of what? Presumably not of a miraculous cure in the case of a well-informed and rational patient? More probably the one hope remaining to such a patient will be for a peaceful death, preferably while still able to recognise and say good-bye to chosen family members.

It may be that one of the unspoken medical objections is an unwillingness to respond to the patient's wish to discuss his or her approaching death. This is absolutely necessary before voluntary euthanasia can be decided upon. The discussions provide an opportunity for shared anticipatory grieving which is helpful to the patient and the surviving family. Doctors who lack communication skills and/or the ability to face strong emotions will naturally try to avoid occasions that require both.

Of all these objections Grant Gillett's 'pause',[21] the individual doctor's reluctance to perform an act of voluntary euthanasia, is the only one that commands respect. And, as stated above, proposed legislation will include every doctor's right to refuse to bring about a death by voluntary euthanasia, as well as every patient's right to ask for it. The prospect of change in one's established practices is welcomed by few of those whose settled habits will be affected by the change, but this cannot be a valid argument against permissive legislation.

VOLUNTARY EUTHANASIA IN THE NETHERLANDS

The Netherlands is the only country whose medical profession and courts have openly recognised the widespread desire for the availability of voluntary euthanasia and, by means of case law, developed agreed guidelines for its careful practice. Two of the most important of the provisos are that it is the patient who of his or her own free will makes an explicit and deliberate request for euthanasia, and that a second doctor must check the diagnosis and the patient's refusal of further life-prolonging treatment.

The Dutch Government is also the only one to have commissioned a thorough and detailed study of death and dying, which appeared as the Remmelink Report (1991).[22] One of the reasons for undertaking this study was the barrage of ill-informed criticism which was being published overseas, notably a highly tendentious article in the *Hastings Center Report* (Jan/Feb 1989). A resounding refutation of this article was published in the Nov/Dec issue, and all readers of Dr Fenigsen's original article are recommended also to read the Dutch response to it. The Remmelink Report itself was misrepresented in Britain when it first appeared. For example, the 38% of deaths which involved medical decision-making that might have shortened life were at first regarded as euthanasia deaths. Many of these decisions were made without consulting the patient. It was then realised that nearly all of these (35%) were non-treatment decisions or the alleviation of pain and other symptoms with opioids in such dosages that the patient's life might have been shortened. These are common medical practices everywhere, rarely in consultation with the patient.

Another more serious criticism was that 0.8% of the deaths were the result of life-terminating acts without explicit and persistent request. Half of these people had spoken earlier of their wish for a peaceful death and almost all had been known for long periods by the doctors treating them. They were all close to death and suffering grievously, by suffocation for example. Such deaths occasionally happen everywhere and merciful doctors hasten the end. The Dutch authorities, who are not happy about that 0.8%, do at least know the extent of the problem and are in a position to address it. The same cannot be said of any other country.

At present Dutch doctors who report a voluntary euthanasia death expose the relatives to a police investigation and have themselves to face a long period of suspense during which they do not know whether or not they will be prosecuted. It is small wonder that some record the fatal illness as the cause of death. But the Dutch authorities, again, would prefer to know how many dying patients ask for and receive medical help to die and have taken steps, with encouraging results, to increase the accuracy of these reports.

The opinion of Dutch citizens is over 80% in favour of having this choice legally available at the end of life. It is worth noting that only 40% of those asking for voluntary euthanasia actually secure a doctor's co-operation in receiving it. This does not suggest that doctors are becoming eager or careless in agreeing to perform it, as some opponents have suggested would be inevitable. Carrying out voluntary euthanasia is a rare experience for most Dutch doctors, but when the occasion arises most accept it as their last act of care for their autonomous patient.

VOLUNTARY EUTHANASIA AND RELIGION

The House of Lords Select Committee included four members of the medical profession (one of them the Chairman), four lawyers, two of whom have specific experience of grappling with medical and ethical issues, and four lay members. No mention of religious representation was made, though the committee members included the Archbishop of York, Lord Rawlinson who speaks from a Catholic standpoint and Lord Mishcon who is learned in the Jewish faith. Approximately one-third of the written evidence they considered came from religious organisations or individuals who approach this problem from a religious standpoint. However, it is worth noting that Britain is to-day an overwhelmingly secular society;[23] the church/chapel/synagogue/mosque plays an important part in the lives of very few of its citizens. There is thus a great disparity between the importance attached to religious doctrine in the deliberations of the Select Committee and in the minds of the electorate. There is a similar disparity in the official religious doctrine on voluntary euthanasia and the views of those who nominally belong to one of the major religious groups. When the National Opinion Polls are done those responding are asked their religious affiliation with the following results:[24]

Percentage in favour of legalising voluntary euthanasia

Agnostic	93%	Roman Catholic	73%
Church of Scotland	85%	Jewish	60%
Church of England	80%		

It is also pertinent in estimating the regard that should be paid to orthodox religious doctrine to note that in the Netherlands a priest is always invited to join the preliminary discussions and to be present at the voluntary euthanasia death, if that is the patient's wish. The Dutch doctors involved say they have never known a priest, Roman Catholic or Dutch Reformed, to refuse.

THE PATIENT'S FAMILY

The dying patient and his or her doctor are the central figures in voluntary euthanasia, but we must not forget the welfare of the surviving family. Many Dutch people have spoken of the dignity of their relatives' chosen death. Mrs Boyes' death was far from dignified; nevertheless her sons were grateful that in the end Dr Cox took positive action to curtail her appalling suffering. Relatives frequently make the point, bitterly, that the doctor would have been prosecuted for allowing an animal to suffer as their loved person did. They do not understand why humans are treated with less compassion than animals. None of the voluminous writings on problems that arise at the end of life has dealt satisfactorily with this contradiction.

A few carers, the so-called mercy killers, are driven to the point of themselves ending the sufferer's life – at least we assume it is only a few. Since the two or three that appear in court each year have themselves reported what they have done, there could be other cases that are accepted as natural deaths. When these criminals come to trial, provided they plead 'diminished responsibility', the usual sentence is two years' probation. One man, who did not make that plea, was found guilty of murder and served four years of his sentence of life imprisonment.[25] His wife, like most of the 'victims' of this crime, had begged him to end her life. If this wish could be discussed with the general practitioner is it not possible that the relative would not be driven to such extremity and a great deal of anguish be spared?

STATUTE LAW OR CASE LAW?

We have considered briefly the points of view of the doctor and the family, but it is the welfare of the dying person that must be the central concern of this proposed change in the law. Those who at present die in tranquillity having lived a satisfying life almost to its end will continue to do so. But those who have lost their health and all appetite for life will no longer be additionally deprived of the last exercise of their autonomy.

The opportunity to take the first step in making such a choice legally and honourably available to us all has been missed by the House of Lords Select Committee. The first recommendation of its Report is 'that there should be no change in the law to permit euthanasia', failing to make the distinction, so crucial to the rest of us, between choosing to die oneself and having someone else make that choice.

In his Upjohn Lecture[26] Professor Ian Kennedy argues that the law concerning the competent patient who asks his doctor to assist him to die is so unsatisfactory that it will have to be changed. Since the legislature seems unlikely to do this, judging by the stance taken by the House of Lords Select Committee Report, the only remaining means of change is through the courts. He says that the courts can readily develop the law in this way.

But this is where the Dutch began over twenty years ago; the gradual shaping by case law of legitimate and acceptable medical practice concerning the dying is a very slow process. There is much expense of time, money and, above all, suffering involved for the individual patients and doctors whose cases form the basis of this development.

Those who are trying to secure this change in the law will continue to strive for Parliament to frame a law so that the courts can interpret it. In Britain we have the necessary expertise to do this, we have the experience of the Netherlands to learn from and we have a medical profession with the integrity to act within such a law responsibly. Public understanding of the issue and its wishes on the matter, the increasing importance accorded personal autonomy, the demographic factor of our aging population and the continuing development of medical techniques for extending our dying, all point in the same direction. The general attitude to birth control changed completely within a lifetime; it seems incredible now that public discussion and social approval were denied it so recently. In a few years' time it seems likely that we shall look back with the same kind of incredulity to this era, when we had to deny help to the dying who said, as many do today, 'I've had a wonderful life but it's over now and I long for death.'

NOTES

1 Smith, R. Euthanasia: time for a royal commission. *BMJ* 1992;305:728.
2 Brahams, D. Euthanasia: doctor convicted of attempted murder. *Lancet* 1992; 340:783.
3 Dworkin, R. *Life's Dominion*. Harper Collins, London, 1993, p. 185.
4 Dawson, J. Last rites and wrongs: euthanasia, autonomy and responsibility. *Cambridge Quarterly of Healthcare Ethics* 1992;1:81–83.
5 *Airedale NHS Trust* v. *Bland* [1993] Appeal Cases 789 at 857 *per* Lord Keith of Kinkel.
6 Dyer, C. Patient wins bar on future treatment. *Guardian* 15 October 1993. (For a discussion of the legal status of advance directives, see the chapter by Stuart Hornett elsewhere in this volume.)
7 US Federal Law: Patient Self-Determination Act 1990.
8 National Opinion Poll Survey, April 1993.
9 See note 5.
10 *UK Christian Handbook*. Christian Research Association, London, 1993.
11 Rachels, J. *The End of Life*. Oxford University Press, Oxford, 1986, p. 5.
12 See note 5.
13 E.g. *The Times* 15/16 March 1990.
14 *Compassion in Dying et al.* v. *Washington State*. US District Court, W.D. Wash, 3 May 1994 (No. C94-199R). (For a discussion of this case, see the chapter by Yale Kamisar elsewhere in this volume.)
15 Roscoe, J. *Birmingham Post* 13 November 1991.
16 Chard, A. Teenager cleared of helping MS woman to commit suicide. *Guardian* 23 September 1993.
17 Institute of Medical Ethics Working Party Report. *Lancet* 1990;336:610–614.
18 *The Euthanasia Report*. BMA, London, 1988.
19 Ibid., p. 4.
20 Herth, K. Fostering hope in terminally-ill people. *Journal of Advanced Nursing* 1990:15:1250–1259.
21 Gillett, G. *Reasonable Care*. Bristol Press, Bristol, 1989, p. 99.
22 Remmelink, J. *Report: Enquiry into Medical Practice with Regard to Euthanasia*. 1991 Netherlands Embassy. (For a discussion of this Report, see the chapter by John Keown elsewhere in this volume.)
23 Op. cit., note 10.
24 Op. cit., note 8.
25 *R.* v. *Cocker* . Manchester Crown Court, 25 July 1988.
26 Kennedy I. The Quality of Mercy: Patients, Doctors and Dying. Presented at the Royal Society, London, 25 April 1994.

9

Extracts from the Report of the House of Lords Select Committee on Medical Ethics*

By the Select Committee appointed to consider the ethical, legal and clinical implications of a person's right to withhold consent to life-prolonging treatment, and the position of persons who are no longer able to give or withhold consent;

and to consider whether and in what circumstances actions that have as their intention or a likely consequence the shortening of another person's life may be justified on the grounds that they accord with that person's wishes or with that person's best interests;

and in all the foregoing considerations to pay regard to the likely effects of changes in law or medical practice on society as a whole.

ORDERED TO REPORT

PART 1 INTRODUCTION

BACKGROUND

1. Decisions about medical treatment and the end of life are more complicated now than they have ever been. Such decisions are now more frequent, more difficult and more widely debated than in the past.

2. Perhaps the single most important reason for this is the advances in medicine in recent years, and particularly the application of medical technology. As a result patients live longer, where in the past they would have died at an earlier stage of their illnesses. Conditions which not so long ago would have resulted in certain, and fairly swift, death can now be treated and, if not cured, at least held at bay. For many this has resulted in a welcome prolongation of meaningful life, and avoidance of suffering. But for others the poor quality of life which results may raise the question whether treatment will be a benefit or a burden to the patient.

3. Another reason is demographic. As medicine has overcome many life-threatening conditions, more and more of the population are surviving longer and facing the chronic, degenerative conditions which old age may bring. The social implications of this are enormous, since to care adequately for the resulting large numbers of sick and elderly patients is difficult and costly. For some, too, old age may entail a weariness of living, and a wish not to have life prolonged by medical means. Some people cannot accept that their lives could continue to have meaning and value if overtaken by serious illness, disability or dependence.

4. Another factor is the change in the relationship between doctor and patient. The increased importance attached to individual autonomy, or the freedom to make decisions for oneself, has meant that relationships between state and citizen, between doctor and patient, teacher and pupil, parent and child, have all become less paternalistic. Most individuals wish to take more responsibility for the course of their lives, and this applies equally to decisions about medical treatment. Whereas in the past decisions were often left to the doctor alone, decisions are usually now the result of consultation between the patient and the health-care team, with the patient's relatives generally playing a role as well.

5. For all these reasons, there has been wide debate about medical treatment and the end of life. As part of that debate the practice of euthanasia has been much discussed, and a range of bodies has considered the issue. In 1988 for example the British Medical Association (BMA) set up a working

* HL Paper 21-1 of 1993–94. Ordered to be printed 31 January 1994. Crown Copyright is reproduced with the permission of the Controller of HMSO.

party to review their guidance on euthanasia[1]. The 1993 Stevens lecture at the Royal Society of Medicine, the Society's main annual event for lay people, was also on this subject. Campaigning by various interest groups has intensified.

6. The trial of Dr Nigel Cox in 1992, and his conviction for attempted murder after he administered a lethal dose to a suffering patient, prompted great controversy. Some people were concerned that Dr Cox had been prosecuted at all, since he had acted in accordance with the wishes of the patient and her family and with a merciful motive. Others were concerned that, although having broken the law and breached the ethical code of his profession, he received only a suspended sentence and was merely admonished by the General Medical Council (GMC)[2].

7. Different, but related and no less difficult, questions were raised by the case of Anthony Bland, a young man severely injured in the Hillsborough stadium disaster in 1989 and who survived for several years in a persistent vegetative state[3] (pvs). The local health authority, with the support of his family, sought and received a declaration from the High Court, later confirmed by the Court of Appeal and the House of Lords, to the effect that it would be lawful for the artificial nutrition and hydration on which he depended to be discontinued. Some people welcomed the decision that Bland's body need no longer be kept alive, since they considered that all the functions which had made him an individual had been irretrievably lost. Others felt that nutrition and hydration are such basic elements of care that they should only be withdrawn when the patient is in the final stages of the dying process, and that their discontinuance in this case amounted to deliberate killing. This case too gave rise to much press comment[4] and much public debate. Two of the Lords of Appeal in Ordinary who heard the appeal to the House of Lords called for Parliamentary consideration of the issues involved. Lord Browne-Wilkinson said it was "imperative that the moral, social and legal issues raised by this case should be considered by Parliament...If Parliament fails to act, then judge-made law will of necessity through a gradual and uncertain process provide a legal answer to each new question as it arises. But in my judgment that is not the best way to proceed"[5].

8. Debate on these issues has by no means been confined to the United Kingdom. In Canada the Law Reform Commission has considered them[6] and recently the case of Sue Rodriguez has received wide publicity[7]. In New Zealand the Medical Council has reported on pvs and the withdrawal of food and fluids[8]. In 1991 the European Parliament's Committee on the Environment, Public Health and Consumer Protection adopted a resolution in favour of voluntary euthanasia[9].

9. In the United States of America, in a healthcare environment very different from our own, there have been several legal cases concerning the treatment of patients in pvs[10]. Legislation promoting advance directives has been adopted in many states. The activities of Jack Kervorkian, who has assisted the suicide of a number of women by means of his so-called "suicide machine" which administers various lethal drugs, have given rise to litigation and have been widely

---

1 BMA, *The Euthanasia Report*, 1988.

2 For press comment on the case see for example Sunday Times 20 September; Times 24 September; Spectator 26 September; Financial Times 3 October; Guardian 6 October; New Scientist 24 October; (all 1992).

3 For discussion of this condition see paragraph 156, and Appendix 4.

4 See for example Daily Telegraph, Guardian 5 February; The Lancet 13 February; The Tablet 13 March; (all 1993).

5 [1993] AC. 789.

6 Law Reform Commission of Canada, *Report on Euthanasia, Aiding Suicide and Cessation of Treatment*, 1983.

7 Sue Rodriguez, suffering from amyotrophic lateral sclerosis, sought a court order permitting her doctor to assist her suicide when the disease had advanced to such a degree that she no longer wished to live. She was unsuccessful in the lower courts and the Supreme Court dismissed her appeal by a majority judgment on 30 September 1993.

8 Report by the Bioethics Research Centre, University of Otago, February 1993.

9 DOC EN/RR/108939, PE 146.436/fin.

10 See for example Re Quinlan (1976) 355 A 2d 647, Supreme Court of New Jersey; Cruzan v Harmon (1988) 760 SW 2d 408, Supreme Court of Missouri; Re Doe (1992) 583 NE 2d 1263, Supreme Judicial Court of Massachusetts. See also the discussion at pp 192-3 of the evidence.

debated[1]. He is now indicted and facing prosecution in the state of Michigan. In Washington State in 1991 a proposition in favour of physician aid-in-dying for terminally ill people was supported by 46 per cent of those who voted. A similar proposition in California a year later attracted a similar level of support but an attempt to legalise voluntary euthanasia failed[2].

10. In the Netherlands euthanasia, though still a crime under the Dutch Penal Code, has been openly practised for some time. Since the late 1970s legal precedents have been developed such that, providing specific guidelines are observed, a doctor practising euthanasia will not be prosecuted. Among other conditions, the guidelines require that euthanasia should be voluntary and the decision should be made with the concurrence of a second independent physician. After it has been carried out the act must be notified to the coroner and district attorney who decide whether or not to prosecute. A government commission in 1991 considered the operation of this system and its findings gave rise to much controversy[3]. In 1993 the Dutch parliament enacted provisions to formalise the guidelines and the notification procedure for voluntary euthanasia.

THE COMMITTEE'S ENQUIRY

11. It was against this background that the House decided to appoint a Select Committee to consider certain aspects of medical ethics. Our terms of reference address not only euthanasia but also a number of other difficult issues, where similar implications arise.

12. The first part of our terms of reference raises the issue of when it is appropriate to discontinue, or not to initiate, medical treatment[4]. Different considerations inevitably arise in the case of patients who are legally competent and of sound mind and in the case of those who are unable for whatever reason to express their wishes about treatment and are thus incapable of giving valid consent.

13. The second part raises the issue of euthanasia as commonly understood, meaning a deliberate intervention undertaken with the express intention of ending life. This presents the crucial question of whether deliberate killing can ever be justified by the wish of the person killed or by an intention to be merciful.

14. The final part of our terms of reference reminds us that we must consider these matters not only from the point of view of the interests of the individual, or of the medical and allied health professions, or indeed of any other specific group, but of society as a whole.

15. Our terms of reference embrace a wide spectrum of different medical conditions, yet it is the two extremes that come most often to mind when people discuss matters of life and death. At one end of the spectrum is the terminally-ill cancer patient, who is conscious and able to participate in decisions about treatment and for whom the priority is likely to be to achieve the best possible quality of life for the time remaining, by the relief of painful or distressing symptoms. At the other end of the spectrum is the pvs patient, who has no cognitive functions, is not dying, as far as we can tell suffers no pain, but on whom medical treatment appears to confer little if any benefit. In between these two examples lies a whole range of circumstances: the patient with advanced Alzheimer's disease whose relatives may suggest that continued life in such a condition is not what the patient would have wished; the patient with progressive multiple sclerosis who fears continuing to live in an increasingly disabled state; and many others.

16. After some preliminary consideration, we published a report[5] which set out the issues which we felt our terms of reference required us to consider. These were—

---

1 For a discussion of this case see p 204 of the evidence.

2 For details of the two propositions see p 205 of the evidence.

3 Some of the commission's findings are summarised in paragraphs 121 and 122.

4 The expression "medical treatment" was not defined in our terms of reference, but its scope was much discussed by witnesses (see paragraphs 60 to 65).

5 Select Committee on Medical Ethics, Special Report Session 1992-93, HL Paper 67.

— the respective weight to be attached to the sometimes conflicting moral principles of the sanctity of life and the right to personal autonomy

— the extent of a doctor's duty of care to a patient

— the distinction between the withholding or withdrawal of medical treatment, and deliberate intervention to end life

— the different considerations arising in the case of patients who are legally competent and of sound mind, and of patients who are unable to express their own wishes about treatment

— the role of advance directives and proxy decision-makers

— the role of the courts in interpreting the law in the light of changing medical technology and practice

— the case for change in the existing law, and the nature and extent of such change

— the role of the hospice movement and advances in the care of the terminally ill

— the experience of other countries, in particular in Western Europe and the USA.

17. Our report also contained an open invitation for written evidence. We are most grateful to all those who responded to that invitation. The evidence which is printed is listed in the Table of Contents. We also received letters from many individuals, and their views are discussed in Appendix 2. We were greatly assisted at the beginning of our enquiry by the private advice of Professor Ian Kennedy, Director of the Centre of Medical Law and Ethics, King's College, London. We are grateful to him for his assistance.

18. Towards the end of our enquiry we made a visit to the Netherlands, to discuss experience there. We record our warm thanks to those who assisted us. An account of our visit is set out in Appendix 3.

TERMINOLOGY

19. In the course of our report we shall use a number of terms which are either not in common use, or are not always used consistently. In order to avoid misunderstanding we set out here the terms which we have adopted, and the meanings which we attach to them. However many of the concepts which we discuss are elusive. They do not readily lend themselves to precise definition and we recognise that our working definitions are unlikely to be accepted by all commentators.

20. The word **euthanasia** originally meant nothing more than gentle and easy death. In the context of our enquiry, however, we use it to mean a deliberate intervention undertaken with the express intention of ending a life to relieve intractable suffering.

21. The term **passive euthanasia** is often used to describe the withdrawal or withholding of some treatment necessary for the continuance of the patient's life. We consider this term to be misleading. There is plenty of scope for argument over the ethical equivalence of killing and letting die in certain circumstances. In the case of a patient terminally ill with cancer and expected to die very shortly, few people would think it obligatory that antibiotics should be used to treat pneumonia (unless necessary to relieve distressing symptoms), although the patient's life might thereby be prolonged for a few days. We therefore speak of **withdrawing or not initiating treatment** or of a **treatment-limiting decision**.

22. Some people also use the term passive euthanasia to describe the act of a doctor or other person who prescribes or administers pain-killers or other (eg sedative) drugs necessary for the relief of a patient's pain or severe distress, but in the knowledge that a probable consequence of the

prescription is a shortening of the patient's life. Again we think that this usage is incorrect. We speak instead of the **double effect**.

23. The state of mind of the person whose death might be brought about by an act of euthanasia, as we have defined it, is of course significant. **Voluntary euthanasia** occurs when the patient's death is brought about at his or her own request. **Non-voluntary euthanasia** may be used to describe the killing of a patient who does not have the capacity to understand what euthanasia means and cannot therefore form a request or withhold consent. **Involuntary euthanasia** has been used to describe the killing of a patient who is competent to request or consent to the act, but does not do so.

24. The need for society to offer special protection to those who are in any way disadvantaged makes the consideration of competence or capacity particularly important in these matters. We describe as **competent** those patients who are able to understand the available information about their conditions, to consider with medical advice the risks, benefits and burdens of different treatments or courses of action, and thus to make informed decisions. We describe as **incompetent** those patients who are unable, whether permanently or temporarily, to make decisions about their medical care.

25. The group of incompetent patients covers a wide range of individuals with varying medical histories. Incompetence may be the result of mental illness or handicap, of disease or of accident. Patients may be conscious but unable to make or communicate a decision; or they may be unconscious. Many people who were formerly competent to make their own decisions about medical treatment become incompetent in the last stages of their lives as their capacity is impaired by, for example, advanced dementia or the effects of other illness.

26. **Assisted suicide** is the term we use when a competent patient has formed a desire to end his or her life but requires help to perform the act, perhaps because of physical disability. When the help requested is given by a doctor, the act is called **physician-assisted suicide**. A common form of assistance might be providing a lethal dose of a drug for the patient to swallow.

27. We use the term **advance directive** (in preference to the equally common **living will**) to describe a document executed while a patient is competent, concerning his or her preferences about medical treatment in the event of becoming incompetent. The document may specify the types of treatment which the patient would or would not find acceptable in certain circumstances.

28. We use the term **proxy decision-maker** to refer to someone who is appointed to make decisions on behalf of someone who is unable to make decisions for him or herself. A proxy decision-maker may be nominated in advance by the patient while competent, or (as is common in the United States of America) may be appointed by the court.

29. In the case of an incompetent patient, decisions about medical treatment may be made by a doctor in the patient's **best interests**. This is a difficult term to define, since it is used by different people to mean different things in different circumstances. The principle was articulated in the case of *In re F (Mental Patient:Sterilisation)*[1], where it was held that no-one could consent to medical treatment on behalf of an incompetent patient, but that a doctor could treat if it were in the patient's best interests to do so. In determining the patient's best interests, the doctor should act in accordance with a responsible and competent body of relevant professional opinion.

30. **Terminal illness** may be defined as an illness which is inevitably progressive, the effects of which cannot be reversed by treatment (although treatment may be successful in relieving symptoms temporarily) and which will inevitably result in death within a few months at most. It may be distinguished first from an **irreversible condition** (such as, for example, cerebral palsy or spina bifida) which is not progressive and does not necessarily lead to death and secondly from

---

[1] [1990] 2 A.C. 1-84.

chronic progressive disease (such as, for example, rheumatoid arthritis or multiple sclerosis) in which early death is not inevitable, though deterioration is. Definitions of **persistent vegetative state** are discussed in Appendix 4.

31. We use the expression **health-care team** to mean the doctors, nurses and other professionals involved in the care and medical treatment of the individual patient.

32. For a patient who is terminally ill, **palliative care** may be the most appropriate course which the health-care team can offer. The World Health Organisation has described palliative care as "a form of care that recognises that cure or long-term control is not possible; is concerned with the quality rather than quantity of life; and cloaks troublesome and distressing symptoms with treatments whose primary or sole aim is the highest possible measure of patient comfort"[1]. The Department of Health said "palliative care is active total care provided to a patient when it is recognised that the illness is no longer curable. Palliative care concentrates on the quality of life and on alleviating pain and other distressing symptoms, and is intended neither to hasten nor postpone death" (P 2)[2].

STRUCTURE OF THE REPORT

33. Our report continues with a series of sections in which we consider the issues as presented by the evidence we have received and by the other material available to us. We end with an account of our conclusions and recommendations.

---

1 World Health Organization. *Palliative cancer care*. 1989.

2 For the definition given by the Association for Palliative Medicine, see P 190.

PART 3 OPINION OF THE COMMITTEE

PATIENT'S CONSENT

233. The concept of patient's informed consent[1] is nowadays at the heart of the relationship between doctor and patient, and governs decisions about medical treatment. As well as giving appropriate weight to the wishes of the individual the issue of consent, if properly approached, encourages full and open communication between doctor and patient in a consultative partnership. This is much to be welcomed.

234. We strongly endorse the right of the competent patient to refuse consent to any medical treatment, for whatever reason. The doctor must ensure that the patient understands the likely consequences of such refusal, and the reasons for proposing a particular treatment, but no member of the health-care team may overrule the patient's decision.

235. In some exceptional circumstances there may be a public interest in the outcome of a treatment decision relating to a competent patient which is thought to surpass the interest of the individual. Such a decision must be taken by the High Court, and may not be taken by the health-care team. We do not consider it appropriate to comment on the specific facts of the case in *Re S*, to which witnesses drew our attention[2]. But we urge that, if an individual refusal of treatment by a competent patient is overruled by the Court, full reasons should be given. Only thus can patients be assured that their right to refuse consent to treatment is protected, and that they will not be subjected to medical procedures against their will.

VOLUNTARY EUTHANASIA

236. The right to refuse medical treatment is far removed from the right to request assistance in dying. We spent a long time considering the very strongly held and sincerely expressed views of those witnesses who advocated voluntary euthanasia[3]. Many of us have had experience of relatives or friends whose dying days or weeks were less than peaceful or uplifting, or whose final stages of life were so disfigured that the loved one seemed already lost to us, or who were simply weary of life. Our thinking must inevitably be coloured by such experience. The accounts we received from individual members of the public about such experiences were particularly moving, as were the letters from those who themselves longed for the release of an early death. Our thinking must also be coloured by the wish of every individual for a peaceful and easy death, without prolonged suffering, and by a reluctance to contemplate the possibility of severe dementia or dependence. We gave much thought too to Professor Dworkin's opinion that, for those without religious belief, the individual is best able to decide what manner of death is fitting to the life which has been lived.

237. Ultimately, however, we do not believe that these arguments are sufficient reason to weaken society's prohibition of intentional killing. That prohibition is the cornerstone of law and of social relationships. It protects each one of us impartially, embodying the belief that all are equal. We do not wish that protection to be diminished and we therefore recommend that there should be no change in the law to permit euthanasia. We acknowledge that there are individual cases in which euthanasia may be seen by some to be appropriate. But individual cases cannot reasonably establish the foundation of a policy which would have such serious and widespread repercussions. Moreover dying is not only a personal or individual affair. The death of a person affects the lives of others, often in ways and to an extent which cannot be foreseen. We believe that the issue of euthanasia is one in which the interest of the individual cannot be separated from the interest of society as a whole.

---

1 See paragraphs 40-49 above.

2 See paragraphs 46 and 47 above.

3 See in particular paragraphs 92-94, 98-100, 102, 105, 109 and 111 above.

238. One reason for this conclusion is that we do not think it possible to set secure limits on voluntary euthanasia. Some witnesses told us that to legalise voluntary euthanasia was a discrete step which need have no other consequences. But as we said in our introduction, issues of life and death do not lend themselves to clear definition, and without that it would not be possible to frame adequate safeguards against non-voluntary euthanasia if voluntary euthanasia were to be legalised. It would be next to impossible to ensure that all acts of euthanasia were truly voluntary, and that any liberalisation of the law was not abused. Moreover to create an exception to the general prohibition of intentional killing would inevitably open the way to its further erosion whether by design, by inadvertence, or by the human tendency to test the limits of any regulation. These dangers are such that we believe that any decriminalisation of voluntary euthanasia would give rise to more, and more grave, problems than those it sought to address. Fear of what some witnesses referred to as a "slippery slope" could in itself be damaging.

239. We are also concerned that vulnerable people—the elderly, lonely, sick or distressed—would feel pressure, whether real or imagined, to request early death. We accept that, for the most part, requests resulting from such pressure or from remediable depressive illness would be identified as such by doctors and managed appropriately. Nevertheless we believe that the message which society sends to vulnerable and disadvantaged people should not, however obliquely, encourage them to seek death, but should assure them of our care and support in life.

240. Some of those who advocated voluntary euthanasia did so because they feared that lives were being prolonged by aggressive medical treatment beyond the point at which the individual felt that continued life was no longer a benefit but a burden. But, in the light of the consensus which is steadily emerging over the circumstances in which life-prolonging treatment may be withdrawn or not initiated, we consider that such fears may increasingly be allayed. We welcome moves[1] by the medical professional bodies to ensure more senior oversight of practice in casualty departments, as a step towards discouraging inappropriately aggressive treatment by less experienced practitioners.

241. Furthermore, there is good evidence that, through the outstanding achievements of those who work in the field of palliative care[2], the pain and distress of terminal illness can be adequately relieved in the vast majority of cases. Such care is available not only within hospices: thanks to the increasing dissemination of best practice by means of home-care teams and training for general practitioners, palliative care is becoming more widely available in the health service, in hospitals and in the community, although much remains to be done. With the necessary political will such care could be made available to all who could benefit from it. We strongly commend the development and growth of palliative care services.

DOUBLE EFFECT

242. In the small and diminishing number of cases in which pain and distress cannot be satisfactorily controlled, we are satisfied that the professional judgment of the health-care team can be exercised to enable increasing doses of medication (whether of analgesics or sedatives) to be given in order to provide relief, even if this shortens life. The adequate relief of pain and suffering in terminally ill patients depends on doctors being able to do all that is necessary and possible. In many cases this will mean the use of opiates or sedative drugs in increasing doses. In some cases patients may in consequence die sooner than they would otherwise have done but this is not in our view a reason for withholding treatment that would give relief, as long as the doctor acts in accordance with responsible medical practice with the objective of relieving pain or distress, and with no intention to kill.

---

1 See for example the discussion document of the British Association of Accident and Emergency Medicine, March 1991. Since then the Churchill John Radcliffe Hospital, Oxford, has introduced 24-hour shift working by accident and emergency consultants (press reports 31 December 1993).

2 See paragraphs 136 to 145 above.

243. Some witnesses suggested that the double effect[1] of some therapeutic drugs when given in large doses was being used as a cloak for what in effect amounted to widespread euthanasia, and suggested that this implied medical hypocrisy. We reject that charge while acknowledging that the doctor's intention, and evaluation of the pain and distress suffered by the patient, are of crucial significance in judging double effect. If this intention is the relief of severe pain or distress, and the treatment given is appropriate to that end, then the possible double effect should be no obstacle to such treatment being given. Some may suggest that intention is not readily ascertainable. But juries are asked every day to assess intention in all sorts of cases, and could do so in respect of double effect if in a particular instance there was any reason to suspect that the doctor's primary intention was to kill the patient rather than to relieve pain and suffering. They would no doubt consider the actions of the doctor, how they compared with usual medical practice directed towards the relief of pain and distress, and all the circumstances of the case. We have confidence in the ability of the medical profession to discern when the administration of drugs has been inappropriate or excessive. An additional safeguard is that increased emphasis on team working makes it improbable that doctors could deliberately and recklessly shorten the lives of their patients without their actions arousing suspicion.

244. We would add that the effects of opiates (the drugs most commonly involved in double effect) and of some other pain-relieving and sedative drugs are so uncertain that the outcome of a particular dose can never be predicted with total confidence. The body weight, metabolism, habituation and general condition of the individual patient all affect the response. There have been cases where an error in dispensing resulted in the administration of a dose which seemed likely to be lethal, yet the patient flourished. A doctor called to testify in the case of Dr Bodkin Adams asserted that a particular dose must certainly kill, only to be told that the patient had previously been given that dose and had survived. The primary effect (relief of pain and distress) can be predicted with reasonable confidence but there can be no certainty that the secondary effect (shortening of life) will result. Decisions about dosage are not easy, but the practice of medicine is all about the weighing of risks and benefits.

DECISION-MAKING FOR INCOMPETENT PATIENTS

245. The need for society to offer special protection to those who are vulnerable means that special provision should be made for medical decision-making in respect of incompetent patients. We therefore support the proposal of the Law Commission that a new judicial forum should be established with power to authorise the commencement, withholding or withdrawal of treatment where this is in the patient's best interests. Such a forum would have power to choose between alternatives, rather than simply to declare that a proposed course of action would or would not be lawful, as the courts do at present. We do not envisage that application to the forum would be a routine event: in most cases consultation among the health-care team and the family or other people closest to the patient will result in agreement on an appropriate course. But in the event of dispute as to what is in the patient's best interests, or doubt as to the legality of what is proposed, recourse to an authoritative forum would be of advantage. We also support the proposal of the Law Commission that certain "special category" procedures should always require the authority of the forum.

246. We understand that the Law Commission are likely to recommend that the new jurisdiction should be exercised by a reconstructed and enlarged Court of Protection, with nominated judges of the High Court and nominated circuit judges and district judges. The court would have power to appoint experts to give advice. We are not, of course, acquainted with all the details of the recommendations which the Law Commission will make. We should not, therefore, be regarded as endorsing in advance every aspect of their proposals. However in broad terms we support the creation of a new court along the lines which we understand them to be likely to propose, subject to certain qualifications set out below.

---

[1] See paragraphs 22 and 73 to 79 above.

247. We were initially strongly attracted by the idea of local tribunals comprising legal, medical and lay members to fulfil the functions of the new forum for medical decision-making. We felt that a forum so constituted would command greater confidence and would be more accessible to those who had recourse to it, in particular the family or friends of the patient. However we recognise that the Law Commission's intention is that a new court should discharge other functions in respect of decision-making for incompetent people, not only decisions about medical treatment. Those other functions lie outside our terms of reference. But we acknowledge that it would not be practical or desirable to establish two separate systems of decision-making, one for medical matters and another for dealing with, say, an incompetent person's financial affairs. Indeed it would no doubt sometimes be difficult to distinguish between different types of decision, or to separate one element of a person's affairs from others.

248. We regret however that an entirely judicial forum will not have the same degree of medical or lay input as a tribunal system would permit. We recommend therefore that some mechanism should be adopted whereby the new court will make full use of appropriate independent medical and ethical advice. We also recommend that the new court should be locally based and that its procedures should be as informal and accessible as possible. It should be enabled to deal promptly with emergency applications.

249. We recognise that the range of decisions which the new court will be required to take will be wide, and that some minor matters can appropriately be dealt with at quite a low level. But the type of life or death decision which is the subject of our report should be considered only by judges of appropriate status and experience. In addition to provision for appeal in individual cases we recommend that there should also be provision for monitoring decisions of the court to ensure consistency of ethical standards and direction. We recognise that other considerations may make it desirable that, at least in some cases, the proceedings of the court take place in private. Wherever possible, however, we would recommend public hearings. In any event the judgments of the court should be published.

250. In this connection we note that some witnesses suggested that use of the term "next of kin" in a medical or legal setting was misleading, often being interpreted by patients as requiring them to name their spouse or nearest blood relative when they might prefer to specify a partner or friend. Since the object is surely to identify the individual most closely associated with the patient, we recommend that the new legal forum, and the health-care professions, should adopt an expression more in keeping with current social realities.

TREATMENT-LIMITING DECISIONS

251. The issue of treatment-limiting decisions[1] is crucial to many of the concerns which our witnesses raised with us. For most practical purposes we do not discern any significant ethical difference between those decisions which involve discontinuing a treatment already begun and those which involve not starting a treatment. To make such a distinction could result in patients being subjected to the continuation of unnecessary and burdensome procedures simply because they had been started previously; or it could restrict a doctor's freedom to do everything possible for the patient in an emergency or when diagnosis is uncertain. We do not therefore distinguish between withholding and withdrawal of treatment, in our discussion of treatment-limiting decisions. However, we acknowledge that, in the case of neonates particularly, the withdrawal of treatment becomes harder as time passes, as more love and commitment are invested in the child as an individual.

252. All our witnesses agreed that there is a point at which the duty to try to save a patient's life is exhausted, and at which continued treatment may be inappropriate. But this is not a point which can be readily defined, since it must be identified in the light of each patient's individual condition and circumstances. Obviously it is inappropriate to give treatment which is futile in the

---

[1] See paragraphs 50 to 59 above.

sense that it fails to achieve the hoped for physical result. Indeed to continue a treatment in such circumstances could be irresponsible. A decision not to do so will rarely be controversial.

253. In other cases, a decision to limit treatment may depend on the balance between the burdens which the treatment will impose and the benefits which it is likely to produce. Competent patients can often, with medical advice and after full discussion, make such decisions themselves, perhaps for example foregoing the possibility of a few extra weeks of life because the possible side-effects of the proposed treatment might necessitate being in hospital rather than at home. Such a decision is made on the basis of the quality rather than the length of life, but few would dispute the right of the patient to choose in that way.

254. Controversy arises when treatment-limiting decisions based on the balance of burdens and benefits must be made in respect of incompetent patients. The spectre of one individual judging the quality of life of another gives rise to potent fears. But such decisions, however difficult, must be made if incompetent patients are not to be subjected to the aggressive over-treatment to which competent patients would rightly object.

255. Treatment-limiting decisions in respect of an incompetent patient should be taken jointly by all those involved in his or her care, including the entire health-care team and the family or other people closest to the patient. Their guiding principle should be that a treatment may be judged inappropriate if it will add nothing to the patient's well-being as a person. In most cases full discussion will ultimately lead to agreement on what treatment is appropriate or inappropriate. Where agreement cannot be reached after adequate discussion and time for reflection, provision should be made for a party to the decision-making to apply for a decision from the new forum which we have recommended[1].

256. Some people may suggest that clearer general guidance is needed as to the circumstances in which treatment may be judged inappropriate. But we are not satisfied that this is either possible or desirable. Such a judgment must be made in relation to the condition, circumstances and values of the individual patient. Such matters cannot be defined or legislated for and consensus must be developed on a case-by-case basis, inching forward as best we can. For these reasons we do not favour legislation on the lines of the bill presented by Lord Alport. We are confident that, in making treatment-limiting decisions, doctors who act responsibly, in the way we have described, have adequate protection under existing law.

257. Nor do we think it helpful to attempt a firm distinction between treatment and personal care[2], implying that the former may be limited and the latter not. The two are part of a continuum, and such boundary as there is between them shifts as practice evolves and particularly as the wider role of nursing develops. This boundary is one which the courts were required to try to define in the case of Tony Bland, and that gave rise to much debate about whether nutrition and hydration, even when given by invasive methods, may ever be regarded as a treatment which in certain circumstances it may be inappropriate to initiate or continue. This question has caused us great difficulty, with some members of the Committee taking one view and some another, and we have not been able to reach a conclusion. But where we are agreed is in judging that the question need not, indeed should not, usually be asked. In the case of Tony Bland, it might well have been decided long before application was made to the court that treatment with antibiotics was inappropriate, given that recovery from the inevitable complications of infection could add nothing to his well-being as a person. We consider that, had Tony Bland's health-care team and family been in agreement on this course, it would have been ethically and practically appropriate for such treatment to have been discontinued. Because of his established pvs there was no duty to strive to preserve his life by medical means. We consider that progressive development and ultimate acceptance of the notion that some treatment is inappropriate should make it unnecessary to

---

1 See paragraph 245.

2 See paragraphs 60 to 65 above.

consider the withdrawal of nutrition and hydration, except in circumstances where its administration is in itself evidently burdensome to the patient.

PERSISTENT VEGETATIVE STATE

258. The case of Tony Bland made it clear that, quite apart from questions of nutrition and hydration, treatment-limiting decisions are felt to be particularly difficult in respect of patients in pvs[1]. This seems to be, at least partly, because of widespread misunderstanding of the condition, confusion over diagnosis and misplaced expectations of improvement. We suggest that the development of a generally accepted definition of the condition would assist both the health-care professions and the wider community, and could in time lead to a code of practice for the management of patients in pvs. A similar process occurred in respect of brain stem death. The issue was initially very controversial and hotly debated[2]. But gradually both medical and lay opinion have evolved to a point where there is now almost total acceptance of a single definition of brain stem death and widespread understanding of its implications and management. We consider that a comparable process of evolving a commonly-accepted definition of pvs and a code of practice relating to management would be helpful. We therefore recommend that the colleges and faculties of all the health-care professions, together with other relevant professional bodies, should seek to establish such a definition. We suggest that it might include the following elements—

— that over a period of not less than 12 months there had been no return of cognitive, behaviourial or verbal responses, no purposive motor responses or other evidence of voluntary motor activity

— that the accepted clinical and investigative diagnostic criteria, developed on the basis of those referred to in Appendix 4, were all present

— that the diagnosis of pvs on those criteria should be based on repeated observation by the physician responsible for the care of the patient and should be confirmed by a neurologist of consultant status not previously involved in the case.

"MERCY KILLING"

259. We have considered suggestions that, although deliberate killing should remain a criminal offence, killing to relieve suffering (that is deliberate killing with a merciful motive) should not be murder but that a new offence of "mercy killing" should be created[3]. At present the offence of murder embraces acts of deliberate killing which vary enormously in their character and which most people would agree vary "in degree of moral guilt"[4]. The significant question however is whether the law could or should make a distinction between them.

260. We consider that it should not. To distinguish between murder and "mercy killing" would be to cross the line which prohibits any intentional killing, a line which we think it essential to preserve. Nor do we believe that "mercy killing" could be adequately defined, since it would involve determining precisely what constituted a compassionate motive. For these reasons we do not recommend the creation of a new offence.

PENALTY FOR MURDER

261. Pressure for a new offence of "mercy killing" arises mainly because of the perceived injustice of the mandatory life sentence for murder[5]. We strongly endorse the recommendation of a previous Select Committee[6] that the mandatory life sentence should be abolished. This would

---

1 See paragraphs 156-162 above.

2 See Appendix 5 for a brief discussion of this issue.

3 See paragraphs 127-129 above.

4 Report of the Committee on the Penalty for Homicide, Prison Reform Trust, London 1993, page 21.

5 See paragraphs 130 to 135 above.

6 *Murder and Life Imprisonment*, Report of the Select Committee, Session 1988-89, HL Paper 78-I.

enable the judicial process to take proper account of the circumstances of a case and the motives of the accused. It would avoid the law being brought into disrepute either by the mandatory imposition of a life sentence in respect of an act which was widely thought to be compassionate and (by some) arguably justifiable, or by the inappropriate substitution of lesser charges where it was expected that a jury would not convict for murder because of the mandatory life sentence. It would also give scope for an effective life sentence to be imposed where the circumstances made it appropriate.

ASSISTED SUICIDE

262. As far as assisted suicide is concerned, we see no reason to recommend any change in the law. We identify no circumstances in which assisted suicide should be permitted, nor do we see any reason to distinguish between the act of a doctor or of any other person in this connection.

ADVANCE DIRECTIVES

263. We commend the development of advance directives[1]. They enable patients to express in advance their individual preferences and priorities in respect of medical treatment should they subsequently become incompetent. Their preparation can (and indeed should) stimulate discussion of those preferences between doctors and patients. They can assist the health-care team and other carers in making decisions about appropriate treatment in respect of patients who are no longer able to take part in that debate. Advance directives may express refusal of any treatment or procedure which would require the consent of the patient if competent. We emphasise however that they should not contain requests for any unlawful intervention or omission: nor can they require treatment to be given which the health-care team judge is not clinically appropriate.

264. We have given careful consideration to the terms of Lord Allen of Abbeydale's private member's bill, and to the points which he set out in his two memoranda. We have also considered the arguments of other witnesses who advocated legislation on the subject of advance directives. But we conclude that legislation for advance directives generally is unnecessary. Doctors are increasingly recognising their ethical obligation to comply with advance directives. The development of case law is moving in the same direction. We agree with the assessment of the Crown Prosecution Service[2] and confidently expect that a doctor who acted in accordance with an advance directive, where the clinical circumstances were such as the patient had considered, would not be guilty of negligence or any criminal offence. Adequate protection for doctors exists in terms of the current law and in trends in medical practice. We suggest that it could well be impossible to give advance directives in general greater legal force without depriving patients of the benefit of the doctor's professional expertise and of new treatments and procedures which may have become available since the advance directive was signed. We recognise that it would be possible to specify precisely particular categories of treatment which a patient would find unacceptable in **any** circumstances, such as a blood transfusion in the case of a Jehovah's Witness.

265. Instead of legislation for advance directives generally, we recommend that the colleges and faculties of all the health-care professions should jointly develop a code of practice to guide their members. The BMA's Statement on Advance Directives[3] has much to recommend it as a basis for such a code. The informing premise of the code should be that advance directives must be respected as an authoritative statement of the patient's wishes in respect of treatment. Those wishes should be overruled only where there are reasonable grounds to believe that the clinical circumstances which actually prevail are significantly different from those which the patient had anticipated, or that the patient had changed his or her views since the directive was prepared. A directive may also be overruled if it requests treatment which the doctor judges is not clinically indicated, or if it requests any illegal action. There should be a presumption, in the absence of any explicit instruction to the contrary, in favour of all ordinary care and clinically-indicated treatment

---

[1] See paragraphs 181 to 215 above.

[2] See paragraph 183 above.

[3] Published in April 1992 and printed at PP 33-39.

being given. A doctor who treats a patient in genuine ignorance of the provisions of a directive should not be considered culpable if the treatment proves to have been contrary to the wishes therein expressed, and there should be no expectation that treatment in an emergency should be delayed while enquiry is made about a possible advance directive. Doctors who anticipate having conscientious objections to complying with the directives of their patients should make this clear at an early stage in their preparation, so that patients may transfer to other doctors if they wish.

266. The code of practice should also encourage professionals to disseminate information about advance directives. It should establish procedures for a directive to be lodged by a patient with the general practitioner, who should be required to produce it to any other health-care professional who has care of the patient, for example on the patient's admission to hospital. The existence of an advance directive could be indicated by a card which the patient would carry, and the code should make provision for such a practice.

267. We also recommend that the proposed code of practice should encourage, though not require, regular review and re-endorsement by patients of the provisions of their advance directives. This would not only go some way towards eliminating the danger of a directive becoming out of line both with medical practice and with the patient's current wishes but would also demonstrate the patient's continuing commitment to the directive, which would reinforce its value as a statement of the patient's wishes.

PROXY DECISION-MAKING[1]

268. Whilst the idea of the patient-appointed proxy is in many ways attractive, it is vulnerable to the same problems as advanced directives, and indeed to a greater degree. Whilst the intentions of a mature adult may remain tolerably stable for many years, the same cannot be said about the person whom the future patient regards as most suitable to reflect in a sympathetic and sensitive manner the particular mixture of ethical, social, religious and emotional premises which would have determined any choice made by the patient. Personal relationships are not immutable, and the choice of proxy might become out of date within quite a short time. Thus, unless the advanced choice is repeatedly revised, something which (life being what it is) may well not happen, there is a risk that when the time for decision arrives it will fall to be made by someone who has lost the close rapport with the patient that once existed, and who may indeed through changes in relationships be someone whom the patient would no longer wish to represent him or her.

269. Furthermore, the two types of substituted decision-making[2] are open to objections, both conceptual and practical, which have been widely discussed in the literature. The conceptual difficulties are particularly prominent in relation to surrogates of the second kind, where the appointment is made, not by the patient himself, but on an *ad hoc* basis by an external agency once the question of withholding or withdrawing treatment has arisen. Thus, for example, the appointment of a surrogate to act for a patient who, through mental infirmity, has never been competent to form a reasoned judgment, seems to stretch the concept of patient autonomy to breaking point. This would also be the case if the patient were a carefree young adult, living solely in the present, with no thought for the morrow and no true understanding that life may change for the worse, and having no taste or capacity for addressing the wider and deeper issues raised by grave illness, inability to communicate, destruction of personal dignity and erosion of the quality of life. It may be said with force that it is no more than a fiction to suppose that a surrogate in choosing between life or death is making a choice as the representative of the patient when it is a choice which the patient never had the occasion to contemplate.

270. The practical difficulties of ascertaining what choice the patient would have made if capable of doing so have been widely recognised. Even a thoughtful and articulate person, discussing the question in depth with relatives or peers, may not have foreseen the kind of bodily

---

[1] See paragraphs 216 to 221 above.

[2] See paragraph 217 above.

or mental extremity which puts the continuation of life in issue; and in the majority of cases, no such discussions will have taken place, so that the putative intentions of the patient would have to be gleaned from random previous statements, coupled with a general appreciation of the patient's moral and social convictions. It has been asserted that as the sole basis for decision, divorced from wider consideration of "best interest", this type of material is unreliable for three reasons. First, "verbal expressions of preferences lack the indicia of commitment and thoughtfulness attributable to actual choices. Second, because a person's preferences can change radically over time, use of prior statements ignores the possibility that the person may have incorporated revised goals, values, and definitions of personal well-being into the decision he would make. Finally, informal oral statements are likely to be so general as to provide little guidance in concrete treatment decisions[1]."

271. The fact that even a decision made by the surrogate in complete good faith may lack objectivity cannot be ignored. As the prolongation of life becomes ever more successful, and more expensive, a surrogate (who may often be either paying the bills or be entitled to benefit from the patient's estate which is being depleted by the bills) cannot be unaware of the financial detriment which prolongation carries in its train - a problem which the patient himself might not have foreseen. Conversely, the psychological pressure on a surrogate who is also a member of the family may cause him or her to insist on the maintenance of life beyond the point at which the patient, if competent, would have wished the struggle to be abandoned. Whilst acknowledging the strong current of opinion in favour of proxy decision-making, for all these reasons we do not favour the more widespread development of such a system. There is however no reason why an advance directive should not contain a request to doctors to consult if practicable with a third party, without the doctors being necessarily bound by that third party's opinion.

PROFESSIONAL RESPONSIBILITY

272. Some people may consider that our conclusions overall give too much weight to the role of accepted medical practice, and that we advocate leaving too much responsibility in the hands of doctors and other members of the health-care team. They may argue that doctors and their colleagues are no better qualified than any other group of people to take ethical decisions about life and death which ultimately have a bearing not only on individual patients but on society as a whole. But no other group of people is better qualified to do so. Doctors and their colleagues are versed in what is medically possible, and are therefore best placed to evaluate the likely outcomes of different courses of action in the very different circumstances of each individual case. By virtue of their vocation, training and professional integrity they may be expected to act with rectitude and compassion.

273. Moreover, health-care professionals are by no means a homogeneous group: they bring to their practice a variety of philosophical and religious views which make it unlikely that any single ethos is likely to dominate accepted practice in a way which might prejudice the interests of an individual patient. In any event, few decisions of the kind which we have discussed are any longer taken by a practitioner acting alone. The increasing emphasis on discussion with the patient or, in the case of an incompetent patient, on consultation with the patient's family or friends, means that the values and priorities of the individual are given proper weight in the decision-making process. This is further reinforced by the growing importance attached to collective decision-making by the health-care team as a whole, and in particular, the greater participation of nurses in the decision-making process. This is another way in which a further point of view, informed by the close, constant contacts which nurses have with the patient or relatives, is involved in deciding appropriate courses of action. The breadth of experience of a hospital chaplain or other spiritual adviser is another resource which may be drawn upon.

---

1 Harvard Law Review, Vol. 103 No. 7, May 1990, "Developments - Medical Technology and the Law," page 1650.

HEALTH-CARE RESOURCES

274. Obviously, resources for health-care are not infinite. There are limits to what society is able and willing to afford and rationing of resources has become a fact of life in all developed societies. As medical technology becomes more sophisticated and therefore more expensive, difficult and at times controversial decisions must be made about priorities. An element of inequity is inevitable. The development of new treatments for example is particularly costly, and the very latest options will be available to few patients, though it may be hoped that they will lead the way for others.

275. Nonetheless health-care teams should not be put in a position of having to make such decisions in the course of their day-to-day clinical practice. Their concern must be for the welfare of the individual patient. Decisions about the treatments which society can afford should be made elsewhere than in the hospital ward or the doctor's consulting room, and they should be made on the basis that such treatments as society does wish to fund must be available equally to all who can benefit from them. In particular we would emphasise that treatment-limiting decisions of the kind which we have discussed should depend on the condition of the individual patient and on the appropriateness to that patient of whatever treatment or methods of management are generally available, and should not be determined by considerations of resource availability.

276. Despite the inevitable continuing constraints on health-care resources, the rejection of euthanasia as an option for the individual, in the interest of our wider social good, entails a compelling social responsibility to care adequately for those who are elderly, dying or disabled. Such a responsibility is costly to discharge, but is not one which we can afford to neglect. In this connection therefore we make the following recommendations—

- high-quality palliative care should be made more widely available by improving public support for the existing hospice movement, ensuring that all general practitioners and hospital doctors have access to specialist advice, and providing more support for relevant training at all levels

- research into new and improved methods of pain relief and symptom control should be adequately supported and the results effectively disseminated

- training of health-care professionals should do more to prepare them for the weighty ethical responsibilities which they carry, by giving greater priority to health-care ethics and counselling and communication skills

- more formal and regular consideration of health care ethics at a national level would be helpful

- long-term care of those whose disability or dementia makes them dependent should have special regard to the need to maintain the dignity of the individual to the highest possible degree.

CONCLUSION

277. In conclusion, we wish to thank all those who devoted much time and effort to presenting to us their sincerely held opinions. The task of formulating our opinion in the light of their arguments has been a difficult and demanding one. But in the end we have been able to achieve a consensus, and are unanimous in making this report to the House.

PART 4 SUMMARY OF CONCLUSIONS

278. We recommend that there should be no change in the law to permit euthanasia (para. 237).

279. We strongly endorse the right of the competent patient to refuse consent to any medical treatment (para. 234).

280. If an individual refusal of treatment by a competent patient is overruled by the Court, full reasons should be given (para. 235).

281. We strongly commend the development and growth of palliative care services in hospices, in hospitals and in the community (para. 241).

282. Double effect is not in our view a reason for withholding treatment that would give relief, as long as the doctor acts in accordance with responsible medical practice with the objective of relieving pain or distress, and without the intention to kill (para. 242).

283. Treatment-limiting decisions should be made jointly by all involved in the care of a patient, on the basis that treatment may be judged inappropriate if it will add nothing to the patient's well-being as a person (para. 255).

284. We recommend that a definition of pvs and a code of practice relating to its management should be developed (para. 258).

285. Development and acceptance of the idea that, in certain circumstances, some treatments may be inappropriate and need not be given, should make it unnecessary in future to consider the withdrawal of nutrition and hydration, except where its administration is in itself evidently burdensome to the patient (para. 257).

286. Treatment-limiting decisions should not be determined by considerations of resource availability (para. 275).

287. Rejection of euthanasia as an option for the individual entails a compelling social responsibility to care adequately for those who are elderly, dying or disabled (para. 276).

288. Palliative care should be made more widely available (para. 276).

289. Research into pain relief and symptom control should be adequately supported (para. 276).

290. Training of health-care professionals should prepare them for ethical responsibilities (para. 276).

291. Long-term care of dependent people should have special regard to maintenance of individual dignity (para. 276).

292. We support proposals for a new judicial forum with power to make decisions about medical treatment for incompetent patients (paras. 245, 246).

293. We do not recommend the creation of a new offence of "mercy killing" (para. 260).

294. We strongly endorse the recommendation of a previous Select Committee that the mandatory life sentence for murder should be abolished (para. 261).

295. We recommend no change in the law on assisted suicide (para. 262).

296. We commend the development of advance directives, but conclude that legislation for advance directives generally is unnecessary (paras. 263, 264).

297. We recommend that a code of practice on advance directives should be developed (paras. 265-267).

298. We do not favour the more widespread development of a system of proxy decision-making (para. 271).

10

Walton, Davies, Boyd and the legalization of euthanasia

LUKE GORMALLY

1. INTRODUCTION

THIS CHAPTER ESSAYS a critique of a mixed bag of contributions to the contemporary debate about the legalization of euthanasia. 'Walton' in the title designates the Report of the House of Lords Select Committee on Medical Ethics, a Committee chaired by Lord Walton of Detchant; the Committee's Report was published on 17 February 1994 (for convenience I shall refer to the Committee as the Walton Committee and its report as the Walton Report). Davies and Boyd refer to the contributions to the present volume by Jean Davies and Kenneth Boyd.

The Walton Report is a very different document from the writings of Davies and Boyd which are to be considered here. It is the product of a little less than twelve months work by a distinguished Committee whose members heard, pondered and debated evidence from representatives of a fairly wide range of views. The debate within the Committee was clearly at times vigorous and sometimes evidently polarized on fundamental issues. That the Committee produced a unanimous Report is at least in part owing to two facts: the first, that certain issues were either not addressed or left unresolved; the second, that certain recommendations had a significance in the minds of some members which they lacked in the minds of others.[1]

In assessing a report such as that of the Walton Committee, the recommendations of which relate to legislation and public policy, it is not reasonable to expect a developed argument for its recommendations. What one looks for is the consistency of those recommendations with what one takes to be a sound view of what law and public policy should be. So an assessment of the Walton Report requires some exposition of the view that forms the basis of one's assessment.

In responding to Davies' and Boyd's contributions, however, one's critical approach is bound to be different. They are both contributors to the public debate, seeking to persuade the rest of us that we should find some accommodation within the law for the practice of euthanasia. So the questions to be asked about those contributions are in the main about the soundness of the arguments they advance for the conclusions they wish us to embrace, and about their ability to rebut major counterarguments to their positions.

I turn first, then, to a summary exposition of the position which I think can and should be defended about the legalization of euthanasia.[2] This will serve both as the basis for my assessment of the Walton Report and as a statement of the counterposition which Davies and Boyd should be able to dispose of if the position they advocate is to win the intellectual argument.

2. A FRAMEWORK OF MORAL UNDERSTANDING

The moral understanding we need in considering euthanasia and its legalization can begin, I think, from a fundamental intuition about justice. The intuition is that we should not determine in an arbitrary way who are the *subjects* of justice, i.e. who are entitled to be treated justly. A widespread approach, influential in medical ethics, to determining which human beings possess human rights and are to be respected as such, falls foul of this fundamental intuition. For this approach maintains that the value and dignity associated with the possession of basic human rights depends upon human beings first developing psychological abilities which they retain as presently exercisable abilities. But if actual possession of such abilities is a necessary condition of the claim to be treated justly, questions have to be faced about precisely *which* abilities must be possessed, and how developed they must be, before one enjoys this claim to be treated justly. And these questions can be answered only by *choosing* which to count as the relevant abilities and precisely how developed they must be to count. But any such choices are bound to be arbitrary. If I say, for example, that one necessary ability is 'understanding', what exercisable mastery of concepts do I require? Wherever I draw the line, the human beings who fall just below it will differ little in mastery of concepts from those just above the line, and may, in any case, be close in time to achieving the same level of ability. Nonetheless, it is said that they do not possess the fundamental dignity and value in virtue of which one possesses basic human rights.

The only alternative to such arbitrary determinations of who are the subjects of justice is the assumption that every human being – simply in virtue of being human – has the dignity and value recognition of which entails acknowledgement of their basic human rights. And this means that if we are to treat people justly we must regard that dignity and value as an *ineliminable* attribute of human beings.

That proposition is of basic importance when we come to consider when planned killing of a human being may be justified. Voluntary and non-voluntary euthanasia are both types of planned killing.

The most elementary requirement a justification of killing has to meet is that the reason given for the killing is compatible with recognition of the ineliminable dignity and value of the human being who is to be killed.

Does the justification of voluntary euthanasia meet this test? Well, what purports to justify killing a patient at his request? Not just the fact of the request. Requests can be motivated by depression and misinformation, for example. A doctor recognizing that there is a worthwhile life still to be lived is not going to accede to a request for euthanasia even if he has no objections in principle to the practice. He will accede if he can agree that the continuing life of this patient is on balance no longer worthwhile. So it is this judgement – *that the patient lacks a worthwhile life* – which does the real work of justifying the killing of the patient. But such a justification is incompatible with recognizing the ineliminable dignity and value of the patient's life.

This analysis shows that there is very little separating justification of voluntary from justification of non-voluntary euthanasia. In the latter kind of case people are more likely to be open with the judgement that the patient's life is no longer worthwhile; it is because they so think that they believe that putting an end to that life is a benefit to the patient, or at least does him no harm.

The justifications of both voluntary and non-voluntary euthanasia are incompatible, then, with recognition of the ineliminable dignity of every human being; voluntary and non-voluntary euthanasia are radically incompatible with what we need to acknowledge if we are to live well with each other. And since recognition of that dignity is necessary to the very existence of justice in society, the criminal law should not accommodate, either by statute or judicial decision, the practice of either voluntary or non-voluntary euthanasia.

The significance of our equality-in-dignity as human beings for justice in society is the fundamental reason, also, for maintaining criminal sanctions on aiding and abetting suicide. A person who aims to end his own life is clearly persuaded that that life is no longer worth living. The criminal law cannot, consistent with its moral foundations, go along with that estimate of a person's own worth. It does not prosecute those who *attempt* suicide, because of the prudential judgement that in so doing it would be likely further to undermine their prospects of recovering some sense of the worthwhileness of their lives. But it rightly prosecutes the one who aids and abets suicide and who, in doing so, in effect tells the would-be suicide that his life is indeed without value.

If the law should not accommodate euthanasia and aiding and abetting suicide, we need to be clear what is to count as euthanasia and what is to count as suicide.

The fundamental objection to euthanasia which we have identified is an objection to aiming to cause someone's death in order to put an end to a life judged no longer worthwhile. Both the causation of death and the objective achieved in causing death are the *reasons* the agent has in acting.

Both may be present in a course of conduct in which what precisely causes death is not a positive act, such as the injecting of potassium chloride, but the omission of something necessary to sustain life, such as insulin for an insulin-dependent diabetic or food for any human being. Of course, not just *any* person's failure to provide what is necessary to sustain someone's life is a culpable omission, only the failure of those who have some duty to provide what is omitted.

So one can carry out euthanasia by deliberate omissions; and one can deliberately aid and abet suicide by omitting, at the request of the person who desires to die, what is necessary to sustain life, when one knows that the request is (or has been) motivated by the desire of the person making the request to put an end to his own life.

The account I have offered of what is fundamentally objectionable in euthanasiast killing (and, by parity of reasoning, in aiding and abetting suicide) identifies it as any deliberate course of conduct aimed at bringing about a patient's death on the grounds that that patient's life is no longer worthwhile.

This account shows why not *any* causing of a patient's death as a result of, for example, medication aimed at controlling pain is to be counted as euthanasia. For such a causation of death wholly lacks what is essential to euthanasia: for what brings death about is not done *in order* to cause it and, *a fortiori*, not done to put an end to an existence judged no longer worthwhile; causation of death is no part of the agent's *reason for acting*. The doctrine of double effect, that foreseeable but unintended causations of death are not culpable if the good effect one aims to achieve warrants one's chosen conduct, is an integral part of any moral framework which recognizes the crucial moral significance of intention (and reasons for action) to the evaluation of action.

For like reasons, the causation of death is not culpable if it results from a failure to do what one had good and sufficient reason not to do.

This brings us to the consideration (integral to the discussion of euthanasia) of what good reasons a doctor may have for omitting life-saving treatment when the omission may or will cause death. Here we need to consider both reasons grounding the decisions of competent patients and reasons bearing on what is owing to the incompetent patient.

The background against which we should consider such reasons is a clear understanding of the limited purpose of medicine. 'The purpose of medicine is the restoration and maintenance of health (or of some approximation to health) or the palliation of symptoms. Health is that condition of the body in virtue of which it functions well as an organic whole, so that the individual both enjoys physical vitality in itself and is well-placed to achieve some of the other goods intrinsic to human well-being. *Health is valued as inseparably an intrinsic and an instrumental good*. The palliation of symptoms (when cure is not achievable) aims precisely to control those impediments to participation in other human goods which arise from organic malfunctioning; in other words, given that not even an approximation to health can be achieved, one aims to secure as *tolerable* a state of the organism as possible so that conscious living (with family and friends and others) may continue. Thus, palliative medicine, in deploying techniques of pain control, is focused just like other forms of medicine, on the organic component of our aptitude to share in other human goods' (Gormally 1994*a*: 134).

One implication of this understanding of the purpose of medicine is that if a living human body has been so severely damaged that it no longer makes sense to speak of a continuing capacity to share in human goods other than life itself, then what is integral to what we value in health is no longer achievable. But once the good of health, so understood, ceases to be achievable doctors are under no obligation to employ *medical treatment* with a view simply to prolonging life. Prolongation of life is not an independent goal of medicine; it makes sense as long as one can sustain a degree of organic well-functioning sufficient to allow for some sharing, however minimal, in other human goods.

The fact that the specific purpose of medicine is not achievable in a patient does not, however, absolve a doctor from the duties of ordinary care for that patient – the provision of food and fluids, warmth, shelter, and so on. The provision of these is an elementary expression of our recognition of the inherent dignity of the patient, who is not to be abandoned or treated as disposable.

The distinction I have made between the basis of duties to provide medical treatment and the basis of duties to provide ordinary care explains why, for example, it may be reasonable to withdraw antibiotic treatment but not reasonable to withdraw tubefeeding from a patient. (For a fuller treatment of this issue see Gormally 1993*a*.)

I have been discussing a kind of circumstance in which any kind of strictly medical intervention is no longer required because any would be futile in relation to the proper purpose of medicine. 'Futility' names a general reason why treatments may be deemed inappropriate and so withheld or withdrawn: the treatments can no longer achieve the purpose for which they are designed.

But treatments may be withheld or withdrawn – and reasonably refused by a competent patient – not only because they may be futile, but also because, though promising some benefit, they have unduly burdensome consequences for the patient: they are excessively taxing for the patient physically, or psychologically, or spiritually, prevent one from achieving certain important goals, unduly cramp one's lifestyle, impose inordinate financial burdens on others.

Despite much contemporary talk about our new-found liberation from the oppressive grip of medical paternalism, discussion of the rights of the competent patient goes back centuries in the long-established Catholic tradition of reflection and teaching about medical ethics. There were two fundamental reasons recognized in that tradition for the assertion of those rights, which continue, I believe, to be valid. The first is that an adult individual's health is in the first instance *his* responsibility. 'The doctor's responsibility to aid and abet the restoration of health can best be discharged if the basic responsibility of the patient is recognized and respected. This means that the doctor must, within limits, respect the competent patient's choice' (Gormally 1994*a*: 136).

The second reason is that the restoration or maintenance of health in one's life can be constrained by other commitments. Hence the place it has in one's life, and what one can agree to in the way of treatment, must be decided by reference to one's other responsibilities.

Much contemporary assertion of patient's rights, however, rests on more comprehensive claims about the import of respect for autonomy, in the sense of the right of self-determination. Those claims as they are advanced by some are grossly inflated.

To be autonomous means to be self-governed or self-determining in the conduct of one's life. But what exercises of this capacity are genuinely valuable and, as such, to be respected? Only those exercises of the capacity which really make for our flourishing and well-being. Of course this answer assumes that there are objective, knowable conditions of human flourishing, so that it can be shown that some of our choices undermine rather than make for human well-being. That assumption is I believe true (and if it is not then first-order ethical discussion is vacuous). There is nothing, then, in the character of self-destructive choices which commands our respect.

Self-determination is, of course, an integral feature of our well-being: my flourishing as a human being requires that *I* make choices, that what I do is my doing, and what I achieve my achievement. And if the capacity for self-determination is to develop it is evident that there must be some scope for erroneous choices. But given that autonomy is to be valued precisely in so far as it makes for our genuine fulfilment, there are no general grounds for respecting every kind of self-destructive choice (whether the morally self-destructive or the physically self-destructive).

Have we got reason to respect the anticipatory exercise of self-determination that we find in advance directives? It depends on what has been specified.

Advance directives can be useful devices for informing a doctor of the kinds of consequence of treatment that a patient is likely to find unduly burdensome. And a doctor may have good reason to take this information into account when considering whether the treatment he has in mind for a now incompetent patient would be sufficiently beneficial to warrant certain burdensome consequences of the treatment. But the concern which gives point to such deliberations is concern for the *good* of the patient, not concern to respect the patient's autonomy. An incompetent patient no longer possesses autonomy, which requires a present capacity for forming intentions and making choices. It is only those who believe that the dignity and value of a now incompetent patient's life derives wholly from the choices he made when competent who even *appear* to have a case for allowing those choices to override other considerations. But it is false to believe that the dignity and value of an incompetent patient's life rest on such an infirm foundation. His fundamental dignity as a human being exists independently of the character of his prior choices. And what that dignity requires of those who care for him is that they act for his good or, as is commonly said, in his 'best interests'.

However, it will be clear that the notion of 'best interests' as applied to the care of patients has an objective interpretation within the moral framework I am articulating. What *medically* serves a patient's best interests is what secures either a patient's restoration to health, or some approximation to health, or, if the patient is dying, effectively controls distressing symptoms. And what is further required in the best interests of a patient is that he be cared for in ways expressive of the carer's recognition of his human dignity, a recognition incompatible with aiming to end the patient's life.

The above is an outline of the framework of moral understanding I believe we should bring to consideration of the practice of euthanasia and to the question of its legalization, as well as to questions about the ethics of withholding treatment and care which are so closely associated with the topic of euthanasia. We can now turn first of all to an assessment of the Walton Committee's response to the questions which fell to be considered by it.[3]

3. THE WALTON REPORT

3.1. Background to the Report

The main questions which confronted the Committee had been brought into focus by a number of judicial decisions handed down in the first years of this decade and by two cases in particular which attracted considerable public attention. The first of these was the trial and conviction of Dr Nigel Cox for attempted murder after he had injected with potassium chloride his patient Mrs Lillian Boyes who was suffering excruciating pain. The second case was that of Tony Bland, one of the victims of the Hillsborough football ground disaster on 15 April 1989. When he died on 3 March 1993 he had been in what is termed a 'persistent vegetative state' for almost four years. Tony Bland was cared for in the Airedale General Hospital, and the Airedale NHS Trust sought from the High Court 'declarations that the Trust and their responsible physicians may lawfully discontinue all life sustaining treatment and medical support measures designed to keep Anthony Bland alive . . . and that they may lawfully discontinue and thereafter need not furnish medical treatment to Anthony Bland except for such purpose of enabling Anthony Bland to end his life and die peacefully with the greatest dignity and the least of pain, suffering and distress.'

With a minor change of wording these declarations were granted by the High Court and upheld by the Court of Appeal and finally by the House of Lords on 4 February 1993 (*Airedale NHS Trust* v. *Bland* [1993] Appeal Cases 789).

Counsel for the Official Solicitor, representing Tony Bland, had argued that stopping his tubefeeding would be murder because the doctor would be intentionally causing death. Three Law Lords accepted the contention that it was indeed intended to kill Tony Bland (and the remaining two did not reject the contention). As Lord Browne-Wilkinson put it: 'What is proposed in the present case is to adopt a course with the intention of bringing about Anthony Bland's death. As to the element of intention or *mens rea*, in my judgement there can be no real doubt that it is present in this case: the whole purpose of stopping artificial feeding is to bring about the death of Anthony Bland.'

Nonetheless, their Lordships decided that stopping feeding would not be murder, since it is not murder to cause death by an omission if there is no legal duty to carry out the act which is omitted. In the case of Tony Bland, they decided

- that stopping feeding was an omission and
- that the doctor was under *no duty to continue feeding* because
- the feeding was *medical treatment*, which was
- *not in the patient's best interests* as it was
- *futile*, because
- *a responsible body of medical opinion did not regard existence in Tony Bland's condition as a benefit*.

There is much in this judgement that is contestable:

- the classification of tubefeeding as 'medical treatment';
- the view that it was futile;
- the reason given for judging it futile, namely that 'a responsible body of medical opinion did not regard existence in Tony Bland's condition as a benefit'. In other words, because a responsible body of medical opinion would deem Tony Bland's continued existence no longer worthwhile, it was lawful to end his life by stopping tubefeeding;
- and finally, the ruling by a majority of the Law Lords that bringing about a patient's death by deliberate omissions is for a doctor a lawful (and sometimes obligatory) part of carrying out a duty of care for that patient.[4]

Some of the Law Lords explicitly recognized that this ruling relies on a morally indefensible distinction which renders the English law of homicide incoherent. For that law, after *Bland*, treats as criminal a death-causing *act* while treating as lawful a death-causing *omission* decided upon, with the very same intention of causing death, by a doctor who has a duty to care for the patient whose life is thereby terminated.

The *Cox* case and the *Bland* case and earlier cases concerned both with the rights of the competent to refuse treatment and with the proper grounds for decisions to treat the incompetent, were the judicial background to the Walton Committee. Those cases, together with the activities of pressure groups (particularly the Voluntary Euthanasia Society) to secure statutory recognition of advance directives and the legalization of voluntary euthanasia, help explain the terms of reference of the Committee:

> to consider the ethical, legal and clinical implications of a person's right to withhold consent to life-prolonging treatment, and the position of persons who are no longer able to give or withhold consent;
>
> and to consider whether and in what circumstances actions that have as their intention or a likely consequence the shortening of another person's life may be justified on the grounds that they accord with that person's wishes or with that person's best interests;
>
> and in all the foregoing considerations to pay regard to the likely effects of changes in law or medical practice on society as a whole.

Those terms of reference in fact encompass a very large number of questions. It would be beyond the scope of this chapter to assess the Walton Committee's response to all the questions that fell to be considered by it. But the Committee's answers to (or failures to answer) certain questions have a fundamental bearing on their recommendations about what the law and public policy should be in regard to euthanasia. It is on their response to those questions that I shall base my assessment of the Walton Report.

The fundamental questions I take to be the following:

- What counts as euthanasia? And, specifically, is there euthanasia only where there is a *positive* act intended to terminate the life of the patient for, as it is thought, the patient's benefit?
- Is the foreseen causation of a patient's death, brought about in consequence of measures intended to control pain, indistinguishable from euthanasia, or is it clearly distinguishable? (The question about double effect.)
- Is there a justification for voluntary euthanasia which would warrant its legalization?
- Is there a justification for non-voluntary euthanasia (i.e. euthanasia of those incapable of asking to be killed) in terms of their 'best interests'?
- What ethical limits are there (and what legal limits should there be) to a competent person's right to withhold consent to life-prolonging treatment?
- Can one as a doctor be guilty of aiding and abetting suicide by omitting life-prolonging treatment declined by a competent patient?
- How much authority should anticipatory decisions (or advance directives) have in respect of one's treatment when incompetent? What practical limits should there be to their influence on clinical decisions?
- Is it possible to aid and abet suicide in complying with an advance directive?
- How should one determine what are the 'best interests' of an incompetent patient?

I have already presented in section 2 broadly sketched answers, consistent with the tradition of common morality, to these questions. And that will be the basis on which I evaluate the Walton Report's answers.

3.2. The Walton Report

The Report's recommendations begin well with the recommendation that there should be no change in the law to permit euthanasia. A number of strong reasons are offered for this recommendation, but the most fundamental is expressed as follows:

> we do not believe that these arguments [for legalizing euthanasia] are sufficient reason to weaken society's prohibition of intentional killing. That prohibition is the cornerstone of law and social relationships. It protects each of us impartially, embodying the belief that all are equal. (para. 237)

This formulation is notable for two things: first, it makes clear that what is prohibited is intentional killing. Secondly, it links that prohibition to that which gives us an equal claim to just treatment – our ineliminable equality-in-dignity as human beings.

Because the prohibition bears on *intentional* killing, the Report rightly goes on to defend the notion of double effect from two charges:

- first, that it erroneously seeks to attach moral significance to the distinction between intentional and foreseen causations of death, and thereby accommodates the 'hypocritical' practice of euthanasia accomplished as a foreseeable side-effect of administering opiates;
- secondly, that the distinction it makes between foreseen and intended causations of death is in fact indiscernible.

As the Report points out: 'juries are asked every day to assess intention in all sorts of cases, and could do so in respect of double effect if in a particular instance there was any reason to suspect that the doctor's primary intention was to kill the patient rather than to relieve pain and suffering' (para. 243).

Consistent with their emphasis on intentional killing, the Committee is rightly opposed to the creation of a new offence of 'mercy killing': 'To distinguish' (they say)

> between murder and 'mercy killing' would be to cross the line which prohibits any intentional killing, a line which we think it essential to preserve. Nor do we believe that 'mercy killing' could be adequately defined, since it would involve determining precisely what constituted a compassionate motive. (para. 260)

Equally welcome is the Committee's view that

> As far as assisted suicide is concerned, we see no reason to recommend any change in the law. We identify no circumstances in which assisted suicide should be permitted, nor do we see any reason to distinguish between the act of a doctor or of any other person in this connection. (para. 262)

So far so good. There is, however, a major drawback to these welcome recommendations on euthanasia and suicide: the Report is radically unsatisfactory on what *counts* as euthanasia and suicide. The fault is not immediately apparent in the Committee's recommendations but goes right back to the stipulative definition of euthanasia which seems to have controlled the Committee's deliberations and which is stated at the outset of the Report at paragraph 20. Euthanasia is defined as 'a deliberate *intervention* undertaken with the express intention of ending a life to relieve intractable pain' (emphasis added). This definition, in suggesting that euthanasia exists only where there is a *positive act* intended to end a life has a decisive and shaping influence on the entire Report.[5] Because of this definitional move the Committee manages to avoid confronting the reality of intentional killing *by omission*. In doing so they also evade the urgent need to confront the intellectually incoherent condition of the English law of homicide following the *Bland* judgement. As I remarked earlier, this was well recognized by some of the Law Lords at the time of the judgement, and it quite clearly remained a preoccupation of one of them, Lord Mustill, throughout his time on the Committee. This makes the Committee's failure to recommend any resolution of the incoherence all the more puzzling. The proper direction resolution of the incoherence should take is reversal of that part of the judgement which held that terminating a patient's life by planned omission may be a lawful (and, indeed, obligatory) part of carrying out a duty of care.

As long as we are stuck with the indefensible doctrine that you may not intentionally cause a patient's death by a positive act but that you may (and sometimes ought) to cause a patient's death by a course of planned omissions embarked on precisely because a 'responsible body of medical opinion' judges that the patient no longer has a worthwhile life, then the law is saying both 'Yes' and 'No' to euthanasia. It did not say 'Yes' to euthanasia before *Bland*, and the Walton Committee's apparent 'No' contributes nothing to reversing the judicially contrived 'Yes'.

The Report's recommendations on euthanasia would leave us, then, with a profoundly unsatisfactory legal framework for the practice of medicine.

Related to the Report's systematic oversights about euthanasia by planned omission is its blindness to the reality of suicide by planned omission and the way this can implicate doctors in aiding and abetting such suicide.

There are two reasons, I think, why the law should not seek to have doctors override apparently suicidal refusals of treatment by competent patients. The first reason is that it is not always easy to distinguish a suicidal refusal of treatment from one reasonably motivated by consideration of the burdens of treatment. The second reason is that, because of the positive value of encouraging the exercise of self-determination by competent patients in regard to health, public policy must leave some scope for choices contrary to a person's interests.

But these reasons do not justify the Report's 'strong endorsement' at paragraph 234 of 'the right of the competent patient to refuse consent to any medical treatment, for whatever reason'. What this formulation fails to recognize is that 'a refusal which is motivated by suicidal intent is unlawful even though suicide itself is not a criminal offence' (Finnis 1994: 168). If suicidal intent were not unlawful, it is difficult to see how it could be maintained that assistance, and agreements to assist, in suicide are serious criminal offences.

The value of a present exercise of self-determination in regard to health is *not* a consideration with any application to the incompetent. Consequently, if a doctor has good reason to think that the advance directive of a once competent patient is motivated by suicidal intent in directing the withdrawal of treatment or basic care (such as nutrition) he has good reason to override that directive. The Committee do emphasize that advance directives 'should not contain requests for any unlawful intervention or *omission*' (emphasis added), but since there is no recognition in the Report of *omission motivated by suicidal intent*, the Report makes no recommendation that directives which require assistance in suicide by omission of treatment or care should be made illegal (if they are not already).[6]

In discussing treatment of the incompetent the Committee are inclined to recommend a 'best interests' standard. But they make determinative of a patient's 'best interests' – following judicial precedent – 'a responsible and competent body of relevant professional opinion'. This does not offer an objective criterion of 'best interests', but a formal device which on occasion has shown itself to be a vehicle for advancing euthanasiast decisions to withdraw or withhold treatment or care, supposedly in the 'best interests' of patients, on the ground that the patient would be better off dead.

In discussing decisions to limit treatment of incompetent patients the Committee recommend that:

> The[ir] guiding principle should be that a treatment may be judged inappropriate *if it will add nothing to the patient's well-being as a person.* (para. 255) [Emphasis added]

This formulation, read – as it will be read by many – in the light of positions advanced by a number of contemporary writers in medical ethics, seems manifestly dangerous. For if so read, the application of the 'guiding principle' will be decided by the consideration that the life of the patient is so irretrievably *subpersonal* in character that nothing could count as adding to 'the patient's well-being as a person'. So understood, the formula allows considerable scope for variants on the judgement that, since patients no longer have worthwhile lives, it is reasonable to withhold treatment and/or care precisely to end those lives. The Committee's formula offers no safeguard against policies of euthanasia by planned omission.

It should be clear, then, that euthanasia by planned omission is neither clearly identified nor opposed by the Report. And in recommending abolition of the mandatory life sentence for murder (para. 261) the Committee may seem to have wished to mitigate the sanctions of the criminal law for those who carry out euthanasia by positive act. If Parliament were to accept this recommendation we may find that sentencing policy has the effect of further encouraging active euthanasia.

3.3 Conclusion

In relation to the precise question of whether euthanasia should be legalized, the position of the Walton Report can be summarized as follows:

- It makes recommendations opposing the legalization of both euthanasia and assisted suicide by positive act. In doing so, the Report may be said to have held the line against further erosion of respect for human dignity beyond the point reached in the *Bland* judgement.
- The Report makes no recommendations which would resolve the incoherent state of the law created by the *Bland* judgement. Consequently the framework of the law for the practice of medicine will remain, as far as the influence of the Report goes, inherently instable.
- The Report seems unaware of the moral reality of suicide by planned omission, and is bereft of recommendations for how the law or codes of practice might enable doctors appropriately to respond to such suicidal proposals as they may be found in advance directives.
- The Report's recommendations on treatment of the incompetent and treatment-limiting decisions for the incompetent seem hospitable to policies of euthanasia by planned omission.

Given the composition of the Walton Committee, it is reasonable to acclaim the achievement of those of its members who successfully resisted recommendations which might further have eroded respect and protection for vulnerable human beings. But there was an urgent need to address the law's present incoherence in prohibiting euthanasia by positive act while permitting (and sometimes enjoining) euthanasia by planned omission. The Report gives little sign of recognizing the need, let alone addressing it. It remains, therefore, that there is everything still to play for in the public policy debate over how the incoherence should be resolved. Jean Davies and Kenneth Boyd are clearly among those who would like to see the law accommodate active euthanasia. What do their chapters in this book have to offer in the way of persuasive argument for such accommodation?

4. JEAN DAVIES

Despite Mrs Davies' experience as a leading figure, nationally and internationally, in the voluntary euthanasia movement, she has little to offer in the way of serious moral argument for the radical changes in law she would like to see. She seems to *assume* she belongs to the party of enlightenment and, as such, has no need to work at making her case. It is characteristic of her confidence that she thinks of the UK as 'lagging' behind other countries – behind the United States over giving statutory force to advance directives, and behind Holland, of course, in its judicial and legislative accommodation of euthanasia.

While Mrs Davies does not undertake to argue a case she does have a number of points she asserts and which might be thought to tell in favour of legalizing euthanasia. I will take them up and comment on them.

> the voluntary euthanasia movement is not concerned with involuntary euthanasia. The arguments supporting the former are very different from those that would justify the latter. (page 84)

There is, of course, a distinction between voluntary and non-voluntary euthanasia, but what distinguishes them (the request of the patient) is not what is decisive in justifying voluntary euthanasia. As I have already explained (section 2), what bears the main weight of justifying voluntary euthanasia also justifies non-voluntary euthanasia. If it is reasonable to claim that killing a person is a benefit to him only if that person no longer has a worthwhile life, then the incompetent as well as the competent stand to be benefited. Why should the inability of the incompetent to request the benefit be deemed a reason for depriving them of it? The difference, then, between voluntary and non-voluntary euthanasia while obvious enough is neither deep nor very significant. Hence there is no reason in principle to accept Mrs Davies' confident assertion that proposed legislation would 'sharply distinguish between them and confine itself entirely to medical help to die given at the patient's considered and enduring request'. (page 84) I will briefly comment later on the empirical evidence suggesting that whatever *legislation* may confine itself to, doctors will not in practice be staying within the confines.

Given what offers itself as the decisive consideration in the justification of voluntary euthanasia, the voluntary euthanasia movement cannot confidently dissociate itself (as Mrs Davies assumes) from Nazi euthanasia. The connection is not an accident of linguistic association but intrinsic, arising from what can be seen to be decisive to the justification of killing in both voluntary and Nazi euthanasia.

The Nazi practice of euthanasia had its intellectual roots in the eugenics movement which became increasingly influential in German medical circles from the end of the nineteenth century. The movement grew in part as a response to the severe economic conditions in Germany, particularly after defeat in the 1914–18 War. When the jurist Karl Binding and the psychiatrist Alfred Hoche published their tract *The Permission to Destroy Life That Is Not Worth Living* in 1920 (Hoche and Binding 1920), their *motive* was to rid society of the 'human ballast and enormous economic burden' of care for the mentally ill, the handicapped, retarded and deformed children, and the incurably ill. But the *reason* they invoked to *justify* the killing of human beings who fell into these categories was that the lives of such human beings were 'not worth living', were 'devoid of value'.

Once it is accepted that one may justify the killing of a human being on the grounds that he lacks a worthwhile life, one has in effect repudiated recognition of the ineliminable dignity and worth of every human being. And with that repudiation goes repudiation of the indispensable foundation of justice in society.

It seems clear that Mrs Davies would associate herself with those whose view of human worth and dignity does entail a denial of basic human rights to many human beings. She thinks that the principle of the sanctity of life is too tainted by its religious roots to have a role in determining law and public policy in a secular society. But the principle of the sanctity of life is nothing more than the principle of the inviolability of innocent human life, i.e. the inviolability of the lives of those who could not be said to deserve death. If you kill someone because you think that for some reason he *deserves* death your reason for killing him is at least not inconsistent with recognition of his dignity as a human being. Indeed the thought that someone may deserve to be so treated assumes a high view of the dignity of that person for one thinks of him as answerable either for the capital crime he commits (for which he deserves capital punishment) or for the grave threat to the common good he is party to in taking up arms against the state (for which he has no right to expect not to be killed) (Gormally 1993*b*: 766).

There seems to be no place in Mrs Davies' outlook for the inviolability of innocent human life, for she appears to associate herself with the discriminatory division of human beings (advocated in one form or another by Singer, Kuhse, Warnock, Dworkin and others) into those who enjoy 'the specifically human consciousness of having a life to live' and those who are 'simply alive'. Only the lives of the former possess distinctive value, because it is only in the consciousness of having a life to live and in the exercise of the abilities to live it that one gives value to one's life. Those who lack that consciousness and the associated abilities simply lack valuable lives; in themselves they represent no compelling reason why we should not end their lives (Gormally 1994*a*: 120–6).

In alluding to the distinction between 'being alive' and 'having a life to live', Jean Davies refers to Tony Bland and other patients in a 'persistent vegetative state' (PVS). But it would be a mistake to think that it is only PVS patients who might be described as not having a 'life to live'. The distinction when applied is necessarily arbitrary in determining who shall and who shall not be deemed to have lives to live (see section 2). At various times the distinction has been employed to exclude from the scope of justice the unborn child, the newborn child, infants before they acquire a concept of themselves as perduring entities, the mentally handicapped, and those with senile dementia. The distinction is all too apt for employment as a convenient device for rationalizing the killing of the weak and the vulnerable by those who find their existence inconvenient.

Jean Davies takes it that the legalization of euthanasia is warranted by what she supposes to be the dominant social understanding of the claims of autonomy. And she takes the claims of autonomy to override other moral principles. She quotes in support of this view observations made by judges in the *Bland* case, particularly Lord Goff's view that 'the principle of the sanctity of human life must yield to the principle of self-determination'. But this dictum must be read in the light of the fact that Lord Goff is in the context giving a quite unconventional interpretation to the principle of the sanctity of human life, for he takes it to encompass two quite distinct principles, neither of which is the principle of the sanctity of human life. The principles which underlie and explain Lord Goff's observations are: (i) 'It is always unlawful to kill (take another man's life)'; (ii) 'Human life should be preserved if at all possible, by any available means, regardless of circumstances'. Neither is the principle of the sanctity of human life as traditionally understood, which stipulates that 'It is always wrong intentionally to kill an innocent human being' (Gormally 1994*a*: 119 footnote). If Mrs Davies thinks *this* principle may be overridden by the claims of autonomy then it should be quite evident that her position offers no defence for the weak in face of the will of the powerful. It is a high price to pay for advocacy of euthanasia.

Mrs Davies seems to think that the claims of autonomy give an overriding authority to advance directives. She invokes in support of this view the evidence given by the Crown Prosecution Service (CPS) to the Walton Committee. The CPS's evidence is not, however, a satisfactory basis for evaluating the force of advance directives. The evidence states:

> 3.13 If an insensate patient has expressed his wishes *vis-à-vis* not consenting to medical treatment in the future (so called 'living wills'), doctors must abide by the terms of that previous expression of intention or wish, though a special care may be necessary to ensure that any prior refusal of consent to medical treatment is still properly to be regarded as applicable in the circumstances which have subsequently occurred. (Walton III: 81; Walton I: 39, para. 183)[7]

But that is not the only care in respect of an advance directive which a doctor needs to have. Though the Walton Committee say that 'We agree with the assessment of the Crown Prosecution Service' (Walton I: 54, para. 264), what they say a paragraph earlier (para. 263) is more basic for defining the concern a doctor should have. 'We emphasise . . . that they [advance directives] should not contain requests for any unlawful intervention or *omission*' [emphasis added]. As I have earlier noted (section 2) an omission motivated by euthanasiast or suicidal *intent* is unlawful.

There is some evidence in Mrs Davies' chapter of two pieces of confusion which frequently feature in advocacy of euthanasia.

She confidently assures her readers that 'Most philosophers agree that allowing to die and helping to die are morally equivalent behaviour for the doctor'. If the types of conduct she has in mind are (i) acting with a view to ending the patient's life and (ii) deciding upon a course of omissions (of treatment or care) also precisely with a view to ending the patient's life, then she would be right to think them morally equivalent. But neither (i) nor (ii) is morally equivalent to: (iii) allowing a patient to die precisely because one has no good reason to seek to prolong his life and has good reason to treat or care for him in ways which will foreseeably result in his death (though what one is aiming at is, e.g., control of pain or the avoidance of the burdens of a form of possibly life-prolonging treatment). Proponents of euthanasia characteristically advance the view that (i) and (ii) are morally equivalent to (iii) because (iii) is a kind of choice which is widely recognized as morally acceptable.

The fact that Mrs Davies quotes global figures from the Remmelink Report for deaths resulting both from the withdrawal of treatment and from the giving of opiates, without referring to the distinction the Remmelink researchers made between intended and merely *foreseen* causation of death, suggests that she wants to regard any 'allowing to die' as morally equivalent to euthanasiast killing. Her reading of philosophers on this topic has perhaps been confined to an unbalanced diet of utilitarians. Admittedly, bioethics is something of a philosophical slum, overcrowded with utilitarian philosophers seeking refuge from the intractable foundational problems that arise from the utilitarian undertaking to reconstruct morality. In the mouths of utilitarians the claim that 'letting die' and 'killing' are morally equivalent merely expresses the theoretical prejudice that the moral significance of our choices derives solely from their consequences. Since the central consequence of both killing and allowing to die is that someone is indeed dead, it is supposed that little of importance exists to distinguish them.

If, however, human action is centrally characterized by intention (i.e. by precisely what it is we propose to do with a view to securing our purpose), then we should observe that while we always have reason not intentionally to kill the innocent we do not always have reason to seek to prolong their lives; indeed we may have good reason to allow them to die (see section 2). So there is no moral equivalence between, on the one hand, my allowing someone to die precisely because life-prolonging treatment would be excessively taxing to him, and, on the other, my deliberately omitting insulin for an insulin-dependent diabetic precisely to bring about his death, or deliberately bringing about someone's death with an injection of potassium chloride. In the first case what I propose in behaving as I do is to avoid the burdens of treatment; bringing about the patient's death is no part of my means or my purpose. In the second and third cases bringing about the death of the patient is what I aim to achieve.

A second confusion characteristic of advocacy of euthanasia emerges in Mrs Davies' view that doctors are perhaps resistant to euthanasia because it means leaving the decision in the hands of the patient. The explanation cannot be true but the assumption that underlies it is widespread. Euthanasia is not a form of suicide. What euthanasiasts like Mrs Davies want is doctors *killing* patients. The doctor is a responsible agent. Any undertaking on his part to kill involves him in responsibility for that course of action – *he* has to answer for what he does. So the doctor has to have what appears to be a good reason for ending the patient's life. Fundamentally, as we have seen, the reason will be some variant of the judgement that the patient no longer has a worthwhile life. Of course the doctor may think there are no objective criteria for assessing the worth of a life, that the only person in a position to say whether a life is worthwhile is the person whose life it is, because it is down to that person to *give* worth to his life. But in concurring with the evaluative viewpoint of the aspirant to euthanasia the doctor is, in practice, making the reason for *his own action* the patient's judgement on his life: that reason is now the doctor's reason, even if it is derivative in the way suggested. It is a muddle, then, to suggest that 'in voluntary euthanasia the patient is the decision-maker'. The patient can decide to ask, but the doctor has to decide whether or not to kill, and he has to have what seems *to him* a good reason for killing. The alternative to overly paternalistic doctors is not medical automata.

Mrs Davies keeps referring to voluntary euthanasia as something the practice of which would be 'carefully controlled', and therefore as very unlikely to give rise to non-voluntary euthanasia, which we unreasonably fear because we imagine doctors will be heedless of the requirements of patient autonomy. The fear is not at all unreasonable as the morally disastrous experience of the Netherlands shows.[8] But Mrs Davies' sanitized account of what happens there prevents her from acknowledging this truth. I shall not tarry over trying to correct her rosy picture of Dutch practice, since elsewhere in this volume John Keown provides an accurate picture of what is happening in Holland, and specifically of the slide from voluntary to non-voluntary euthanasia.

In general Mrs Davies seems to have somewhat relaxed standards in the presentation of empirical data. Along with her colleagues in the Voluntary Euthanasia Society she persists in saying that 79% of the population would like to see voluntary euthanasia legalized. She appears annoyed that the Walton Committee took this claim with a pinch of salt. But as they pointed out to John Oliver, the Secretary of the Society, when he was giving evidence to the Committee, the question 'Should the law allow adults to receive medical help to a peaceful death' is not well designed to elicit information about whether people believe doctors should be allowed to kill their patients (Walton II: 92).

I concluded the previous section by saying that there is much to play for in the public debate about how the present inconsistency in the law should be resolved over euthanasia by action and omission. There is little cogent argument in Mrs Davies' chapter to provide good reasons for resolving the inconsistency in the way she would wish – by legalizing active euthanasia. What is most remarkable about her chapter is the apparent unawareness of just how radical the change is for which she pleads, and of the consequent need to face and answer the fundamental objections to that change.

5. KENNETH BOYD

Two thirds of the way through his chapter Kenneth Boyd writes:

> I have argued that deconstruction of deontological arguments condemning and criminalising suicide means that the proper place for debating the ethics of suicide is in the individual conscience of the person concerned. (page 78)

Boyd's chapter is ostensibly about euthanasia, and it is not to be assumed that the issues raised for morality and the law by A killing B coincide with the issues raised by B killing himself. Nonetheless, the sentence quoted is helpful since many a reader of his chapter may have failed to detect any very clear argument. Indeed, it seems to me that the modish references to deconstructing an argument have nothing to do with showing the falsity of any premises or the invalidity of any inference which has been employed to show the wrongness of suicide, but they have everything to do with advertising the fact that if you swallow some of the dominant intellectual assumptions of our age you will fail to make much sense of traditional Christian reasoning about suicide. Whether that tells against the reasoning or against the assumptions of our age is a question that does not seem to occur to Boyd.

The suspicion that Boyd is not arguing, but simply advertising his realization that there is no support to be found for traditional Christian thinking about suicide if you start from a particular set of philosophical prejudices, is reinforced if we turn to Boyd's invocation of Hume early in his paper.

What Boyd quotes from Hume is not precisely (as he says) Hume's 'rebuttal of the claim that suicide usurps God's role'; it is, rather, part of Hume's attempted rebuttal of the view that suicide is wrong because it 'encroaches on God's established order', where that claim is understood to mean, under one interpretation considered by Hume: it is wrong to disrupt the operation of any general causal law, since the divine order of the universe is constituted precisely by the totality of causal laws.

This démarche of Hume's targets an absurd strawman, and his attack on it involves him in making a number of plainly silly assumptions; their silliness ought, at any rate, to be plain to anyone claiming to be a theologian. Hume talks as though human life just were 'a few ounces of blood' following 'their natural channel' and suicide no more than diverting those 'few ounces . . . from their natural channel'; as such, suicide would be simply a particular instance of that prudent diversion 'from their ordinary course [of] the general laws of motion' without which there would be no durability to our existence.

(We divert rivers from their course to prevent floods and we block the movement of avalanches.)

The life of man is indeed 'submitted . . . to human prudence', but since human life is more than a 'few ounces of blood' prudence, rightly understood, is itself 'submitted' to certain norms – norms observance of which enables us to respect the goods and values which are foundational to our flourishing as human beings. Central to those goods and values is the ineliminable worth of human life itself, a worth which the potential suicide is tempted to deny. Hume's 'argument' simply fails to engage with considerations of this order.

Boyd's carelessness in invoking Hume is repeated in his invocation of the name of St Thomas More who, we are told, 'by implication' called into question 'the traditional Christian condemnation . . . of suicide'. It requires considerable hermeneutical naivety (ill befitting a deconstructionist) to get this conclusion out of a reading of More's *Utopia*. More's *A Dialogue of Comfort Against Tribulation* makes it clear that he regards suicide as a 'wicked temptation'. But even without that evidence it should be clear to anyone sensitive to the *genre* of *Utopia* that its reference to suicide and euthanasia should not be read at face value. The book is a satire on the institutions of sixteenth-century Europe. The vehicle for the satire is More's picture of a society informed by *pagan* virtue. The institutions of a nominally Christian Europe leave it falling far short of pagan virtue. But the assumption behind the device is that pagan virtue too is radically defective, and the institutions of pagan society are corrupted by pride. Even so, they are evidently less corrupt than the institutions of 'Christian Europe'. What the volume is arguing for is radical conversions of heart so that society may be informed by grace rather than pride.[9]

If there is truth in this account of More's intent in *Utopia* it should be clear how misconceived is the attempt to co-opt his name in any attack on traditional Christian teaching about suicide and euthanasia.

More grievous than Boyd's misuse of 'authorities' is the conceptual confusion he weaves around the notion of suicide. It is not properly distinguished from self-sacrifice by reference to *motive* (as Boyd would have it) but rather by reference to *intention*. A man who swallows a cyanide tablet to protect national secrets he fears he would divulge to an enemy under torture is not acting in a self-regarding fashion but he is committing suicide. For suicide involves one aiming (i.e. intending) to end one's own life, whereas what we call self-sacrifice involves no such intention, but rather the willingness to accept that one's death may be caused as a consequence of one's choosing to act (or refrain from acting) in a way required by one's commitment to some purpose, persons or cause. The distinction can be made without psychoanalytic discernment of motives, such as Boyd thinks necessary. Of course a psychoanalytic discernment of motives may suggest that a given individual's suicide is not culpable. But the fact that a particular act is not culpable does not mean that it was not a bad kind of act to have done – contrary to what is required of us if we are to act well with a view to our flourishing as human beings.

Boyd's mistaken proposal that the nature of suicide is to be analysed by reference to motive sets him on a false trail which is the *Leitmotif* of the paper: 'the ethics of suicide . . . is a matter of individual conscience'. There are two key questions for an ethics of suicide: (i) What counts as suicide? (ii) Is it ever justified? Neither of these questions in their general form is to be answered by 'consulting one's own conscience'. Of course there may be a need to clarify one's conscience about the nature of the proposal one has in mind in, say, refusing treatment: Am I doing it because the treatment is unduly onerous or because I want to put an end to my life? And if the answer to the question 'Is suicide ever justified? is 'Yes – sometimes', then, if I have suicide in mind, I should be clear that *my* reasons for committing it are among those which can justify it (i.e. that my conscience and my deliberations are in line with the truth about suicide). But those enquiries (which might be called matters for individual conscience) presume that one has settled the general questions, which are not to be settled by some exercise in the introspection of personal motives.

Boyd's focus shifts from discussing suicide to discussing euthanasia without taking account of the fact that the case for justifying euthanasia does not coincide with the case for justifying suicide. In particular, if we are to legalize euthanasia we need to be satisfied that there is a kind of justification for a doctor killing a patient which is consistent with the valuation of human life which any society must uphold if it is to meet the most basic requirements of justice.

As far as I can make out, Boyd's thinking on finding a legal accommodation for euthanasia seems to proceed as follows:

1 There is reason to acknowledge that straightforward legalization of euthanasia may well expose the frail and the elderly to the dangers of non-voluntary euthanasia.
2 But the protection actually afforded them is by a law which does not distinguish between murder and euthanasia and which has no rational basis as a ground for its enforcement.
3 There are 'groups for whom voluntary euthanasia *may* be justified'.
4 The law is inadequate to this situation because the law crudely assimilates types of activity the specificity of which should be recognized

and respected. If it did, then doctors could sensitively engage in dialogue with patients who ask for euthanasia without looking over their shoulders in fear of a looming charge of murder.

5 Whether a given euthanasia request is *justified* can emerge only in a dialogue between patient and doctor in which the role of the doctor is to so immerse himself in the first-person perspective of the patient as to be able to recognize when 'justification' exists.

6 There is some need to monitor the decisions doctors make to accede to patients' requests for euthanasia, and this is a task which might be carried out by a review committee. (It is not clear exactly what they would be reviewing: the *doctor's* account *post-mortem* of what the patient had thought justified his killing?)

It is hard to imagine what protection Boyd believes his scheme would afford the vulnerable and the frail elderly, utilitarian pressures (as he himself acknowledges) being what they are. But I shall not concentrate on that feature of his proposal but on two key points in his background thinking – (2) and (5) above.

Boyd's view that there is no rational basis for assimilating euthanasia to murder is simply asserted, if somewhat obliquely by way of a quotation from Derrida. If Boyd were to recognize that the core of the concept of murder is 'intentional killing of the innocent', that it is not defined by reference to motives (the character of which is difficult to establish), and that the most fundamental duty of the state is the protection of innocent human life, then he might appreciate the formidable difficulties in the way of detaching the notion of euthanasia from that of murder. Recognition of the difficulties should lead a proponent of the legalization of euthanasia to confront them straightforwardly.

I have argued in section 2 that euthanasia relies for its justification as killing on a valuation of the life of the patient which is simply inadmissible in the law.[10] It is this fact we should keep firmly in focus and, accordingly, we should continue to treat euthanasia as a grave crime which is not in practice to be distinguished in kind from murder.

When turning to consider Boyd's point (5) it becomes apparent that his discussion is obscured by a systematic confusion of problems of understanding with problems of justification. Boyd admits that he finds it 'difficult to specify . . . precise criteria for determining whether or not a particular request [for euthanasia] can be *justified*' [emphasis added]. But his discussion then swings to the problem of acquiring a certain inward *comprehension* of the first-person perspective of the other – specifically, the other who requests euthanasia. This swing seems to be motivated by the thought that justifications of euthanasia are difficult to pin down just in so far as the meaning of the other is inaccessible. But the search for the meaning of the 'other' must presuppose a language of shared meanings. And the question of whether the understood utterances of the 'other' establish a justification of euthanasia in his case in turn *presupposes* criteria of justification, which have some standing independently of the particularities of this conversation with this aspirant to euthanasia.

There is a general need, then, to settle questions about criteria of justification, questions which are clearly separable from questions about whether what any given person says is (i) sufficiently clear to be understood, and (ii) satisfies the proposed criteria for justification. What appears to be Boyd's approach to questions of justification makes the answer unique to each conversation. But that could not yield criteria and, as an approach to seeking justifications, is indistinguishable, for all Boyd has to say in explanation of it, from the arbitrariness of Humpty Dumpty in *Alice Through the Looking-Glass*. Traditional Christian teaching about euthanasia, which Boyd represents as the enemy of sound morality, seems positively liberating in comparison with such oppressive arbitrariness, which has nothing coherent to offer in defence of the weak and the vulnerable.

Boyd's essay prompts a question which, naturally enough, it does not itself raise: Why is someone, who claims to be a theologian, so accepting of the conventional assumptions of his age and so incomprehending of the tradition from which he comes? Indeed, Boyd has so little sense of any moral tradition that he simply side-steps questions about criteria of moral justification and retreats into a picture of unique 'justifications' recognizable in the struggle to articulate the first-person perspective of one's interlocutor. Like a typical post-Nietzschean modernist who has lost faith in the capacity of human discourse to articulate truth and identify falsehood, and who thinks the language of common morality an ideological figleaf for the lust for power, Boyd rises to the claims of the individual as one defending every person's right to self-assertion. But if there are no general criteria of justification – and so of justice – against which to judge exercises of power and self-assertion, what defence have moralists after the style of Boyd against being manoeuvred into the role of apologists for powerful establishments?

6 CONCLUSION

Walton leaves untouched the 'morally and intellectually misshapen' state of the law in regard to euthanasia (Lord Mustill) created by the *Bland* judgement. Jean Davies and Kenneth Boyd would like to see the law rendered consistent by the legalization of active euthanasia. But like most apologists for such a position they do not even begin to rise to the intellectual challenge of making a good case for it.

What we in fact need for the sake of moral truth, intellectual consistency, and the protection of the vulnerable, is a restored recognition of the criminal character of both euthanasia and assisted suicide when carried out by planned omission.

REFERENCES

Finnis, John 1994. Living will legislation. In *Euthanasia, Clinical Practice and the Law*, ed. L. Gormally, pp. 167–176. London: The Linacre Centre.

Gormally, Luke 1992. The living will: the ethical framework of a recent report. In *The Dependent Elderly: Autonomy, Justice and Quality of Care*, ed. L. Gormally, pp. 53–69. Cambridge: Cambridge University Press.

Gormally, Luke 1993*a*. Definitions of personhood: implications for the care of PVS patients. *Catholic Medical Quarterly* 44/4: 7–12.

Gormally, Luke 1993*b*. Against voluntary euthanasia. In *Principles of Health Care Ethics*. ed. Raanan Gillon, pp. 763–774. Chichester: John Wiley.

Gormally, Luke (ed.) 1994*a*. *Euthanasia, Clinical Practice and the Law*. London: The Linacre Centre.

Gormally Luke 1994*b*. the BMA Report on Euthanasia and the case against legalization. In *Euthanasia, Clinical Practice and the Law*, ed. L. Gormally, pp. 177–192. London: The Linacre Centre.

Hoche, Alfred and Binding, Rudolf 1920. *Die Freigabe der Vernichtung lebensunwerten Lebens*. Leipzig: Verlag von Felix Meiner.

Kennedy, Ian [chairman] 1988. *The Living Will: Consent to Treatment at the End of Life. A Working Party Report*. London: Edward Arnold.

Keown, John 1993. Hard case, bad law, 'new' ethics. *Cambridge Law Journal* 52: 209–212. [Now see also (1997) 113 *Law Quarterly Review* 481–503 – Ed.]

[Walton I] House of Lords, Session 1993–94. *Report of the Select Committee on Medical Ethics*, Vol. 1, *Report*. London: HMSO.

[Walton II] House of Lords, Session 1993–94. *Select Committee on Medical Ethics*, Vol. 2, *Oral Evidence*. London: HMSO.

[Walton III] House of Lords, Session 1993–94. *Select Committee on Medical Ethics*, Vol. 3, *Written Evidence*. London: HMSO.

NOTES

1 See, for example, Baroness Warnock's expression of disappointment at the Government's refusal to accept the Select Committee's recommendation that the mandatory life sentence should be removed for the crime of murder. In the House of Lords debate on the Select Committe Report on 9 May 1994 she concluded her

speech by saying: 'In my view it is at the stage of sentencing that the motive of pity or perhaps a desire to do what the sufferer deeply wants, should be taken into account if such a motive is ascertained. In my own view paragraph 261 in our report in which we argued that the mandatory life sentence should be abolished, is one of the most important in our report. Surely the Government's expressed view that 'prison works' cannot be called in aid in such cases as those we are considering' [*Hansard* vol. 554 (No. 83) cols. 1377–8]. I think it improbable that every member of the Committee felt the same way about paragraph 261 as Baroness Warnock.

2 The position is more fully expounded in Gormally, 1994*a*: 111–165, and in Gormally, 1993*b*.

3 For a detailed submission on many of the questions which fell to be considered by the Walton Committee see 'Submission to the Select Committee of The House of Lords on Medical Ethics by The Linacre Centre for Health Care Ethics, June 1993' in Gormally, 1994*a*: 111–165.

4 In this and the two previous paragraphs I follow closely, in parts verbatim, an unpublished analysis of the Law Lords' judgement in *Bland* by Dr John Keown. See also Keown, 1993.

5 Restricting euthanasia to positive acts is inconsistent with the rationale of defining it by reference to intention, that is by reference to one's reasoning about one's chosen purpose in acting and the means chosen precisely with a view to achieving that purpose. Euthanasia is bringing about someone's death with a view to putting an end to a life judged no longer worthwhile; if it were to be judged worthwhile there would be no case for saying that the person killed is benefited, or at least not harmed, by being killed. But in seeking to bring about someone's death for such a reason omission of treatment or care may be in many circumstances a more eligible means of accomplishing one's end than a positive act such as injecting a toxic substance.

The indefensible habit of invoking a distinction between killing by positive act (judged wrong) and allowing someone to die, judged acceptable even when the choice of such conduct is intended to cause death, seems to have become almost ineradicable in medical circles, particularly in BMA publications. (On its presence in the 1988 BMA Report on Euthanasia see Gormally, 1994*b*.) More worrying still is the increasing extent to which lawyers are embracing the distinction, despite the fact that it has no warrant in the law of homicide (see Finnis, 1994: 168–9). Reference has already been made in the main body of the text to the disastrous way in which the Law Lords in *Bland* stumbled into a reliance on this distinction, while acknowledging that in doing so they had rendered the law 'misshapen'.

There are academic medical lawyers, however, who, because of their failure to grasp the role of intention in identifying the character of conduct and its moral significance, have long relied on a supposedly straightforward distinction between acts and omissions. An influential case in point is Professor Ian Kennedy, Professor of Medical Law and Ethics at King's College, London. The distinction is integral to the moral framework of the Report of the Working Party chaired by Kennedy on *The Living Will: Consent to Treatment at the End of Life* which was published in 1988 (Kennedy, 1988; for an extended critique of the Report see Gormally, 1992*b*, and more briefly and incisively, Finnis, 1994). The logic of Kennedy's failure to grasp the significance of intention has recently come home to roost in his 1994 Upjohn Lecture in which he advocates judicial 'development' of the law to permit active euthanasia by doctors. What he presents as the 'legal rationale' for this advocacy is based on inferences which rest on a radically unsound analysis of the notion of intention (which conflates foresight with intention), as well as on a failure sufficiently to distinguish problems in the analysis of intention from problems about what is to count as admissible *evidence* for intention. The use of an essentially lethal substance provides the sort of *prima facie* evidence of an intention to kill which is not so clearly available when planned killing is by an opiate which has palliative uses. But in so far as standards of medical practice are established in the control of pain, a doctor whose intention (i.e. aim) is to kill a patient by the use of pain-control medication is likely to become more readily detectable. Nonetheless, there is bound to remain a grey area in practice. But difficulties over establishing a person's intention should not lead to confusion over what intention is. Nor should those difficulties, as they arise in relation to the doctor who dissembles his intention, lead us to conclude (as Kennedy concludes) that 'the law endorses, indeed entrenches, hypocrisy'.

Apart from the confusions about intention, Kennedy's lecture is marred by his obfuscation of issues in naming the activity he wishes to have legalized 'doctor-assisted suicide', when what he is discussing is not suicide but the killing of patients by doctors for the supposed benefit of the patient. The description of what is under discussion as 'suicide' gives, however, an air of plausibility to Kennedy's moral case ('non-legal argument') for active euthanasia, namely that the legal prohibition of it is an indefensible restraint on a patient's right to freedom in the determination of his life. The naive inadequacy of this moral case is sufficiently indicated by pointing out, first, that since there is no such thing as an unrestrained right to self-determination one needs to demonstrate why having someone kill one is a reasonable exercise of a limited right to self-determination; and, secondly, that the killing of patients by doctors in any case clearly raises issues other than those of patient self-determination, since the principal agent is the doctor.

6 The provisional proposals of the Law Commission recommending legislation to give advance directives statutory force contain nothing to prohibit non-treatment with intent to shorten life. *Medically Incapacitated Adults and Decision-Making: Medical Treatment and Research*. Consultation Paper No. 129. London: HMSO, 1993.

7 The CPS's authority for this evidence is *obiter dicta* about advance directives in *Bland*. But advance directives were wholly irrelevant to the *Bland* case and the judges presented no argument for their force and limits.

8 What Mrs Davies calls a 'resounding refutation' of Fenigsen's 1989 exposé of what was happening in Holland was little more than a manifestation of collective pique by a group of pro-euthanasia Dutch academics that the truth had got out despite their efforts to control data by stipulative definition: non-voluntary euthanasia became an unmentionable phenomenon because euthanasia was decreed to be voluntary by definition! The uncritical support for euthanasia by many Dutch bioethicists and medical lawyers, and the absence of any genuinely open and informed debate on the practice of euthanasia in Holland, have played a major part in ensuring the acceptance of euthanasia there and its consequent corruption of Dutch medicine. The role of the Dutch political and academic establishment in promoting euthanasia is a topic meriting close study.

9 I am grateful for what I learned in conversation about More's *Utopia* from the Rev. Dr Dermot Fenlon of the Birmingham Oratory.

10 So for the most part does suicide in a medical context. Boyd has a passing observation on what he supposes to be Trollope's exposure of 'the flank of religious positions which prohibit suicide while being prepared to defend just wars and capital punishment'. I have already briefly explained in section 4 why the two latter may not be exposed to the fundamental objection which may be levelled against euthanasia and suicide.

11

Where there is hope, there is life: a view from the hospice

ROBERT G. TWYCROSS

INTRODUCTION

IN THIS CHAPTER, 'euthanasia' is used to describe:

> The compassion-motivated, deliberate, rapid and painless termination of the life of someone afflicted with an incurable and progressive disease. A suffering and terminally ill person is not allowed to die – his or her life is terminated.
>
> (Roy and Rapin 1994)

In the course of the chapter, I shall make the following points:

- Patients do not always receive adequate pain and symptom relief or, with their families, adequate psychological and practical support.
- Hope is an essential part of hospice/palliative care, and stretches far beyond cure and survival.
- Provided there is 'good enough' pain and symptom relief, suicide and a desire 'to end it all' are generally associated with a transient mood disorder, a depressive illness or delirium (confusion).
- Careful evaluation is necessary whenever a patient expresses suicidal thoughts or a desire 'to end it all'.
- 'Good enough' pain relief is virtually always possible in patients with incurable cancer. In patients where pain persists, the goal becomes 'mastery over pain'.
- Other distressing symptoms can also be alleviated, often considerably. Changes in the patient's way of life, however, may well be necessary.
- At the end of life, allowing nature to take its course and not intervening with 'heroic' measures is good practice both medically and ethically.

- AIDS patients, although often younger and with different social support structures, are similar to cancer patients in their attitudes to euthanasia.
- Many elderly people are concerned that legalized euthanasia would exert subtle and not-so-subtle pressures on them to 'get out of the way'.
- Almost all people who request euthanasia within the setting of a specialist palliative care service change their minds after days or weeks.
- Estimating survival (prognosis) is not easy and doctors are sometimes *years* out in their original estimate.
- Doctors are often more fearful of death than patients and physically fit people. This has implications when evaluating medical attitudes towards euthanasia.
- It is generally accepted that it is not possible to contain voluntary euthanasia within secure limits. Evidence from the Netherlands confirms this.
- There is considerable misinformation in circulation about euthanasia and the use of drugs such as morphine and diamorphine.
- Within the setting of a specialist palliative care service, intolerable distress is usually psychospiritual in origin and not physical.
- On rare occasions it may be necessary to sedate a patient heavily in order to relieve intolerable distress. Here, although the patient's life may be shortened, the intent is to relieve suffering and not to kill.
- The way forward is not legalized euthanasia but better palliative care, particularly when the interests of society as a whole are taken into account.

A PATIENT'S TESTIMONY

Eight months after cancer was diagnosed, and 6 months after his general practitioner had indicated that he would die a painful death in less than 3 months, Sidney Cohen wrote:

> My cancer was diagnosed in November and my health deteriorated rapidly thereafter. By January I was bedbound by pain and weakness, having been able to drink only water for six weeks . . . I felt desperate, isolated and frightened and at that time I truly wished that euthanasia could have been administered.
>
> I now know that only my death is inevitable and since coming under the care of the Macmillan Service [hospice homecare] my pain has been relieved completely, my ability to enjoy life restored and my fears of an agonizing end allayed. As you can see, I'm still alive today. My weight and strength have increased since treatment made it possible to eat normally and I feel that I'm living a full life, worth living. My wife and I have come to accept that I'm dying and we can now discuss it openly between ourselves and with the staff of the Macmillan Service, which does much to ease our anxieties.

> My experiences have served to convince me that euthanasia, even if voluntary, is fundamentally wrong and I'm now staunchly against it on religious, moral, intellectual and spiritual grounds. My wife's views have changed similarly.

What made the Sidney Cohen who wished for euthanasia change and become the Sidney Cohen who is 'staunchly against it on religious, moral, intellectual and spiritual grounds'? I suggest that the following factors collectively led to his profound change of attitude:

> my pain has been relieved completely;
> it is possible to eat normally;
> my weight and strength have increased;
> my fears of an agonizing end have been allayed;
> my ability to enjoy life has been restored;
> my wife and I have come to accept that I'm dying and we can now discuss it openly;
> the Macmillan Service does much to ease our anxieties.

Sidney Cohen and his wife discovered, as many others have, that 'the two extremes of dying in agony and being killed do not exhaust the possibilities for the stricken patient'. In doing so, they moved from a vicious circle of hopelessness and despair to an onward journey sustained by hope.

THE MEANING OF HOPE

Hope is an essential part of hospice care. A traditional saying states, 'While there's life, there's hope'. In my experience this is not so. The reverse is, however; namely, 'Where there is hope, there is life'.

Hope can be defined as an expectation greater than zero of achieving a goal. Goal-setting is an integral part of hospice care. In one study, doctors and nurses in two hospices in the UK set almost twice as many goals as doctors and nurses in a District General Hospital (Lunt and Neale 1987). Goal-setting explains why a patient may say, 'Now I know there's hope' when, for example, he is told that it is possible to relieve his pain, and that sleep and appetite can be improved, even though he may also have just learned that he has terminal cancer. It is a useful opening gambit to ask a new patient, 'What do you hope will come out of this consultation?' In this way, the patient 'sets the agenda', and the doctor is given an immediate focus based on the patient's order of priorities.

Research has demonstrated that hope may increase in patients close to

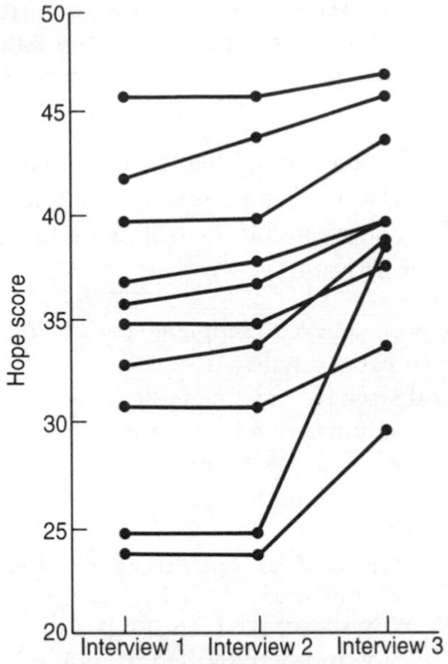

Figure 1. Hope scores in 10 home-care patients shortly after referral to a hospice programme (interview 1); when ability to complete activities of daily living became severely impaired (2); and when death was thought likely within 2 weeks. Reproduced from Herth 1990.

death – provided they are receiving adequate symptom relief (Figure 1). A group of 30 hospice patients were asked in a structured interview what factors affected hope (Table 1). The importance of a meaningful relationship, reminiscence (making sense of one's personal life-story) and humour provide an explanation as to why hope can increase when someone is close to death; a time when 'doing' (achieving) becomes impossible and 'being' (just being myself) becomes the mode of existence.

These data possibly explain why people generally do not ask for euthanasia but are content to let nature take its course. After all, the most fundamental hope of all humans must surely be, 'I will not be abandoned'. If this is so, then the basic message we need to convey to the dying is, 'We will not abandon you. You are important to us' – a message conveyed more by actions than by words.

CANCER AND THE DESIRE TO DIE

A number of studies have shown that almost all people who commit suicide have a mental disorder at the time (Stengel and Cook 1958; Barraclough *et al.*

Table 1. *Factors which influence hope in the terminally ill*

Decrease	Increase
Feeling devalued	Feeling valued
	Reminiscence
Abandonment and isolation	Meaningful relationship(s)
	Humour
Lack of direction	Realistic goals
Uncontrolled pain and discomfort	Pain and symptom relief

From Herth 1990.

Table 2. *Desire for death among 44 terminal cancer patients*

Number with depression (n = 11)	
Suicidal thoughts (past)	2
Suicidal thoughts (current)	1
Wished for death (but not suicide)	7
Never wished for death/suicide	1
Number not depressed (n = 33)	
Never wished for death/suicide	33

From Brown *et al.* 1986.

1974; Winokur and Tsuang 1975). It has also been shown that cancer patients who commit suicide have fewer psychological resources and have made a poorer adjustment to their illness than other cancer patients (Farberow *et al.* 1971).

Data from the Memorial Sloan-Kettering Cancer Center in New York indicate that in suicidal cancer patients (Breitbart 1989, 1990): one-fifth were delirious (confused), one-third had a major depression and over half had an adjustment disorder, usually associated with a very anxious and/or depressed mood. In another study, hospice patients were screened for depression and interviewed to see whether they actively wished for death (Brown *et al.* 1986). Patients were considered to be depressed if they fulfilled DSM-III criteria for major depression or had a Beck depression inventory (short version) score of 15 or more. Patients with symptoms of delirium or dementia were excluded. Eleven of 44 patients were found to be severely depressed. All 10 patients who desired death or had had suicidal thoughts were in this subgroup (Table 2). No patient who was not depressed had thoughts of suicide or wished death to come early, once again demonstrating the association between suicidal thoughts and actions and identifiable psychological disturbances (Sainsbury 1973). It is clearly incumbent on doctors to identify correctable psychiatric or adjustment disorders in physically ill patients who express suicidal ideas or a desire 'to end it all'.

ELICITING THE ISSUES BEHIND REQUESTS FOR EUTHANASIA

A 62-year-old hospital administrator had a lymphoma which did not respond well to chemotherapy. As the disease spread, he spent increasingly more time in hospital. One day the man said he could take no more chemotherapy and asked his oncologist to kill him: 'You can give me a drug and no one would know. I am in much agony and will die soon anyway.'

A psychiatric assessment was requested. The patient was found to be exhausted and depressed. He asked the psychiatrist for a lethal drug 'to put me out of my misery' but added that he could not kill himself. When asked to discuss this further, the patient began to present a rational argument for ending his life because of his suffering, the expense, and the burden on his family and medical carers. He said he felt ashamed and embarrassed by his dependence, and by letting others down by not continuing chemotherapy.

The psychiatrist recommended that the patient, the oncologist, and the patient's wife clarify the issues of prognosis, chemotherapy, and other treatment options. The oncologist acknowledged that he may have pushed the patient too hard in relation to chemotherapy. The patient and his wife began discussing his possible death and reaffirmed their love and respect for each other. It was agreed that the patient should participate more in his daily care, and he and the oncologist began to discuss comfort rather than cure.

The patient began to feel more optimistic as his fever, erythema and pruritus abated as part of the disease's fluctuating course and, to his wife's chagrin, he asked his oncologist about more aggressive care. He felt stronger, slept better, and began to eat solid food. He went home for one month, during which time he was relatively symptom-free. He was then readmitted with pneumonia, deteriorated rapidly and died three weeks later. (Weddington 1981)

The methodical exploration of underlying issues in patients who request euthanasia should include (Block 1990):

- adequacy of pain and symptom management;

- the psychological status of the patient, with particular reference to depression;
- the context and the meaning of the request to the patient.

Psychological well-being is impossible if the patient is troubled by severe physical symptoms. Satisfactory symptom control is of paramount importance. No patient should be forced to request euthanasia because of unrelieved pain or other distressing symptoms such as vomiting or shortness of breath. Methods exist to control such symptoms, either completely or to a great extent (Twycross 1995).

UNRELIEVED PAIN

Admiraal, a well-known Dutch anaesthetist and euthanasiast, has stated that pain is never a legitimate reason for euthanasia because methods exist to relieve it (Dawson 1986). Estimates of unrelieved cancer pain vary. The figure of 50–80% quoted for developed countries includes data from over 30 years ago (WHO 1986). A lot has happened since then, including the emergence of the hospice movement and the introduction of the World Health Organization's Method for Relief of Cancer Pain (WHO 1986). Recent data are more encouraging. For example, in some 200 cancer pain patients treated in accordance with WHO recommendations, the results were as follows (Takeda 1989): complete relief, 86%; adequate relief, 11%; poor relief, 3%. The reasons for poor relief were not specified but included several patients with major psychological distress (Takeda, personal communication). The negative impact of continuing psychological distress on pain relief is one which requires much time and skilled counselling to resolve (see case history p. 162).

Reviewing nearly 3400 case notes at St Christopher's Hospice, London, Saunders reported that pain was 'difficult to control' in 1% (Saunders 1981). The Macmillan Home Care Service at St Joseph's Hospice, London, reported an incidence of unrelieved pain in patients cared for at home of 10% (Lamerton 1978). The higher percentage possibly relates partly to the reluctance of some patients to take medication. Other patients decline the offer of admission to hospital or hospice for further treatment, preferring to 'soldier on' at home even though with incompletely controlled pain.

A 66-year-old man with intra-pelvic spread of a bladder cancer was referred for outpatient assessment at the local hospice. He was exhausted and in great distress because of insomnia caused by round-the-clock frequency of micturition and by pain in the lower abdomen and legs. The frequency of micturition and insomnia were both corrected by drug therapy. On the other hand, he continued to experience a 'golf ball' sensation in the perineum ('but it's not really painful') and an intermittent nerve pain in the right lower leg. This was usually mild but, on occasion, could be more troublesome. As lowering the dose of morphine did not make the pain worse, it was concluded that this particular pain was probably at best only partly opioid responsive. This residual pain had only minimal impact on the patient's activity and enjoyment of life. Therefore, because nerve blocks sometimes cause leg weakness and/or urinary incontinence, it was decided not to recommend one at this stage.

The contrast between the man's condition at his initial assessment and subsequent reviews continued to be considerable, despite occasional trouble with constipation or frayed emotions. So, was his pain controlled or was it not? In absolute terms, no: but, in his estimation, yes.

At St Christopher's Hospice, when assessing pain control, patients are divided into two broad categories (Haram 1978): those in whom there is 'good relief from pain' and those in whom 'pain is difficult to control'. Considering the many factors that can influence pain relief, either for good or for ill, this is in fact a sensible way of summarizing the relief obtained. When considering pain control, one has to bear in mind that:

- pain relief is not an 'all or none' phenomenon;
- all pains are not equally responsive to analgesics;
- some pains continue to be brought on by activity and/or weightbearing;
- relief is not generally a 'once only' exercise; old pains may re-emerge as the disease progresses or new pains develop.

It is only occasionally necessary to admit a patient to hospice/hospital to achieve adequate relief, notably in those whose pain is associated with major psychological distress.

When these factors are taken into account, one can re-state the primary goal of pain management as seeking to help a patient move from a position in which he is mastered by the pain to one in which he establishes mastery over the pain. When a patient is mastered by pain, the pain is overwhelming and all-embracing. When sufficiently improved, a patient may say:

> I still have the pain, but it doesn't worry me now.
> It's still there, but it's not what you'd call pain.
> I can get on with things and forget it now.

Of course, the ideal remains complete relief. But, in practice, partial relief is acceptable provided the patient is significantly more comfortable, physically and mentally rested, and both patient and family are demonstrating their mastery of the situation. There is then little need to pursue relentlessly the ultimate goal using invasive (surgical) techniques which do not guarantee success and may well be complicated by weakness, numbness or incontinence.

The concept of 'mastery over pain' has been validated by the Wisconsin Brief Pain Inventory (Daut and Cleeland 1982). When using this inventory, patients score both pain intensity and activity interference (Figure 2). Parameters are scored on a scale of 0 to 10. Patients with pain rated 1–3 record little impact by the pain on either activity or enjoyment of life (Table 3). In other words, there is mastery over the pain and, from a pain perspective, the patient is enjoying a good quality of life.

On the other hand, many cancer patients with persistent pain have expectations which are far lower than they need be. All patients must be assured, when first seen, that the situation can be improved and that it is possible to relieve most, if not all, of their pain. It is always possible to achieve at least some improvement within 48 hours. It is often wise, however, to aim at 'graded relief'. As some pains respond more readily to treatment than others, improvement must be assessed in relation to each pain. The initial target is a pain-free, sleep-full night. Some patients have not had a good night's rest for weeks or months and are exhausted and demoralized. To sleep through the night pain-free and wake refreshed is a boost to both the doctor's and the patient's morale. Next, one aims for relief at rest in bed or chair during the day; finally, for freedom from pain on movement. The former is always eventually possible; the latter sometimes not. Relief at night and when resting during the day, however, gives the patient new hope and incentive, and enables him to begin to live again despite limited mobility. Freed from the nightmare of constant pain, his last weeks or months take on a new look.

The doctor must be determined to succeed, however, and be prepared to spend time assessing and reassessing the patient's pain and other distressing symptoms. In addition, a balance is needed, learned only from experience, between marking time therapeutically so as to capitalize on the beneficial effect of better sleep and improved morale, and pressing on decisively to avoid the situation such as that recorded of a 90-year-old man admitted to a London Hospital with bone pain and who died still in pain 3 months later (Hunt *et al.* 1977).

BREATHLESSNESS

Although many symptoms respond to a combination of drug and non-drug measures, it is sometimes necessary to compromise in order to avoid

Circle the one number that describes how, during the past week, pain has interfered with your:

A. General activity

0	1	2	3	4	5	6	7	8	9	10
Does not interfere										Completely interferes

B. Mood

0	1	2	3	4	5	6	7	8	9	10
Does not interfere										Completely interferes

C. Walking ability

0	1	2	3	4	5	6	7	8	9	10
Does not interfere										Completely interferes

D. Normal work (includes both work outside the home and housework)

0	1	2	3	4	5	6	7	8	9	10
Does not interfere										Completely interferes

E. Relations with other people

0	1	2	3	4	5	6	7	8	9	10
Does not interfere										Completely interferes

F. Sleep

0	1	2	3	4	5	6	7	8	9	10
Does not interfere										Completely interferes

G. Enjoyment of life

0	1	2	3	4	5	6	7	8	9	10
Does not interfere										Completely interferes

Figure 2. Wisconsin Brief Pain Inventory: interference factors.

unacceptable adverse effects. For example, atropine-like effects such as dry mouth or visual disturbance may be limiting factors. With intestinal obstruction, it is often better to aim to reduce the incidence of vomiting to once or twice a day rather than to seek absolute control.

Specific mention should be made of shortness of breath. It is unusual to be able to control this completely, particularly if it is caused by cancer spreading

Table 3. *Relationship between worst pain rating and interference ratings of cancer patients*

Worst pain rating	No. of patients	Activity interference (mean)	Enjoyment interference (mean)
1	13	0.2	0.8
2	16	1.5	1.9
3	33	1.4	1.6
4	41	2.6	2.8
5	100	4.4	4.4
6	45	5.4	5.0
7	54	6.2	5.7
8	39	6.2	5.8
9	17	7.5	6.3
10	49	7.1	6.8

in the lungs. In this situation, management is comparable to incompletely relieved pain; the aim is re-defined as mastery over breathlessness.

As yet, the management of breathlessness is not as well understood by doctors as the relief of pain. Even so, the answer is *not* euthanasia but better education. As with all symptoms, *explanation* is vital to management. Guidance about helping to abort 'respiratory panic attacks' (usually by a physiotherapist) and the teaching of simple relaxation techniques based on controlled breathing are important. Many patients benefit by the use of a regular small dose of anti-anxiety drug (e.g. diazepam 5–10 mg at bedtime). The use of regular small doses of oral morphine yields considerable benefit in many patients by reducing the rate of breathing at rest from, say, 35–40/minute to 18–20/minute (with a corresponding reduction of breathing rate when walking short distances from 60/minute to 30–35/minute). Advice about modifying one's way of life is also important – for example, asking a friend to collect one's pension from the post-office, having a home-help to do the heavy housework, having a commode available downstairs if the only toilet in the house is upstairs, or moving one's bed downstairs. The benefits of these sorts of measures have been attested by others (Lichter and Hunt 1990; Twycross and Lichter 1993).

MINDLESS MEDICINE

Many people are afraid of not being allowed to die when at the natural end of their lives because of the 'heroic' use of high-technology medical interventions (such as were used on General Franco and Emperor Hirohito). This fear leads some people to support euthanasia. There is no guarantee, however, that a euthanasia statute would solve this problem. What is called for is *better medical education.*

Thus, although hospice care and euthanasia are mutually exclusive philosophies, both abhor mindless medicine. For example, for an octogenarian to say 'I've lived a good life and I am ready to go' is, in my opinion, neither immoral nor anti-life. It is merely a recognition of the biological fact of life that eventually we must all die and that, with the onset of progressive disability, the burden of living has become too demanding. In consequence, because death is ultimately inevitable, a doctor must practise his skills accordingly. The claim that a doctor must preserve life at all costs is biologically as well as ethically untenable.

In palliative care there are perhaps many occasions when, having weighed up the relative benefits and burdens of a proposed course of action, the right initial step seems to be 'to give death a chance' – in other words, not to prescribe an antibiotic in a terminally ill moribund patient who has developed pneumonia or not to blood transfuse a patient whose dying is complicated by acute blood loss (Figures 3 and 4).

AIDS AND EUTHANASIA

AIDS is a relatively rare disease in the United Kingdom. Deaths from AIDS in 1990 amounted to less than 1% of those from cancer. My own experience of caring for AIDS patients is therefore slight. In consequence, I shall refer to data from a series of 110 patients with AIDS cared for in London by either AIDS Community Care in Bloomsbury and the Middlesex Hospital or the AIDS Hospice at the Mildmay Mission Hospital (George 1990). At these centres, dying and death are addressed specifically as part of care. This means that, *inter alia*, suicide and euthanasia are discussed with all patients.

As a result of this policy, euthanasia has been addressed 'in significant terms with approximately 10% of people' (George 1990). Only 2 of 110 patients have pursued euthanasia as a realistic option. With one, the issue had only just arisen at the time of the report, so the outcome was not known. With the other, the offer of contact with the Voluntary Euthanasia Society was not pursued and, after an inpatient admission to a hospice, this patient 'dispensed with euthanasia altogether'. George states that within the context of good palliative care:

> In the last month of life, euthanasia is a serious option in only a small minority, and in our experience this is symptomatic of an unresolved agenda, rather than a considered and clear choice. (George 1990)

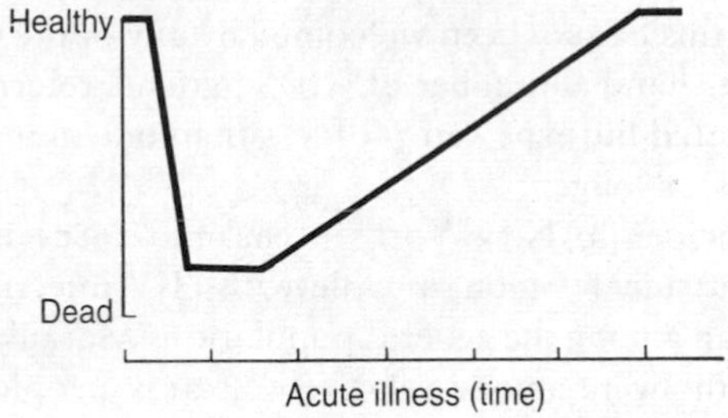

Figure 3. A graphical representation of acute illness. Biological prospects are generally good. Acute resuscitative measures are important and enable the patient to survive the initial crisis. Recovery is aided by the natural forces of healing; rehabilitation is completed by the patient on his own, without continued medical support.

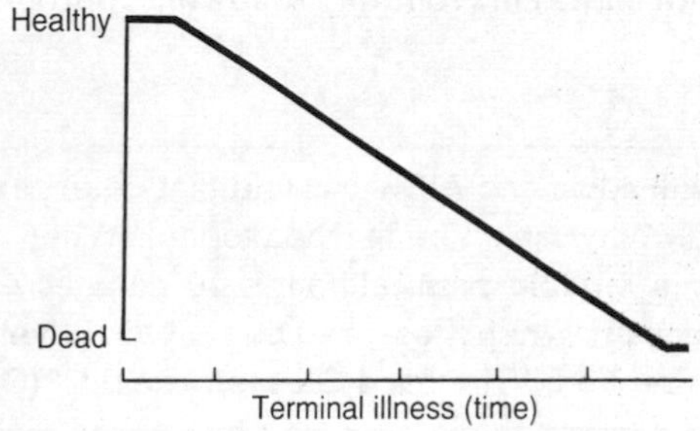

Figure 4. A graphical representation of terminal illness. Biological prospects progressively worsen. Acute and terminal illnesses are therefore distinct pathophysiological entities. Therapeutic interventions that can best be described as prolonging the distress of dying are both futile and inappropriate.

These figures contrast markedly with those from the Netherlands where 30% of AIDS patients receive euthanasia (Z. Zylicz, personal communication).

About 50% of patients have a significant change in attitude and world view in the last 3 months of life, moving from the desire for acute intervention and the postponement of death towards acceptance, and psychological and spiritual peace:

> The introduction of voluntary euthanasia [would] mean that many people will be denying themselves this crucial time when half of them are likely to have major shifts in their emotional and spiritual attitudes. (George 1990)

It should be stressed that prognostication in AIDS is very difficult. About 25% of AIDS patients move with unexpected rapidity towards an earlier than anticipated death; this has *not* been welcomed by any of the patients (George 1990). On the other hand, a number of AIDS patients referred for palliative care with an estimated life expectancy of less than one month have survived for several months or longer.

What about suicide? In New York in the mid-1980s it was estimated retrospectively that suicide among people with HIV infection was 36 times more prevalent than among the general population (Marzuk *et al.* 1988). But most of these deaths were among relatively healthy people, and related to being told the diagnosis rather than the onset of distressing symptoms or disability.

Of the 47 deaths with the Bloomsbury Community Care Team, two have been suicide. One was a bereaved lover, also with AIDS, who killed himself two weeks after the death of his partner. The second occurred on the day of referral. One patient who attempted to take his own life subsequently came to view suicide and euthanasia unfavourably following appropriate care within a hospice setting.

> When a patient with advanced AIDS was told that deterioration was now imminent, he said, 'Why can't it be finished today?' When asked why, he said that he was in terrible pain, although 10 minutes earlier he had denied having any pain. When reassured that, if pain developed, it could be controlled, he replied, 'Oh, that's OK then, isn't it?' (George 1990)

THE ELDERLY

I have not discussed the issues surrounding dementia and other degenerative diseases in the elderly (e.g. cerebral atherosclerosis, Parkinsonism) because I was asked to comment as a hospice physician. I am aware that, with these conditions, the time-scale is years rather than months, and that the potential for chronic psychological distress in both patient and family may well be greater. However, I cannot see how one could have euthanasia for geriatric patients but not for cancer and AIDS patients. If euthanasia is wrong for cancer and AIDS patients, it must also be wrong for elderly patients. A geriatric nurse has written:

> Over and over again I have seen a patient change her mind; it is different if you are well from when you are incapacitated . . . While healthy, dependency and confusion might feel abhorrent; it might not be so when you are there. (Hirschfeld and Ziv 1989)

> Agnes was in a geriatric continuing care ward. She was mentally alert but crippled with arthritis. This confined her to bed or electric wheelchair. She had no close relatives. I used to see her on my evening and weekend rounds of the hospital, and we had the same conversation each time: 'I want to be put away. There is no point in being alive. I am a nuisance to the nurses. I wish euthanasia were legal'. My reply was always the same: 'You know I can't "finish you off" and I wouldn't want to. You keep us all going with your quips and jokes. The nurses enjoy looking after you.' After some months she was transferred to a nursing home. She had her own room, she liked the communal facilities, and the home cooking. She was able to plan her own day rather than have it dictated by ward routine. She now enjoyed living and no longer spoke of euthanasia. (Whitfield 1990)

And what of the elderly themselves? Two hundred and sixty randomly selected elderly people in a medium-sized city in the Netherlands were approached by letter; 132 agreed to be interviewed. Seventy-six were living independently and 56 were living in six different nursing homes. The interviews comprised 10 questions, ranging from 'How is your contact with your children and other family members?' to 'What would you think of it if the government were to allow euthanasia?' Of those living independently, 66% were against such a move; of those living in nursing homes, *95% were against*. About one-third of the respondents opted to make a further comment ('Do you have anything further to say in connection with these questions?'). Some of their comments are contained in Table 4.

A CHANGE OF MIND

In my experience, patients who request euthanasia almost invariably change their minds. The reason for this varies. Often, it relates to good palliative care; they obtain relief from distressing symptoms, the depression is treated, and/or they no longer feel abandoned and alone.

> Mr BL, a 62-year-old divorcee, developed jaundice. A laparotomy the following month confirmed carcinoma of the head of the pancreas and by-pass surgery was undertaken, when it was noted that there were liver secondaries. The postoperative course was complicated by an intra-abdominal abscess, which delayed the start of a course of chemotherapy.

Meanwhile, he left hospital to be cared for by close friends. A few weeks later, when they went on holiday, he returned to his own home and began to drink heavily. He neglected himself and soon was in a very poor condition. This pattern continued even after the friends returned from their holiday and invited him back into their home.

After the first pulse of chemotherapy, he declined any more. He was referred to the local hospice because of abusive behaviour and intractable abdominal pain. He was seen as an outpatient and admitted the following day.

Both in clinic and after inpatient admission he said he just wanted to be left alone and to curl up and die. Ideally he wanted an injection to finish things off 'but nobody will do that for me'. He remained withdrawn and was verbally aggressive at times. The pain was readily controlled with a small dose of morphine (30 mg twice a day). He was encouraged to sit out of bed and, subsequently, to get dressed and go out for short walks. His mood improved steadily.

Two weeks later he was asked about his earlier requests for 'an injection to finish things off'. He replied, 'Oh, that wasn't me, doctor; that was the alcohol speaking.' He subsequently went home and, a few weeks later, asked if he could recommence chemotherapy. Initially he did well but, a few months later, began to deteriorate again. He died in comfort at home cared for by a daughter and his friends. He did not ask for euthanasia.

A man aged 58 with disseminated cancer and paraplegia, who continued to experience distressing pain on movement, wrote:

> Only last year I read Exit's *Guide to Self-Deliverance*. Approved of it. Obvious, isn't it? Finish now, with dignity . . . Save me the agony. Astonishingly, I don't want to take or lose my life. Glad there's no Euthanasia Bill through Parliament. If there were, I'd be even more suspicious of the people who look after me. I'd think each pill designed to kill me . . . Each nursing act carried out to shorten life. (Warburg 1988)

A patient told me that her general practitioner had reacted negatively when she told him she was a member of the Voluntary Euthanasia Society. I explained that this was probably because euthanasia is not only illegal but also proscribed by traditional medical ethics. I also said that I was glad she had told me that she was a member, even though I was constrained by the same limitations as her general practitioner. I went on to say that, although I would never intentionally kill a patient, I would certainly not stand by and let

Table 4. *Comments by elderly Dutch people interviewed about euthanasia*

People must be allowed greater freedom in the matter of euthanasia
The unnecessary stretching of human life is inhumane
If you want to die, then do it yourself, but don't burden other people with the matter
People must have a living will made while they are well
The doctor is an expert. He will be able to decide whether euthanasia is really necessary and permissible
I find it difficult, but good just the same, to be compelled to reflect on these matters
It has frightened me
Euthanasia may not become a law, but there must be open discussion about it
I hope that people will have a change of heart, the Netherlands is leading the way, that is frightening
When government officials get older, they will get their turn
If euthanasia is passed, then things can become difficult for believers
We still want to live long and happily
See to it that someone comes by once again
Older people are shoved into a corner, they certainly also have a right to live!
There is a great danger that euthanasia will be misused
What are we up to?

From Segers 1988.

her suffer unbearably. I urged her to talk to me again should she feel that she had reached the point when she wanted euthanasia, so that I could reassess the situation with her. A few months later she was admitted to Sobell House in a very weak condition. She was, however, *compos mentis* and, although she had opportunities to say, 'Please give me a lethal injection', she did not. Instead, she slid gently into coma and died peacefully several days later, with her daughter beside her.

'HOW LONG HAVE I GOT, DOCTOR?'

Predicting survival in advanced cancer is a matter of 'informed guesswork'. Not surprisingly, such 'guestimates' are often inaccurate (Parkes 1972). Usually, the best a doctor can say is:

> If you can see deterioration on a month-by-month basis, survival is likely to be months.
>
> If you can see deterioration on a week-by-week basis, survival is likely to be weeks.
>
> If you can see deterioration on a day-by-day basis, survival is likely to be days.

But how long is 'months', 'weeks' or 'days'? An acute infection or a hypercalcaemic crisis can seemingly move a patient into the 'days' category until a successful and appropriate therapeutic intervention prevents further deterioration, and the patient begins to improve again.

Mr SC was diagnosed as having carcinoma of the prostate when 68 years of age. He received the usual anti-cancer therapies for this condition over the next 4–5 years. He was seen as an outpatient at the local hospice because of general deterioration and intractable pain. His general practitioner considered him terminal. The Macmillan nurse assisting in the clinic described him as 'all grot and crumble'.

Three days later the pain worsened markedly and, when subsequently admitted, an X-ray confirmed the presence of a fracture of the right femur. He was transferred to the Accident Service and a dynamic hip screw was inserted. He went home after about 2 weeks, and continued to improve gradually.

Three months later, he developed symptomatic anaemia; blood tests suggested cancerous infiltration of the bone marrow. He received blood transfusions every 10–12 weeks for about a year, after which the intervals extended up to 6 months. He continued to be self-caring at home. Finally, he died of an acute fulminating infection nearly 3 years after his initial referral.

In this case, the underestimated prognosis did not have any serious sequelae. But that is not always so:

Mr CJ, aged 48, was diagnosed as having cancer of the right maxillary antrum in October 1989. He was given 2 months to live and told that he would go blind. Thirteen months later he had not gone blind and had improved sufficiently to return to work.

Mr GL was diagnosed as having carcinoma of the pancreas and recurrence of multiple myeloma. Eight years previously, when aged 47, he had been given 2 years to live when the myeloma was originally diagnosed. When given this prognosis Mr GL cut himself off socially from his family and began to drink excessively. Eight years later his wife was still angry about the false prognosis and stated than an error of this magnitude by a doctor is unforgivable.

DOCTORS' ATTITUDES

Compared with patients and physically fit people, doctors have been noted to express a greater fear of death, more rejection of personal death and significantly more negative death imagery (Feifel 1963). It is not clear whether the more marked fear of death reflects a determinant of original entry into the medical profession, or is attributable to medical training and experience, or to greater honesty, or to being more in touch with one's emotions. It does, however, add another dimension to the euthanasia debate.

About 10 years ago, a retired general practitioner in Oxfordshire who helped out by doing holiday locums for other doctors told me that he had resigned from the Voluntary Euthanasia Society because he had come to realize that patients did not want euthanasia. He went on to say that he was wondering how best to prevent a drawn-out death. He said that perhaps the way forward was to prescribe a cortisone-like drug in high doses and, when the body was dependent on it, to stop it abruptly in the hope that the patient would die rapidly of cortisone deprivation. This is a helpful anecdote in that it reveals that it was the doctor who had the problem, and not the patients.

> Perhaps many of the desperate treatments in medicine can be justified by expediency, but history has an awkward habit of judging some as fashions, more helpful to the therapist than to the patient. (Main 1957)

Patients tend to be sedated when the carers have reached the limit of their resources and are no longer able to stand the patient's problems without anxiety, impatience, guilt, anger or despair (Main 1957). A sedative will alter the situation and produce a patient who, if not dead, is at least quiet.

Helping doctors and nurses understand their own negative emotions towards death, and to cope with them, is part of the aim of training in palliative care. In the Netherlands, where euthanasia is practised, there is little education in this field. For example, only about a quarter of all Dutch doctors have been trained in cancer pain management (Dorrepaal 1989). This lack is reflected in pain relief data. A survey in a large teaching hospital in Amsterdam showed that only about a quarter of cancer patients received optimal treatment for their pain, and that over half were treated inappropriately (Dorrepaal *et al.* 1989). Forty per cent of doctors were unaware of the pain (sometimes severe) which their cancer patients were experiencing.

Further, one is left wondering why approximately 30% of cancer patients in the Netherlands use less morphine than prescribed or even discontinue it after discharge from hospital (Dorrepaal 1989). Could it be that they fear the misuse of morphine by their doctors more than the pain?

THE SLIPPERY SLOPE

The 'slippery slope' argument takes several forms (Lamb 1988). In the context of euthanasia, it refers to the danger of voluntary euthanasia leading to imposed euthanasia (either involuntary or non-voluntary). Protagonists for voluntary euthanasia argue strongly against such a likelihood. However, the Report of a Commission set up by the Dutch Government (the Remmelink Report) demonstrates beyond doubt that in the Netherlands the slippery slope is already a reality (Gunning 1991). *Imposed euthanasia already occurs in the Netherlands*; indeed, a majority of cases of euthanasia involves no explicit request by the patient (Keown 1994).

It is disturbing, therefore, that nearly half of a group of doctors recently surveyed in the UK would welcome the liberties extended to the medical profession in the Netherlands in relation to voluntary euthanasia (Ward and Tate 1994). Reference to the House of Lords Select Committee on Medical Ethics (1994) is apposite:

> We do not think it is possible to set secure limits on voluntary euthanasia . . . We took account of the present situation in the Netherlands; indeed some of us visited that country and talked to doctors, lawyers and others. We returned feeling uncomfortable, especially in the light of evidence indicating that non-voluntary euthanasia . . . was commonly performed, admittedly in incompetent terminally ill patients. We also learned of one case in which voluntary euthanasia was accepted by both doctors and lawyers in a physically fit 50-year-old woman alleged to be suffering from intolerable mental stress.
>
> (Walton 1994*a*)

The extension of euthanasia to non-physically ill patients is another example of the slippery slope effect. The woman referred to above was divorced, had had one son die of cancer and the other die by suicide. Euthanasia for morbid grief/depression? This is where the Dutch experience has taken them. In my opinion, to say, 'It could never happen here' is naive. It was the medical profession in the 1920s which introduced imposed euthanasia into Germany (Alexander 1949; Binding and Hoche 1975). All the Nazis did was to extend the concept on political grounds. Two further cases histories from the Netherlands illustrate the dangers (Z. Zylicz, personal communication).

A patient with disseminated breast cancer had severe pain. Morphine was administered by injection once or twice a day and the dose was increased every 2 days in an endeavour to achieve relief. Eventually, she was receiving more than 2 g of morphine a day but was still in pain.

Several weeks previously, at a hospital outpatient visit, she told the doctor she would never choose euthanasia because of her beliefs. She was admitted under the care of the same doctor and treated with intravenous midazolam and morphine. She became unconscious, so the dose of midazolam was decreased. She woke up and stated she was free of pain. She said goodbye to her family and to the doctor. After a weekend on duty, the doctor went home at 0900 on the Monday morning. She died 30 minutes later. Next day, a junior nurse told the weekend duty doctor that another doctor had ordered a twenty-fold increase in the dose of morphine. Her family had been asked to leave the room. The order was given verbally and the doctor refused to confirm it in writing. When the doctor was challenged by the weekend duty doctor he replied 'It could have taken another week before she died: I just needed this bed.'

An old man was dying from disseminated lung cancer. His symptoms were well controlled and he asked if he could go and die at home. When his four children were told about his wish, they would not agree to take care of him. Even after repeated discussion, they refused. Instead, they pointed to their father's suffering and the need to finish things quickly 'in the name of humanity'. When the doctor refused, they threatened to sue him. Because the patient insisted on going home, a social worker went to investigate. She discovered that the patient's house was empty and that every piece of furniture had been taken by the family.

FANTASY AND REALITY

The data from Holland disclose that euthanasia without request is a widespread reality. Yet the fantasy that there is no slippery slope is perpetuated. In the English-language synopsis of the survey commissioned by the Remmelink Commission in the Netherlands, the Dutch authors failed to mention in the summary of the article that 0.8% of deaths (over 1000 cases) occurred as a result of imposed euthanasia (van der Maas *et al.* 1991), and data concerning deliberate drug overdosage with intent to kill were entirely omitted. Further, the fact that many doctors would prefer not to perform euthanasia again was said to 'prove' that there is no evidence of a slippery slope effect – despite the incontrovertible evidence to the contrary marshalled by John Keown in his contribution to this volume.

Another persistent fantasy concerns the effect of strong analgesics such as morphine and diamorphine (heroin). For example, an article about euthanasia in the *Observer* misstated the effects of heroin when used as an analgesic (Collee 1991). It was asserted that 'it is quite normal for doctors to prescribe heroin to terminal cancer patients in dosages which they know to be cumulatively fatal'. In most people, however, half of a dose of heroin is removed from the body in about 2.5 hours. It is usually given every 4 hours and does *not* cumulate in the body unless there is associated kidney failure. Heroin, like morphine, is therefore a very safe analgesic. This is why its use is preferred to a drug with a long 'half-life' such as methadone which could be cumulatively fatal if supervision is inadequate during the initial phase of dose titration (Twycross 1977).

It was also stated that 'patients acquire a tolerance to heroin which requires ever increasing dosages'. Clinical evidence suggests, however, that this is not normally the case – the main reason for dose increments is tumour progression causing more pain (Twycross 1994). However, should tolerance develop, this includes tolerance to the adverse effects of heroin as well as to its analgesic effect. Thus there is no prospect of a 'gradual heroin overdose' unless a doctor deliberately escalates the dose in the absence of either increasing pain or tolerance.

I wrote with two colleagues to the *Observer* to emphasize these points. The letter concluded:

> We should like to reassure any of your readers who may be suffering from incurable cancer that, should they experience distressing pain, either heroin or its principal active metabolite morphine can be safely used in the knowledge that it will *not* cause them to die sooner than would otherwise be the case.

I was not surprised to receive a letter of gratitude from one patient who had been disturbed by the article's inaccuracy, and the author of the article has apologized (privately) for not double-checking his facts before publication.

UNCONTROLLED SUFFERING

As is now generally recognized, most cancer pain can be readily relieved. But what of those whose pain is resistant to routine pain relief measures? Many such patients do not obtain relief initially because their pain is being used as a channel for the expression of mental anguish.

Mrs W, aged 34, was admitted to the hospice suffering from cancer of the breast with widespread metastases. She had lost two children at term and now had a much treasured son aged 3.

While still relatively well she had dealt with her situation intellectually, making all the necessary arrangements for her approaching death. As she weakened it was clear that she still had not come to terms with her illness emotionally. Now she was asking, 'Why all this? Why me?' She grieved over the losses she had already sustained; she wanted to be able to meet her young son at the playschool when he was ready to come home, and to cuddle him, but could no longer do so. She missed her home, but because of her condition could make only brief visits. She lamented her increasing dependence and showed overwhelming despair at the impairments yet to come, fearing especially loss of control over physical functions. Her grief was manifested in crushing, intractable pain. She said, 'I am resigned to the fact that this is my lot. It is the pain I cannot accept. Dying is all right, but there is no reason for this pain, no purpose in it. I am no longer angry with God for my fate, but why this pain?'

Oral morphine in doses reaching 1500 mg over 24 hours was ineffective. Complaints of shattering pain continued and she was miserable and often withdrawn. The slightest movement caused her to cringe in pain. Care to pressure areas was no longer permitted. For relief, large and frequent doses of intravenous diazepam were required. Epidural morphine was commenced at this stage and was continued over a 5-week period.

Gradually she came to terms with her situation. As this occurred, her need for analgesia became less and eventually she was kept pain-free on a dose of 10 mg of oral morphine every 4 hours. She improved to the point where she was able to be wheeled down the road on an ambulance trolley to buy an Easter egg for her son, and to visit the local art gallery the day before she died. (Lichter 1991)

In this deeply moving and tragic account, to have offered euthanasia when the pain was seemingly intractable would have prevented the woman reaching a state of real acceptance and physical comfort. What sort of a legacy would she have left had she received euthanasia at the height of her distress? In the event, what she eventually left was the gift of peace to both husband, son, siblings, parents and friends – the paradoxical gift of peace amidst the chaos and distress of bereavement.

> Of course terminal cancer is unspeakably awful. That aspect needs no emphasis. More difficult to imagine is the blessedness which is the corollary of the awfulness. If music is the food of love, so are the cries of anguish. I think my wife learnt more of our love during those dreadful months than she did at any other time, and we of hers, too. Going quickly in one's sleep, or in a sudden accident, or peacefully in the fullness of years – all these deaths minimize

suffering, and that is one blessing. But the suffering of a long and terminal illness is not all waste. Nothing that creates such tenderness can be all waste.

I truly believe that the way my wife coped with her cancer was a form of love in that it brought out the best not only in her but in us as well. As a destroyer, cancer is second to none. But it is also a healer; or an agent of healing. I believe my wife felt this, and drew satisfaction from this, as she lay dying: conscious that she had made the best of the last few months. (Worsthorne 1990)

IN CONCLUSION

I have been a hospice doctor for over 20 years. During this time, my opinions on many issues both within and outwith clinical practice have changed. One that has not changed, however, is my belief that it would be a disaster for the medical profession to cross the Rubicon and use pharmacological means to precipitate death intentionally. When everything is taken into account (physical, psychological, social and spiritual), euthanasia is *not* the answer, either for the patient, the family, the professional carers or society. Indeed, to espouse euthanasia in the light of all that I have learned and experienced during this time would be to betray the thousands of patients I have looked after over the last 24 years.

If the reasons for my conviction were to be examined, the euthanasiast might well be able to say *of each individual reason*, 'That's no reason for opposing voluntary euthanasia.' In so doing, he would seemingly be able to destroy the logic of my position. But only *seemingly*; because, even if no one objection were deemed sufficient, I believe that, taken together, they add up to an overwhelming case against (Table 5).

This is why I applaud the conclusion of the House of Lords Select Committee on Medical Ethics (1994) that there should be no change in the law to permit euthanasia:

> [There is] not sufficient reason to weaken society's prohibition of intentional killing which is the cornerstone of law and of social relationships. Individual cases cannot reasonably establish the foundation of a policy which would have such serious and widespread repercussions. The issue of euthanasia is one in which the interests of the individual cannot be separated from those of society as a whole. (Walton 1994*a*)

Instead, the Committee urged the development and growth of palliative care services throughout the UK. The same conclusion was reached some years ago by a working party set up by the British Medical Association (1988).

Likewise, I share the sentiments of the Nursing Forum on AIDS of the

Table 5. *Pragmatic reasons for opposing euthanasia*

Reason	Comment
Many requests stem from inadequate symptom relief	Patients no longer ask when their symptoms are adequately relieved
Other requests relate to a sense of uselessness or feeling a burden	Good palliative care restores hope by giving the patient a sense of direction
Persistent requests often reflect a depressive illness	Depression requires specific treatment, not euthanasia
Patients frequently change their minds	Many patients have transient periods of despair through which they pass
Prognosis is often far from certain	Some patients live for years longer than originally anticipated
A 'euthanasia mentality' results in voluntary euthanasia extending to imposed euthanasia	This is indisputably the case in the Netherlands
If voluntary euthanasia were permitted, elderly and terminally ill patients would feel 'at risk'	Anecdotal evidence and the results of a survey of elderly people in the Netherlands lend support to this contention
Pressure on doctors from relatives to impose euthanasia on patients could be irresistible	The Remmelink Report demonstrates that relatives do put pressure on doctors
Doctors who find it hard to cope with 'failure' will tend to impose euthanasia regardless of patients' wishes	Anecdotal evidence from the Netherlands supports this contention
Voluntary euthanasia will remove the incentive to improve standards of palliative care	Palliative care is still in its infancy in the Netherlands; improvements are undoubtedly being hindered by the *de facto* acceptance of voluntary euthanasia

Royal College of Nursing:

> [We are] vehemently opposed to any initiatives which would seek to legalize euthanasia for people with AIDS. Such legalized death would encourage the prevalent ignorance about the condition and decelerate the research being undertaken into this condition. It could also have serious ramifications for other chronically and terminally ill people. Rather, medicine and nursing should grasp the opportunity to pursue education about this condition, and gain information and knowledge so that symptomatic manifestations of AIDS can be relieved, enabling people to live to the full the remainder of their lives, and eventually achieve an easy death without the need for euthanasia. (Fleming 1988)

There are rare occasions when it is necessary to use benzodiazepines, phenothiazines and/or barbiturates to sedate a patient in order to relieve intolerable distress in one whose dying is complicated by, for example, an agitated delirium or tracheal obstruction (Lichter and Hunt 1990). I am still bound, however, by the cardinal ethical principle that I must achieve my treatment goal with the least risk to the patient's life. In this case, rendering the patient unconscious is clearly less of an immediate risk than deliberately killing the patient. Supporters of voluntary euthanasia may well say that I am splitting ethical and therapeutic hairs in as much as the end-points of my action and that of the doctor who would actively assist death are generally identical. I disagree; for me there is a fundamental difference. Even in these extreme and rare circumstances, my *intention* is to alleviate suffering, not to shorten life. The practical, ethical and legal reality of this distinction has been upheld by the Report of the Select Committee on Medical Ethics (House of Lords 1994; Walton 1994*b*).

Further, my approach maintains a necessary measure of humility in the face of the mystery of life and death. The dangers of crossing the Rubicon are so great that, even though I may be forced by extreme circumstances to put one foot into the river, I will continue to respect the necessity of this ultimate barrier (Gaylin *et al.* 1988; Vaux 1988; Reichel and Dyck 1989; Roy 1990).

REFERENCES

Alexander, L. 1949, Medical science under dictatorship. *New England Journal of Medicine* 241(2): 39–47

Barraclough, B., Bunch, J., Nelson, B., *et al.* 1974. A hundred cases of suicide: clinical aspects. *British Journal of Psychiatry* 125: 355–373.

Binding, K. and Hoche, A. 1975. *The Release or Destruction of Life Devoid of Value.* California: Life Quality. (Originally published in German, by Felix Meiner, Leipzig, 1920.)

Block, S. D. 1990. Difficult cases: the request for active euthanasia. Paper presented at the Eighth International Congress on Care of the Terminally Ill, Montreal 1990.

Breitbart, W. 1989. Psychiatric management of cancer pain. *Cancer* 63: 2336–2342.

Breitbart, W. 1990. Cancer pain and suicide. In *Advances in Pain Research and Therapy*, ed. K. M. Foley, J. J. Bonica and V. Ventafridda, pp. 399–412. New York: Raven Press.

British Medical Association. 1988. *Euthanasia*. London: British Medical Association.

Brown, J. H., Henteleff, P., Barakat, S. and Rowe, C. J. 1986. Is it normal for terminally ill patients to desire death? *American Journal of Psychiatry* 143: 208–211.

Collee, J. 1991. A doctor writes. *Observer* 4 August.

Dawson, J. 1986. An open and gentle death? *BMA News Review* January: 22–23.

Daut, R. L. and Cleeland, C. S. 1982. The prevalence and severity of pain in cancer. *Cancer* 50: 1913–1918.

Dorrepaal, K. L., Aaronson, N. K. and Van Dam Fsam. 1989. Pain experience and pain management among hospitalized cancer patients. *Cancer* 63: 593–598.

Dorrepaal, K. L. 1989. *Pijn bij patienten met kanker*. Amsterdam: University of Amsterdam.

Farberow, N. L., Ganzler, S., Cutter, F. *et al.* 1971. An eight-year survey of hospital suicides. *Life-Threatening Behaviour* 1: 184–202.

Feifel, H. 1963. Death. In *Taboo Topics*, ed. N. Farberow, pp. 8–21. New York: Atherton Press.

Fleming, J. 1988. No final solution. *Nursing Standard* 25 June: 11.

Gaylin, W., Kass, L. R., Pellegrino, E. D. and Siegler, M. 1988. Doctors must not kill. *Journal of the American Medical Association* 259: 2139–2140.

George, R. 1990. Euthanasia; the AIDS dimension. In *Death Without Dignity*, ed. N. M. de S. Cameron, pp. 176–195. Edinburgh: Rutherford House Books.

Gunning, K. F. 1991. Euthanasia. *Lancet* 338: 1010–1011.

Haram, B. J. 1978. Facts and figures. In *The Management of Terminal Disease*, ed. C. M. Saunders, pp. 12–18. London: Edward Arnold.

Herth, K. 1990. Fostering hope in terminally-ill people. *Journal of Advanced Nursing* 15: 1250–1259.

Hirschfeld, M. J. H. and Ziv, L. 1989. When a demented patient refuses food: ethical arguments of nurses in Israel. *Palliative Medicine* 4: 25–30.

House of Lords 1994. *Report of the Select Committee on Medical Ethics*. HL Paper 21-I. London: HMSO.

Hunt, J. M., Stollar, T. D., Littlejohns, D. W., Twycross, R. G. and Vere, D. W. 1977. Patients with protracted pain: a survey conducted at the London Hospital. *Journal of Medical Ethics* 3: 61–73.

Keown, J. 1994. Further reflections on euthanasia in the Netherlands in the light of the Remmelink Report and the van der Maas Survey. In *Euthanasia, Clinical Practice and the Law*, ed. L. Gormally, pp. 219–240. London: The Linacre Centre.

Lamb, D. 1988. *Down the Slippery Slope: Arguing in Applied Ethics*. London: Croom Helm.

Lamerton, R. 1978. *Annual Report of Macmillan Home Care Service St Joseph's Hospice*.

Lichter, I. 1991. Some psychological causes of distress in the terminally ill. *Palliative Medicine* 5: 138–146.

Lichter, I. and Hunt, E. 1990. The last 48 hours of life. *Journal of Palliative Care* 6(4): 7–15.

Lunt, B. and Neale, C. 1987. A comparison of hospice and hospital: care goals set by staff. *Palliative Medicine* 1: 136–148.

Main, T. F. 1957. The ailment. *British Journal of Medical Psychology* 30: 129–145.

Marzuk, P. M., Tierney, H., Tardiff, K. *et al.* 1988. Increased risk of suicide in persons with AIDS. *Journal of the American Medical Association* 259: 1333–1337.

Parkes. C. M. 1972. Accuracy of predictions of survival in later stages of cancer. *British Medical Journal* i: 29–31.

Reichel, W. and Dyck, A. J. 1989. Euthanasia: a contemporary moral quandary. *Lancet* ii: 1321–1323

Roy, D. J. 1990. Euthanasia: where to go after taking a stand? *Journal of Palliative Care* 6(2): 3–5.

Roy, D. J. and Rapin, C. H. 1994. Regarding euthanasia. *European Journal of Palliative Care* 1: 57–59.

Sainsbury, P. 1973. Suicide: opinions and facts. *Proceedings of the Royal Society of Medicine* 66: 579–587.

Saunders, C. M. 1981. Current views of pain relief and terminal care. In *The Therapy of Pain*, ed. M. Swerdlow, pp. 215–241. Lancaster: MTP Press.

Segers, J. H. 1988. Elderly persons on the subject of euthanasia. *Issues in Law & Medicine* 3(4): 407–424.

Stengel, E. and Cook, N. G. 1958. *Attempted Suicide: Its Special Significance and Effects*.

London: Chapman and Hall.

Takeda, F. 1989. The management of cancer pain in Japan. In *The Edinburgh Symposium on Pain and Medical Education*, ed. R. G. Twycross, pp. 17–22. London: Royal Society of Medicine.

Twycross, R. G. 1977. A comparison of diamorphine with cocaine and methadone. *British Journal of Clinical Pharmacology* 4: 691–692.

Twycross, R. G. 1982. Euthanasia: a physician's viewpoint. *Journal of Medical Ethics* 8: 86–95.

Twycross, R. G. 1994. *Pain Relief in Advanced Cancer*. Edinburgh: Churchill Livingstone.

Twycross, R. G. 1995. *Symptom Management in Advanced Cancer*. Abingdon: Radcliffe Medical Press.

Twycross, R. G. and Lichter, I. 1993. The terminal phase. In *Oxford Textbook of Palliative Medicine*, ed. D. Doyle, G. W. Hanks and N. MacDonald, pp. 649–661. Oxford: Oxford University Press.

van der Maas, P. J., Van Delden, J. J. M., Pijnenborg, L. and Looman, C. W. N. 1991. Euthanasia and other medical decisions concerning the end of life. *Lancet* 338: 669–674.

Vaux, K. L. 1988. Debbie's death: mercy killing and the good death. *Journal of the American Medical Association* 259: 2140–2141.

Walton, J. 1994*a*. *Medical Ethics: Select Committee Report. Hansard* 9 May, pp. 1344–1349.

Walton, J. 1994*b*. The House of Lords on issues of life and death. *Journal of the Royal College of Physicians of London* 28(3): 235–236.

Warburg, T. L. 1988. *A Voice at Twilight*. London: Owen.

Ward, B. J. and Tate, P. A. 1994. Attitudes among NHS doctors to requests for euthanasia. *British Medical Journal* 308: 1332–1334.

Weddington, W. W. 1981. Euthanasia: clinical issues behind the request. *Journal of the American Medical Association* 246: 1949–1950.

Whitfield, S. 1990. Implications of euthanasia for medical and nursing staff. In *Death without Dignity*, ed. N. M. de S. Cameron. Edinburgh: Rutherford House Books.

WHO. 1986. *Cancer Pain Relief*. Geneva: World Health Organization.

Winokur, G. and Tsuang, M. 1975. The Iowa 500: suicide in mania, depression, and schizophrenia. *America Journal of Psychiatry* 132: 650–651.

Worsthorne, P. 1990. Cries of anguish are the food of love. *Sunday Telegraph* 12 September: 18.

12

Letting vegetative patients die

BRYAN JENNETT

MANY WOULD CONSIDER that the persistent vegetative state and its management has no place in a book on euthanasia. Certainly the very full medical, ethical and legal debates there have been over the past 17 years about managing vegetative patients, largely conducted in the academic journals, the law courts and public press in the United States, have scarcely made reference to the euthanasia issue. The few commentators who have sought to relate the two issues are those whose objections to letting vegetative patients die seem to be based, at least partly, on the fear that to allow this would be seen as a step towards legitimising euthanasia. In Britain, however, some association between the two issues in the public mind became inevitable when two highly publicised legal cases caught the attention of the media in the same week in 1992. In late September Dr Nigel Cox had been convicted of attempted murder for giving a lethal injection to a pain-wracked patient, but in mid-November the General Medical Council decided not to take any disciplinary action against him after which his employing authority agreed to reinstate him subject to certain conditions. That was the same week that the High Court was hearing the case of Anthony Bland, a young man vegetative for three and a half years for whom a declaration was sought to allow withdrawal of life-sustaining treatment – the first such case to come under legal scrutiny in the UK. However, the *Bland* judges emphasised, as had several US judges before them, that a decision to allow withdrawal of life support from a vegetative patient has nothing to do with euthanasia. Moreover, several years previously the Archbishop of Canterbury, quoting a Church report, had stated that it was misleading to extend the term euthanasia to cover decisions not to preserve life by artificial means when it would be better for the patient to be allowed to die (Coggan 1977). Nonetheless an immediate consequence of the *Bland* case was the setting up of a House of Lords Select Committee on Medical Ethics to consider the implications both of withholding life-prolonging treatment and of measures intended to shorten life.

My theme is that the decision to let a vegetative patient die by withdrawing tube-feeding is a logical extension of what has become a widely accepted medical practice that is supported by ethicists and is not challenged by lawyers – namely the withholding or withdrawal of treatment considered of no benefit to a patient and therefore not in his best interests. This practice has been promoted as a public policy issue in the USA for many years as part of the increasing interest in patient-centred medical ethics. This emphasises the importance of respecting the autonomy of patients and on balancing expected benefits and probable burdens to patients when deciding what interventions are appropriate. An important staging post in this movement was the President's Commission on 'Deciding to forego life-sustaining treatment' (1983), which *inter alia* explicitly approved the withdrawal of tube-feeding from vegetative patients. Indeed the word euthanasia did not even feature in the index of this 500 page report. Nonetheless some subsequent commentators have styled deaths from decisions to limit treatment as passive euthanasia. This term is not, however, in common usage and has always been studiously avoided in the Netherlands where decisions at the end of life have been debated by the medical and legal professions and the government for several years. There and elsewhere euthanasia is used only to describe an active intervention intended to bring about the death of the patient. This excludes the incidental hastening of death resulting from drugs given primarily to relieve distressing symptoms.

In order to explain why the management of the vegetative state has posed ethical and legal dilemmas I shall first set out the medical facts about this syndrome. I shall then trace the development in the USA of the acceptance of treatment-limiting decisions (a useful term that covers both withholding and withdrawing) for a wide range of medical conditions. This has resulted in regulations and legislation to facilitate treatment-limiting decisions, and to many cases being decided by State courts, and the involvement of the US Supreme Court in the case of Nancy Cruzan in 1990. I shall then consider the reaction in the UK to developments in America and then deal with the case of Tony Bland. Finally I shall comment on the report of the House of Lords Select Committee on Medical Ethics.

THE MEDICAL FACTS

The vegetative state is a term coined by myself and Professor Plum of New York in 1972 to describe the behavioural features of patients who have suffered severe brain damage that has resulted in the cerebral cortex being out of action. Without the thinking, feeling and motivating part of the brain these patients are unconscious, in the sense that they make no responses that indicate any meaningful interaction with their surroundings, and remain unaware of themselves or their environment. They never obey a command, nor speak a single word. More primitive parts of the brain that are responsible for periodic wakefulness and for a wide range of reflex activities are still functioning, giving the paradox of a patient who is at times awake but always unaware. When open the eyes roam around but do not fix or follow for long, whilst the spastic paralysed limbs never move voluntarily or purposefully. They can, however, withdraw reflexly from a painful stimulus which may provoke a grimace and a groan – but there is no evidence that pain or suffering is experienced. Occasional yawning, smiling, weeping and sometimes laughing can occur but these are unrelated to appropriate stimuli. Reflex swallowing, chewing and gagging occur and breathing is normal with no need for a ventilator.

The diagnosis depends on bedside observation over a period of time by a skilled doctor in a patient who has suffered an appropriate type of brain damage. The medical conclusion is that, in spite of the wide range of reflex activity, there is no evidence of a working mind or of awareness. However, families often claim to observe some responsiveness to their presence or their conversation or ministrations. No reliable laboratory investigations are available to confirm the diagnosis. Computer tomography (CT) or magnetic resonance imaging (MRI) show very marked wasting of the brain, but severe dementia can produce a similar picture without complete unconsciousness. The electroencephalographic (EEG) records vary from case to case, ranging from a flat record in some 5% to one that is near normal in 25%. Usually the EEG is much less responsive than normal to external stimuli, and evoked responses in the cortex to somatic sensory stimuli are usually absent. Studies of the metabolism of the brain involving research techniques that are not available for routine use show that the cerebral cortex is functioning at a very depressed level, equivalent to that of deep barbiturate anaesthesia.

Brain damage that can result in there no longer being enough surviving or connected cerebral cortex to support consciousness can arise from acute insults or chronic conditions. Acute insults may be traumatic (a severe head injury) or non-traumatic. The latter may be due to anoxia from cardiac arrest, low blood pressure or asphyxia, or to hypoglycaemia in diabetics, or to a series of strokes or to intracranial infection or tumour. After severe head injury the main damage is to the subcortical white matter fibres that are disrupted over wide areas, resulting in isolation of the cerebral cortex. After anoxic or hypoglycaemic insult the nerve cells in the cortex and basal ganglia have largely disappeared, due to the lack of oxygen or glucose necessary for their survival. In contrast to these cases resulting from acute insults are patients who become vegetative as a result of chronic dementing conditions such as Alzheimer's disease or, in children, degenerative or metabolic brain disorders or severe developmental abnormalities of the brain, many of them genetic in origin. Some of these chronic conditions cause progressive death of nerve cells within the cerebral cortex, others severe degeneration in the subcortical nerve fibres so that the cortical cells are isolated and unable to function.

After severe head injury patients are usually in sleep-like coma for some 2 weeks before waking up to become vegetative. After non-traumatic insults, without the concussive element that causes coma, patients can become vegetative within a day or so of sustaining brain damage. Most patients who recover consciousness after an acute insult show evidence of an active cortex soon after they open their eyes, and only a minority are temporarily vegetative en route to recovery. How long a patient should have been vegetative before being labelled as in a persistent vegetative state has varied in different reports from 1 to 3 to 6 months. However, recent US consensus statements agree that 1 month should be the defining period (American Neurological Association 1993; Multi-Society Task Force 1994), recognising that this does not mean that the vegetative state will necessarily be permanent.

There is considerable variation in estimates of the frequency or prevalence of vegetative patients. These variations partly reflect differences in how estimates were reached – whether confined to cases from acute insults, to adults or children, or to patients vegetative for 1, 3 or 6 months. Moreover, vegetative patients are found in many different places, including acute hospitals, rehabilitation units, mental institutions, nursing homes and at home with families – and surveys may not include all of these. Estimates in the USA vary from 14 000 to 35 000, a rate per million population (PMP) of 56–140 (The Multi-Society Task Force 1994). About 30% are believed to be children. Estimates in Japan, France and the Netherlands indicate rates considerably lower than in the USA, but may include fewer children or chronic cases. In the UK there are about 23 new cases each year PMP 1 month after an acute insult; many of these will die or recover over the next few months but to those left vegetative must be added patients vegetative from previous years and from chronic conditions. This leads to an estimate of 1000–1500 cases at any one time (18–27 PMP). This is similar to estimates in Japan and France. The much higher American rate probably reflects the 2.5 times greater incidence of severe head injury and perhaps a greater tendency to initiate and continue life-saving and life-sustaining technologies.

In deciding about the appropriate management of vegetative patients the most important consideration is the remaining potential for recovery. A number of patients who are vegetative for a time after an acute insult do regain consciousness. However, a distinction should be made between recovery of some limited degree of consciousness and the restoration of useful function. Many of the patients who recover after being vegetative for several months never speak or are capable of only occasional monosyllabic utterances or of obeying occasional commands; they do not become fully interactive persons with a quality of life that can be enjoyed even at a limited level. Some, however, do regain a degree of independence – although how this term is defined is important. According to the Glasgow Outcome Scale (Jennett and Bond 1975), which is widely used for assessing outcome after acute brain damage, independence indicates the patient's capacity to organise his own life on a day-to-day basis without the support or prompting of family or carers. A more limited degree of independence applies only to activities of daily life, which usually means the capacity for self care within the sick room but requir ing the intervention of others every day for some activities. In the analysis of recovery that follows the social independence of the Glasgow Outcome Scale is implied, rather than this more limited definition of independence.

Several factors determine the potential for recovery, the most important of which is how long the patient has been vegetative. Other factors are the cause of brain damage (traumatic cases recover better than non-traumatic) and the patient's age (children do better than adults, and younger adults better than older, particularly after trauma). The probability of recovery of consciousness and of independence has been analysed by the Multi-Society Task Force (1994) for an aggregate of 754 patients whose outcomes have been published in medical journals. Of patients vegetative 1 month after an acute insult, regardless of age and diagnosis, a third were dead by the end of a year, a quarter were still vegetative, 43% had regained consciousness and 18% had become independent. Of non-traumatic cases, however, only 14% regained consciousness and 2% became independent. After 3 months the chance even of regaining consciousness after non-traumatic damage was only 7% and 3% for adults and children respectively, and only one such patient became independent after being 3 months in a vegetative state. After 6 months only a few children with head injury have ever regained independence. Exceptional cases of late recovery are reported from time to time, often in the non-medical press and with inadequate details to substantiate the claims. Only 5 of 19 such cases were accepted by the US Task Force as valid and all of these patients were left severely disabled without independence.

Several authoritative bodies have now made recommendations about when the possibility of recovery from the vegetative state can be considered as no longer a reasonable prospect (Table 1). When the American Medical Association made its recommendation in 1990 the various late recoveries mentioned above had already all been published, and it was estimated that the error rate in applying its recommendations would be less than 1 in 1000. A more recent report of recoveries after 4 months in the vegetative state from an English rehabilitation centre records that all but one recovered in 12 months. The exception was a patient whose 'recovery' was doubtful in that he still had not spoken nor obeyed commands 5 years after his anoxic insult (Andrews 1993). Obviously the vegetative state that develops at the end stage of progressive dementing processes is not associated with any potential for recovery. However, such patients are sometimes temporarily vegetative during their downward decline, owing to the influence of temporary factors such as toxicity, infection or sedative drugs. These need to be excluded or corrected before accepting that the patient has become permanently vegetative.

Patients who are vegetative have a considerable mortality during the first year, and this is higher after non-traumatic damage and in adults. The average survival in the vegetative state is 3–4 years but cases are recorded living for 10–20 years, one for 37 years and another for 40 years. Once the patient has survived the first year there is a greater chance of prolonged survival. Even patients who become vegetative at the end of a dementing process may live another 3–4 years, some even longer. Death is eventually usually due to pulmonary or urinary tract infection and the duration of survival may depend on how vigorously such complications are treated.

All are agreed that a high standard of supportive nursing care, adequate nutrition and physiotherapy are important in the early months in order to provide the best chance of spontaneous recovery. However, the conclusion of the US Task Force in 1994 was that no treatment actually promotes recovery from the vegetative state, including coma arousal programmes, deep electrical stimulation of the brain and specially designed physical rehabilitation programmes. None of the unexpected late recoveries reported in the literature claim to have resulted from particular treatment regimes.

Table 1. *When is persistent permanent?*

	Non-traumatic	Traumatic	All
1989 Academy of Neurology	1–3 m		
1989 World Medical Association			12 m (6 m if >50 yr of age)
1990 American Medical Association	3 m	12 m (6 m if >50 yr of age)	
1991 Netherlands	1 m	3–6 m	
1993 British Medical Association			12 m
1993 American Neurological Association			6 m
1993 Medical Council of New Zealand			12 m (? less)
1994 Task Force US	3 m	12 m	
1994 Netherlands Health Council	6 m	12 m	
1994 New Zealand Medical Association			Many months

m, months.

ETHICAL ISSUES

The widely accepted ethical approach to the management of patients whose vegetative state is considered to be permanent can be regarded as a logical extension of the increasing acceptance that it is good medical practice to withhold or withdraw treatment considered of no benefit to hopelessly ill patients. The development of life-saving and life-sustaining technologies associated with intensive care units in the late 1950s led to concern that these were sometimes used inappropriately to prolong life or, as some put it, to prolong the process of dying. This led a group of anaesthetists to ask Pope Pius XII in 1957 whether they needed to maintain technological support for patients who were not expected to regain cerebral function. He replied that they were not obliged to use 'extraordinary' measures, by which were meant those that were disproportionately burdensome in relation to expected benefit.

Ten years later the Harvard criteria for brain death emerged, legitimising the withdrawal of ventilator support from heart-beating patients whose brains were deemed irrecoverably damaged (Ad Hoc Committee 1968). That same year intensivists were writing about limiting treatment for other hopelessly ill patients, and the phrase 'death with dignity' first emerged. Speaking to a British Medical Association (BMA) meeting in the year that PVS was described, the Bishop of Durham (1972) questioned 'what degree of respect we should accord vegetative patients as compared with the lives of others who are much more evidently alive and in rapport with other members of society. The so-called principle of respect for life needs to be qualified and married to an explicit concept of personality and linked to ideas about the quality of life.'

A key year in this story was 1976, when the New Jersey Supreme Court allowed the request of the Roman Catholic father of Karen Quinlan, a comatose teenager, to have her ventilator stopped to let her die. The father's request had the support of his parish priest, but the doctors spent months weaning her from the ventilator and she lived for 10 years in a vegetative state. Later in 1976 a single issue of the *New England Journal of Medicine* had papers on do-not-resuscitate orders (Rabkin *et al.* 1976), on living wills (which were given statutory force that year in California) (Bok 1976), on optimum care for the hopelessly ill in intensive care units (Clinical Care Committee 1976), and an editorial entitled 'Terminating life support – out of the closet' (Fried 1976). This last paper was by a lawyer, who noted that lawyers had participated in each of the other three papers in the journal.

The *Quinlan* case opened the way for a succession of court cases in the USA, not only on withdrawing ventilation but on withholding surgery, cancer therapy, and tube-feeding. These cases included a variety of hopelessly ill patients, some of whom were competent and themselves requesting that treatment be limited. These court cases coincided with a burgeoning interest in medical ethics with its four principles of beneficence, non-maleficence, respecting patient autonomy and having consideration for justice in the distribution of health care resources. Notice that these principles do not include saving, preserving or prolonging life. Increasing concern with patient-centred decision making by ethicists, supported by lawyers, led to emphasis on the right of patients to refuse treatment that they considered not to be of benefit – including that which saves or sustains life. The living will and advance directive movements were attempts to extend that autonomy to patients unable when the time came to refuse treatment that in prospect they considered would not be acceptable to them.

The issue of decisions to limit treatment for the hopelessly ill was reviewed at length by the President's Commission (1983) and later the American Medical Association (1986) published guidance on decisions to limit treatment. Both of these authoritative publications specifically approved withdrawal of tube-feeding from vegetative patients. That year also saw the publication of a book *By No Extraordinary Means: The Choice to Forgo Life-Sustaining Food and Water* (Lynn 1986). In 1988 the Office of Technology Assessment of the US Congress published a report on Institutional Protocols for Decisions about Life-Sustaining Treatments. This dealt with five treatments: cardiopulmonary resuscitation, mechanical ventilation, renal dialysis, tube and intravenous feeding and antibiotic therapy. Later that year the Joint Accreditation Board for Hospitals and Nursing Homes made it mandatory for all such institutions in the USA to have agreed protocols for limiting treatment. In 1990 the Patient Self-Determination Act required that all patients on admission to hospital or nursing home be informed of their right to refuse treatment and of their right to make an advance directive. That Federal Act was largely precipitated by the *Cruzan* case – the vegetative patient whose case went to the US Supreme Court. This was because a Missouri Court had denied the right of her family to decide about the withdrawal of tube-feeding in the absence of clear and convincing evidence that the patient herself had expressed a specific wish for this.

Most treatment-limiting decisions are made in the context of acute crises in patients with conditions that threaten imminent death unless there is some medical intervention such as cardiopulmonary resuscitation, emergency surgery, dialysis or artificial feeding. Some such acutely ill patients were previously healthy but affected by sudden illness or accident. Others have chronic progressive diseases, such as advanced cancer, cardiorespiratory failure or AIDS and suffer a predictable episode. Yet others have relatively stable disabilities such as severe dementia or the vegetative state before having a critical illness. In the latter two kinds of case, a prior decision is sometimes made that in the event of such an episode treatment should be withheld – for example, not to resuscitate, perform emergency surgery or admit to intensive care.

With the previously healthy a trial of treatment to establish the possibility of recovery will almost always be necessary. Once such a trial of treatment has failed the question arises of withdrawing treatment. Although most ethicists and lawyers emphasise that there is no difference morally or legally between withdrawing and withholding, health professionals often find it more difficult to withdraw. But unless it is agreed that withdrawal is acceptable once treatment proves futile, there is a risk that doctors may be reluctant to initiate treatment that could be successful for fear that if it were not to succeed a prolonged period of futile treatment would inevitably follow.

It is important to recognise how frequent such treatment-limiting decisions now are. The *Cruzan* court was told that 70% of deaths in US hospitals were in some way planned by patients, families and physicians. A report of 115 deaths in two intensive care units in San Francisco showed that 45% followed a treatment-limiting decision, withdrawing being four times more common than withholding (Smedira *et al.* 1990). Only 5% of the incompetent had living wills. In practice most decisions were therefore made informally by the doctor and the family. More recently it has been reported that two-thirds of deaths in American intensive care units follow a decision to limit treatment. In a review of 9000 deaths in the Netherlands 25% of those that were not sudden were attributed to the side effects of symptom-relieving drugs after active treatment had been stopped, and another 25% resulted from a treatment-limiting decision alone (van der Maas *et al.* 1991). This excluded the 3% of non-sudden deaths that were due to active euthanasia. A survey of deaths in surgical wards in Glasgow showed that 50% occurred without an operation – which presumably had been withheld; of deaths within 30 days of operation 40% had had a treatment-limiting decision in general surgery and in neurosurgery it was over 60%. Another common example of a treatment-limiting decision, although seldom explicitly acknowledged as such, is when a patient with progressive dementia reaches the stage of refusing oral feeds, and it is decided not to institute tube-feeding.

It is clear, therefore, that treatment-limiting decisions are now accepted practice, although in Britain there has been reluctance to formalise these in the American style. Indeed such a development was rejected as inappropriate by a senior British physician (Bayliss 1982). However, his defence of medical paternalism seems out of date a decade later when the principle of patient autonomy is accorded greater importance, and a more recent comment was subtitled 'Learning from America' (Williams 1989). There is now widespread acceptance that it is good ethical medical practice to withdraw or withhold treatment either at the patient's request or because it is considered not of net benefit to the patient – i.e. not in his best interests.

That of course begs the question of what is benefit and who decides that treatment is not of benefit and therefore futile. As already indicated all are agreed that if the patient now or previously has indicated a wish to forego a specific treatment, then that wish must be heeded (see *Airedale NHS Trust* v. *Bland* 1993*a*). Courts in the USA, in Quebec and in New Zealand have each agreed to the withdrawal of ventilation and of tube-feeding at the request of competent patients with advanced neurological disease. Moreover the American Academy of Neurology (1993) has published a position paper spelling out that this is an ethically and legally acceptable course of action. Several American courts, one in South Africa and the *Bland* court in England have all stated specifically that if a vegetative patient had a living will considered valid and relevant that stated a wish to have tube-feeding discontinued, then doctors would be required to withdraw this treatment.

Decisions about stable vegetative patients with no advance directive can seem more difficult. This is because most guidelines on treatment-limiting decisions refer to death being imminent, and on preventing the suffering of dying patients. Neither of these factors applies to the vegetative patient, although in truth many of the patients dying in intensive care units from whom treatment is withdrawn are in fact unconscious and therefore not suffering. The key ethical issue is whether prolonging the life of a patient whose vegetative state is considered permanent brings benefit to that patient. The *Bland* judges explicitly stated that the sanctity of life principle has exceptions and that this could be one. Several religious commentators have also indicated that a life devoid of almost all the attributes of a human being is one that there is no moral obligation to save or prolong. Some may choose to disagree with this and to side with the minority of vitalists who maintain that life of any kind is in itself a benefit. But it does seem that most people, at least in Western countries, believe that prolonging life in a vegetative state is not a benefit. This is evident from the many cases that have been through the courts in several countries, the commentaries of many ethicists, and most public comment on widely reported cases. Another insight into views about vegetative survival comes from advance directives that are made or proposed. When 500 Americans were asked about their wish to be treated by resuscitation, a ventilator, major surgery or artificial nutrition if in a permanent vegetative state, over 80% voted 'no' for each of these treatments (Emanuel *et al.* 1991). More recently doctors and nurses have indicated similar wishes if they themselves were patients (Gillick *et al.* 1993). There are those who discount as invalid the declarations of healthy people about what they would want when seriously disabled or terminally ill, claiming that people's views change. That is to undermine the whole concept of advance directives. In any event it does not seem reasonable to attribute to a vegetative patient the capacity to change his mind. Many formal declarations have now been made about the vegetative state not only by medical bodies but by others that included lawyers and ethicists (Table 2). It is unusual for the diagnosis and management of any medical condition to have been the subject of such a wide and published consensus.

However, the views of relatives of vegetative patients are much more often in favour of continuing life support, and even wishing for new interventions if life-threatening complications develop. Of 33 relatives of mainly elderly vegetative patients in US nursing homes fewer than 1 in 5 would discontinue tube-feeding (Tresch *et al.* 1991). Over two-thirds would want their vegetative relative transferred to an acute hospital for a crisis and would opt for surgery if needed to save life; one-third would want resuscitation or reinstating mechanical ventilation if required to prolong life. Yet none of these relatives held out any hope of recovery. It is therefore important to emphasise that those who support the case for withholding or withdrawing treatment from vegetative patients are doing no more than indicating that this is an ethically and legally acceptable option – not that it is a course of action to be actively recommended. When an American hospital petitioned a court recently to stop the respirator support of an 86-year-old vegetative patient against the wishes of the family, on the basis that there was no right to demand futile treatment, the court found in favour of continuing treatment (Angell 1991). On the other hand several families have successfully sued hospitals in America for prolonging the lives of their vegetative relatives when such treatment had been refused by the patients or their surrogates (Weir and Gostin 1990).

The main ethical reason for withdrawing tube-feeding is therefore lack of benefit once recovery is deemed no longer a reasonable possibility, on the grounds that the reason for initiating tube-feeding had been as a trial of treatment in case recovery did occur. But does prolonging vegetative life do any harm? Some emphasise the indignity of such a state and others that the memory of the patient can be said to be blighted by prolonged vegetative survival. Others counter that the vegetative patient cannot experience indignity. However, we respect the bodies of the dead even though they cannot themselves benefit from this. The question of harm to the relatives is not held to be a relevant ethical consideration, unless it is claimed that the patient would not have wished this burden on them. There are those who say that we should not deny patients this altruism, because patient-centred ethics does not imply that the patient would be concerned only with his own interests.

This raises the difficult issue of determining what a patient's wishes would be, in the absence of an advance directive. In the USA many patients are said to have stated informally that they would not wish to be kept alive in a state like Karen Quinlan, and in this country similar statements may be now made *vis-à-vis* Tony Bland. More often families report the general attitude to life and the values of the patient as a basis for considering what he would have wanted. This is often accepted in the USA as valid for making a 'substituted judgement'. However, this attempt to imagine the patient's own choice has been criticised in the USA as a cruel charade that conceals what is really the decision of the surrogates. In Britain the preference has always been to reach a decision on the basis of the patient's best interests – the balance of benefits and burdens of treatment as weighed by the doctor after consultation with the family.

Table 2. *Declarations on PVS*

1983	President's Commission
1989	Academy of Neurology
	Appleton Conference I
	World Medical Association
1990	American Medical Association
1991	Institute of Medical Ethics
1992	Appleton Conference II
	British Medical Association
1993	American Neurological Association
	Headway
	Medical Council of New Zealand
1994	Multi-Society Task Force
1994	Health Council of the Netherlands
1994	New Zealand Medical Association

Another issue is the relevance of the fourth ethical principle – that of justice in the distribution of health care resources. Those who most often argue this are ethicists, from the Editor of the *Journal of Medical Ethics* (Gillon 1993) to the Appleton Conference (Stanley 1992), as well as those with a specific religious base such as the Bishop of Durham (1972) and Archbishop Coggan (1977). They have all quite explicitly stated that it is difficult to justify the expenditure of resources on prolonging vegetative survival. It is interesting that in the definition of 'extraordinary' or 'disproportionate' treatments by Catholic moralists, both the low probability of benefit and the disproportionate use of resources are usually quoted.

Some Catholic theologians have supported the withdrawal of tube-feeding, notably Paris, a Jesuit who served on the President's Commission and has testified in prominent court cases (Paris and Reardon 1985; Paris and McCormick 1987). There is, however, some disagreement among Catholics on this issue as is acknowledged in the 1992 declaration of the Committee for Pro-Life Activities of the National Conference of the US Catholic Bishops. In Belgium the Catholic University of Louvain (Katholicke Universiteit 1992) has declared that tube-feeding can be withdrawn as it constitutes a disproportionate means of sustaining life in the circumstances of the persistent vegetative state. Commenting on the *Bland* case Kelly (1993) also maintained that treatment withdrawal of this life-sustaining treatment is compatible with Catholic tradition, as did McQueen and Walsh (1992).

Another issue for debate is whether tube-feeding is different from other forms of life-sustaining treatment. Some maintain that supplying food and water represents basic care owed to all people by all people, and that it has symbolic significance in showing care for another human being. They maintain that it is unjustified to classify it as medical treatment because it does nothing to reverse the pathology or to stimulate healing. However, the majority view is that, like ventilation and dialysis, tube-feeding substitutes a lost physiological function – in this case the ability to swallow sufficiently effectively to maintain nutrition. Neither ventilation nor dialysis do anything to restore the loss of function that each substitutes, yet no-one would seriously consider either as other than medical treatment. Medical and ethics groups as well as courts in several countries, including all nine judges who considered *Bland*, all agree that tube-feeding is medical treatment, and that it can therefore be withheld, withdrawn or refused. For their part many ethicists hold that feeding by tube of an unconscious patient is devoid of the symbolic significance of feeding a conscious patient and assuaging his hunger and thirst. They maintain that discontinuing it does not offend any ethical principle, provided that prolongation of life does not hold any prospect of recovery.

Mention has already been made of withholding tube-feeding from elderly demented patients, which is a widely accepted practice, and discussed as such in the geriatric literature (Campbell-Taylor and Fisher 1987). An interesting aspect of the *Cruzan* case was the *Amicus Curiae* brief submitted to the US Supreme Court by the American Geriatrics Society (1990), supporting the view that tube-feeding should be discontinued. Geriatricians were concerned that if the court ruled otherwise for *Cruzan*, they might feel compelled to submit their elderly patients to prolonged periods of tube-feeding.

Yet another issue is whether death after withdrawal of tube-feeding is unpleasant to witness – having accepted that it can cause no suffering to the insentient patient. All the evidence is that this is not so, as set out in several papers. The title of one, 'The sloganism of starvation', referred to the tendency of opponents of withdrawing such feeding to paint a grisly picture of death from dehydration and starvation (Ahronheim and Gasner 1990). The scientific evidence is that imbalance of electrolytes and other biochemicals soon results in coma and that death results from renal failure. The observational evidence from doctors and relatives is that death is peaceful and dignified.

THE BLAND CASE

Anthony Bland (AB) suffered severe anoxic brain damage in April 1989 and following acute treatment in Sheffield was transferred to a medical ward in a district general hospital near his home under the care of Dr Howe, a Consultant Geriatrician who also had training in neurology. When some months later Dr Howe told the family that there was no prospect of recovery AB's parents requested that tube-feeding be discontinued. Concerned with the possible legal repercussions of this Dr Howe sought the advice of the coroner in whose jurisdiction the accident had occurred. He replied that in the event of any type of treatment withdrawal that resulted in AB's death he would have no option but to initiate criminal proceedings. And as evidence of the seriousness of his intent he copied his letter to the Chief Constable. It was 3 years later that the Airedale National Health Service Trust asked the Family Division of the High Court to make a declaration that it would not be unlawful to discontinue tube-feeding for AB.

Soon after this, in September 1992, the Medical Ethics Committee of the BMA issued an extensive discussion document on the treatment of patients in a persistent vegetative state, partly in response to the extensive publicity the *Bland* case was attracting in the media. In accordance with statements previously made in its 1988 Euthanasia Report, it recommended that it was appropriate to withdraw tube-feeding, which was regarded as medical treatment, as soon as recovery was considered no longer possible. It recommended that 1 year was the minimum period to establish irreversibility, and that two additional medical opinions should be sought to confirm the diagnosis and prognosis. The *Bland* judges were to refer frequently to this discussion document as evidence that treatment withdrawal was in accord with 'a body of informed and responsible medical opinion'. This is the so-called *Bolam* test of whether a particular medical action is considered not to be negligent. However, some judges have questioned whether the decision to withdraw treatment, being ethical, is one for doctors alone, either in corporate declarations such as this or in individual cases. The doctor's role is seen by these judges as limited to determining the diagnosis and prognosis and defining what effects or benefits treatment might be expected to have, leaving the ultimate responsibility for determining whether withdrawal is in the patient's best interests to the court.

In November 1992 the Family Division of the High Court heard the case, with medical testimony from Dr Howe and four other experts (two neurologists, a neurosurgeon and a rehabilitation consultant), all of whom agreed about the diagnosis and that there was no prospect of any recovery (*Airedale NHS Trust* v. *Bland* 1993*a*). Counsel for Airedale NHS Trust put the case for discontinuing treatment, and Counsel for the Attorney General as *Amicus Curiae* also advanced a case for discontinuation. Counsel for the Official Solicitor, fulfilling his traditional role of ensuring that the interests of those who cannot speak for themselves do not go by default, argued against treatment withdrawal, which he considered would amount to murder. Sir Stephen Brown, President of the Family Division, granted the declaration that discontinuing treatment would not be unlawful. The case went to the Court of Appeal where the Master of the Rolls and two other judges upheld the High Court decision (*Airedale NHS Trust* v. *Bland* 1993*b*). On further appeal to the House of Lords five Law Lords unanimously upheld the original decision (*Airedale NHS Trust* v. *Bland* 1993*c*).

All nine judges emphasised the importance of consent, and the right of patients to refuse treatment, including that which sustains life – and that such refusal could be in an advance directive. If AB had declared a wish not to have his life prolonged in a vegetative state, the doctors would have been obliged to stop tube-feeding. Absent such a prior statement of views, the correct approach was to consider AB's best interests. All the judges stressed that it was in AB's best interests not to have continued treatment to prolong his life, rather than that it was in his best interest to be allowed to die.

The judges in *Bland* made two other recommendations. One was that future cases of this kind should receive judicial consideration, although some judges hoped that a less formal kind of decision-making might soon emerge. Some judges also expressed concern that they should be expected to develop the law in this difficult field, and recommended that Parliament was the place to debate this issue. As a move towards such a debate the House of Lords set up a Committee to consider not only the problems posed by vegetative patients but the wider issues of all decisions that might shorten life, including passive and active euthanasia. By the time this Committee reported in February 1994 the BMA had issued an agreed set of guidelines based on its earlier discussion paper, and another vegetative case had been referred to the High Court (*Frenchay Healthcare Trust* v. *S* 1994). In this case a percutaneous gastrostomy tube had fallen out and permission was urgently given not to replace it. An appeal, on the grounds that there had not been time to obtain two independent medical reports to confirm the diagnosis and prognosis, as recommended by the BMA guidelines and the *Bland* courts, proved unsuccessful. The wisdom of dispensing with this safeguard has been questioned (Stone 1994).

BMA GUIDELINES

Following consultation by more than 50 contributors on their discussion document, and taking account of the declarations of the courts in *Bland*, the BMA in 1993 issued guidelines, approved by its Council. These stated that all patients should have rehabilitation in the early months, the measures and duration being a matter for clinical judgment. The diagnosis of irreversibility should be made only after 12 months, and with the concurrence of two other independent doctors, one of whom should be a neurologist. Decisions about the patient's best interests should be assessed by doctors, taking account of the views of the families. It was noted that pending further legal pronouncements, a decision to withdraw tube-feeding now required judicial consideration. It was recognised that some doctors might object to treatment withdrawal, and in that event the patient should be transferred to another doctor. If nurses objected to participating in a treatment withdrawal regime, they should be transferred to other duties. Organ donation from vegetative patients was considered inappropriate at present.

REPORT OF THE HOUSE OF LORDS COMMITTEE (1994)

The Report of the House of Lords Committee proved relatively unhelpful in regard to the vegetative state. The Committee was unable to reach a conclusion about whether to regard tube-feeding as a treatment that might under certain circumstances be considered inappropriate to initiate or continue. It went on to suggest that in any event this question need not, indeed should not, usually be asked. In their view an earlier decision to withhold antibiotics for infective complications would make it unnecessary to consider the withdrawal of tube-feeding, except when its administration was evidently burdensome to the patient. This conclusion ignores the fact that survival in a vegetative state can be prolonged even when antibiotics are withheld, hence the need to confront the issue of continuing tube-feeding. On the matter of judicial consideration, the Committee made no specific mention regarding vegetative patients. However, in dealing with the generality of decision-making for incompetent patients it recommended a new judicial forum to authorise the commencement, withholding or withdrawing of treatment, along lines suggested by the Law Commission (1993). The Lords Committee supported the Commission's proposal for 'special category' procedures that would always require the authority of this forum, but without mentioning that one of these categories in the Law Commission's paper was the withdrawal of tube-feeding. This leaves doctors managing vegetative patients in somewhat of a legal limbo. The best they can do, pending the Law Commission's further proposals and any legislation based on these, is to follow the suggestion of the *Bland* courts and of the BMA guidelines.

An editorial accompanying the publication of the Multi-Society Task Force report (1994) discusses two approaches to patients considered to be permanently vegetative (Angell 1994). One is to reach a consensus, similar to that on brain death, about when treatment might be discontinued according to the duration and cause of the vegetative state. If that were done and incorporated into law it would avoid, she asserts, a series of heart-wrenching confrontations between families and others. The decision would be made before the fact and it would be general, not particular. The alternative, favoured by Angell, would be to shift the burden from those who want to discontinue treatment to those who want to continue it. The presumption would be that patients would not wish to be kept alive indefinitely if permanently vegetative. Families taking the idiosyncratic view [*sic*] that treatment should be continued would have to justify their position, perhaps by documenting earlier expressed wishes by the patient. It seems likely, however, to be some time before such a recommendation would be accepted, even in the USA where the dilemma of vegetative survival has been so extensively discussed in the public domain for almost 20 years.

REFERENCES

Ad Hoc Committee of the Harvard Medical School. 1969. Report on the definition of brain death. *Journal of the American Medical Association* 205: 85–88.

Ahronheim, J. C. and Gasner, M. R. 1990. The sloganism of starvation. *Lancet* 335: 278–279.

Airedale NHS Trust v. *Bland* 1993*a*. [1993] Appeal Cases 789.

Airedale NHS Trust v. *Bland* 1993*b*. [1993] Appeal Cases 806.

Airedale NHS Trust v. *Bland* 1993*c*. [1993] Appeal Cases 835.

American Academy of Neurology Ethics and Humanities Sub-committee. 1993. Position statement on certain aspects of the care and management of profoundly and irreversibly paralysed patients with retained consciousness and cognition. *Neurology* 43: 222–223.

American Geriatrics Society. 1990. *Amicus curiae* to the Cruzan Court. *Journal of the American Geriatrics Society* 38: 570–576.

American Medical Association Council on Ethical and Judicial Affairs. 1986. Withholding and withdrawing life prolonging medical treatment. *Journal of the American Medical Association* 256: 471.

American Medical Association Council on Ethical and Judicial Affairs. 1990. Persistent vegetative state and the decision to withdraw or withhold life support. *Journal of the American Medical Association* 263: 426–430.

American Neurological Association Committee on Ethical Affairs. 1993. Persistent vegetative state. *Annals of Neurology* 33: 386–390.

Andrews, K. 1993. Recovery of patients after four months or more in the persistent vegetative state. *British Medical Journal* 206: 1597–1600.

Angell, M. 1991. The case of Helga Wanglie: a new kind of 'right to die' case. *New*

England Journal of Medicine 325: 511–512.
Angell, M. 1994. After Quinlan: the dilemma of the PVS. *New England Journal of Medicine* 330: 1524–1525.
Barlow, P. and Jennett, B. 1991. Decisions to limit treatment in a neurosurgical unit: an aspect of audit of mortality. *Scottish Medical Journal* 36: 109–111.
Bayliss, R. I. S. 1982. Thou shalt not strive officiously. *British Medical Journal* 285: 1373–1375.
Bishop of Durham. 1972. Moral problems facing the medical profession at the present time. *The Bishoprick* 47: 48–61.
Bok, S. 1976. Personal directions for care at the end of life. *New England Journal of Medicine* 295: 367–369.
British Medical Association. 1988. *Report of the Working Party to Review the BMA's Guidance on Euthanasia*. London: BMA.
British Medical Association Medical Ethics Committee. 1992. *Discussion Paper on Treatment of Patients in a Persistent Vegetative State*. London: BMA.
British Medical Association. 1993. Guidelines on treatment decisions for patients in the persistent vegetative state. In *Annual Report 1993*, appendix 7. London: BMA.
Campbell-Taylor, I. and Fisher, R.H. 1987. The clinical case against tube feeding in palliative care of the elderly. *Journal of the American Geriatrics Society* 35: 1100–1114.
Clinical Care Committee of the Massachusetts General Hospital. 1976. Optimum care for hopelessly ill patients. *New England Journal of Medicine* 295: 362–364.
Coggan, D. 1977. On dying and dying well: moral and spiritual aspects. *Journal of the Royal Society of Medicine* 70: 75–76.
Emanuel, L. L., Barry, M. J., Stoeckle, J. D., Ettelson, L. M. and Emanuel, E. J. 1991. Advance directives for medical care: a case for greater use. *New England Journal of Medicine* 324: 889–895.
Frenchay Healthcare NHS Trust v. *S*. 1994. [1994] 2 All England Law Reports 403.
Fried, C. 1976. Terminating life support: out of the closet. *New England Journal of Medicine* 295: 390–391.
Gillick, M. R., Hesse, K. and Mazzapica, N. 1993. Medical technology at the end of life: what would physicians and nurses want for themselves? *Archives of Internal Medicine* 153: 2542–2547.
Gillon, R. 1993. Patients in the persistent vegetative state: a response to Dr Andrews. *British Medical Journal* 306: 1602–1603.
House of Lords. 1994. *Report of Select Committee on Medical Ethics*. HL 21-1. London: HMSO.
Institute of Medical Ethics Working Party Report. 1991. Withdrawing life supporting treatment from patients in a persistent vegetative state after acute brain damage. *Lancet* 337: 96–98.
Jennett, B. and Bond, M. R. 1975. Assessment of outcome after severe brain damage: a practical scale. *Lancet* i: 480–484.
Jennett, B. and Plum, F. 1972. Persistent vegetative state after brain damage: a syndrome in search of a name. *Lancet* i: 734–737.
Katholicke Universiteit Leuven Research Committee on Bioethics. 1992. Ethical considerations on the persistent vegetative state. *Ethischee Perspectieven* 2(3): 14–16.
Kelly, K. 1993. Comment on the Bland case. *The Tablet* 13 March.
Law Commission. 1993. *Mentally Incapacitated Adults and Decision Making: Medical Treatment and Research*. Consultation Paper No. 129. London: HMSO.
Lynn, J. (ed.) 1986. *By No Extraordinary Means: The Choice to Forgo Life-sustaining Food and Water*. Bloomington: Indiana University Press.

McQueen, M. and Walsh, J. L. 1992. Comment on the Bland case. *The Tablet* 19/26 December.
Medical Council of New Zealand Report from Bioethics Research Centre, University of Otago. 1993. *Persistent Vegetative State and the Withdrawal of Food and Fluids*. Wellington: Medical Council of New Zealand.
Medical Council of the Netherlands: Committee on the Vegetative State. 1994. *Patients in a Vegetative State*. Publication 1994/12. The Hague: Health Council of the Netherlands.
National Conference of Catholic Bishops Committee for Pro-Life Activities. 1992. Nutrition and hydration: moral and pastoral reflections. *Issues in Law and Medicine* 8: 387–406.
New Zealand Medical Association Public Issues Advisory Committee. 1994. *Persistent Vegetative State*. Wellington: New Zealand Medical Association.
Office of Technology Assessment. 1988. *Special Report on Institutional Protocols for Decisions about Life-sustaining Treatments*. Washington, DC: Congress of the US.
Paris, J. J. and McCormick, R. A. 1987. The Catholic tradition on the use of nutrition and fluids. *America* 2 May.
Paris, J. J. and Reardon, F. E. 1985. Court responses to withholding or withdrawing artificial nutrition and fluids. *Journal of the American Medical Association* 253: 2243–2245.
Pius XII. 1957. Pope speaks: prolongation of life. *Osservatore Romano* 4: 393–398.
President's Commission for the Study of Ethical Problems in Medicine. 1983. *Deciding to Forego Life-Sustaining Treatment*. Washington, DC: US Government Printing Office.
Rabkin, M. T., Gillerman, G. and Rice, J. D. 1976. Orders not to resuscitate. *New England Journal of Medicine* 295: 364–366.
Smedira, N. G., Evans, B. H., Grais, L. S., Cohen, N. H., Lo, B., Cooke, M. *et al.* 1990. Withholding and withdrawal of life support from the critically ill. *New England Journal of Medicine* 322: 309–315.
Stanley, J. M. 1992. The Appleton International Conference. Developing guidelines for decisions to forgo life-prolonging medical treatment. *Journal of Medical Ethics* 18 [Supplement]: 1–23.
Stone, J. 1994. Withholding life sustaining treatment: the ultimate decision. *New Law Journal* 144: 205–206.
The Multi-Society Task Force on PVS. 1994. Medical aspects of the persistent vegetative state. *New England Journal of Medicine* 330: 1499–1508, 1572–1579.
Tresch, D. D., Sims, F. H., Duthie, E. H. and Goldstein, M. D. 1991. Patients in a persistent vegetative state: attitudes and reactions of family members. *Journal of the American Geriatrics Society* 39: 17–21.
van der Maas, P. J., van Delden, J. M. J., Pijnenborg, L. and Looman, C. N. V. 1991. Euthanasia and other medical decisions concerning the end of life. *Lancet* 338: 669–674.
Weir, R. F. and Gostin, L. 1990. Decisions to abate life-sustaining treatment for non-autonomous patients. *Journal of the American Medical Association* 264: 1846–1853.
Williams, B. T. 1989. Life-sustaining technology: making the decisions: learning from America. *British Medical Journal* 298: 978.
World Medical Association. 1989. *Statement on Persistent Vegetative State*. World Medical Association.

13

A case for sometimes tube-feeding patients in persistent vegetative state

JOSEPH BOYLE

PERSISTENT VEGETATIVE STATE (PVS) is the name, coined by physicians and now widely used, of a specific condition of drastically impaired consciousness. That condition is characterized as 'vegetative' on the basis of the behaviour of patients, not of their underlying neurological disorder or disorders (Jennett 1993: 40). This behaviour includes the following features: The patient has periods of wakefulness and sleep, in contrast to patients in coma who are in a sleep-like condition. During the periods of wakefulness the patient exhibits reflex actions and can swallow small amounts of food and water by mouth, but does not exhibit voluntary action or psychologically meaningful interaction with the environment. Patients in a vegetative state breathe spontaneously (Institute of Medical Ethics Working Party 1991: 96–97).

Vegetative state can be transient, but it can persist. This persistence becomes medically and morally significant when the vegetative state continues long enough to justify an expectation that it will be permanent, that is, if the vegetative state continues to the point that there is no medical prospect that treatment will have any effect on the patient's severely impaired consciousness. The medical judgment that the vegetative state of any given patient is permanent is based on prospective trials and clinical observation; it depends on such considerations as the age and condition of the patient and the cause of the neurological disorder, not on direct observation of this disorder (Institute of Medical Ethics Working Party 1991: 96–97; Jennett 1993: 40–41). I assume that this medical judgment can be confidently made, and that the central moral issues surrounding the treatment of patients in vegetative state arise only when the judgment of permanence has been properly and confidently made.

The persistence of PVS suggests another of its aspects, namely, that patients in this condition can continue to live, some for years, if they are provided with food and water by way of a nasogastric tube or gastrostomy and are provided with other care routinely given to severely disabled persons. In other words, these patients are not dying, at least in one clear sense of that term. In contrast to patients who are expected to die within days or weeks from their illness or injury no matter what steps medical professionals take, many patients in PVS are not likely to die if the care indicated above is provided (Institute of Medical Ethics Working Party 1991: 97).

Another feature of patients in vegetative state is especially relevant to the moral discussion, namely, the belief that they are not capable of experiencing pain. Unlike the behavioural characterization of the vegetative state, this belief is based on anatomical and biochemical evidence concerning neurological activity (Plum 1989: 57–58). While there might be philosophical and evidential questions about the basis for this belief, it is not unreasonable, and I will proceed on the presumption that patients in vegetative state cannot, in any humanly important sense, experience pain.

This brief characterization of PVS leads to the moral questions about the care of patients in PVS which have puzzled medical practitioners and health care decision makers and have led to widespread bioethical debate. On the one hand, the persistence of the vegetative state suggests that efforts to sustain the lives of patients in PVS have about them a kind of futility. But on the other hand, the decision to forgo these efforts, in effect to let these patients die, seems without precedent since the patients can be kept alive without apparent harm to them or excessive burden to others. In short, there is reason to consider withdrawing the care which keeps patients in PVS alive, and there is reason to resist that consideration.

The discussion of the care of patients in PVS has focused upon the artificial provision of food and water by way of either a gastrostomy or a nasogastric tube, which are necessary for prolonged survival (Institute of Medical Ethics Working Party 1991: 97). Plainly, the normative question concerns not only these artificial methods for delivering food and water, but any actions which prolong the patient's life, including spoon-feeding (Finnis 1993: 331). Nevertheless, I will focus upon the provision of food and water by these artificial means, unless I explicitly note otherwise, but I will avoid repeating explicit references to these methods for delivering food and water.

Of course, not all will recognize some reason on each side of the decision to withdraw these forms of care. For the precedents which cause resistance to the consideration of withdrawing them presuppose that withdrawing care and letting people die can be morally distinguished from intentionally killing them, which is taken to be impermissible and presupposes that they are persons. Those who believe that patients in PVS are not persons, or that killing them is permissible even if they are, are not likely to be troubled by the lack of precedents having such presuppositions. Positions on the treatment of patients in PVS have been developed by those accepting such beliefs; they are controversial (Boyle 1992: 32–33).

But these beliefs are marginal to the perplexities and debates about how to care for patients in PVS. These perplexities and debates take place within and between the minds of people sufficiently formed by the assumptions of traditional medical ethics that the lack of precedent for withdrawing food and water from patients in PVS is a consideration to be taken seriously. So, while recognizing that there is a more radical approach to these questions, I will consider the controversies about the care of patients in PVS which arise from within the more traditional perspective of those who assume that patients in PVS are persons who may not be intentionally killed, and therefore believe that withholding this kind of care can be justified only if it can be squared with the precedents according to which doing so is distinguishable from intentional killing (Institute of Medical Ethics Working Party 1991: 97).

Within that perspective a set of possible moral positions on withholding these forms of care emerges. At one end of this spectrum is the position that withdrawing them is a moral obligation, that is, that aspects of the condition of PVS or of the necessary requirements for the care of people in PVS are by themselves sufficient to establish a moral requirement to withdraw food and water. A weaker position is that it is morally permissible to withdraw these forms of care from patients in PVS. Since these two positions are not clearly distinguished in the current discussion, and since the arguments for them are so similar, I will consider only the weaker position according to which withdrawing these forms of care is morally permissible. At the other end of the spectrum is a second position, that it is never permissible to withdraw food and water from a patient in PVS. Between these extreme positions are, thirdly, a spectrum of positions according to which some circumstance of the patient (beyond the fact that he or she is in PVS) or the overall situation of the patient's care (beyond the necessary requirements for caring for such patients) provide reasons why the withdrawal of these forms of care is permissible or even obligatory.

I will consider in detail the first of these normative positions, which I will seek to refute, and then briefly the other two, with a view towards indicating where I believe the correct normative position lies.

THE BENEFITS OF CONTINUED TREATMENT

The reasoning which supports the view that a patient's being in PVS is by itself sufficient morally to justify withdrawing care, and in particular the provision of food and water, starts with the apparent futility of providing such care, and seeks to show that the precedents which cause resistance to that line of reasoning do not in fact do so, but may indeed support it. This reasoning proceeds most simply if there is simply no benefit for these patients in their continued life.

It is clear that, by any estimate, the benefits of keeping a person alive who has no prospect of recovering from the radically impaired consciousness of PVS are small. The condition of these people is one of extreme deprivation; their condition, though stable, is one of radically impaired functioning; and they cannot experience any benefit from their continued existence. However, these uncontroversial judgments are not equivalent to the judgment that continued life is of no benefit to patients in PVS. And the inference from the former to the latter has not been shown to be valid.

If one accepts the view that a person's life has value only instrumentally insofar as it allows the person to engage in further human activities, then this inference would be straightforward. Since the benefit of life is instrumental, it lacks value when the purposes it serves are unachievable. But a person's life cannot simply be instrumental to other goods of that person. For a person's life is not something other than his or her very self, and so the living human organism, however deprived, cannot be separated from the person in the way an instrument can be separated from the purposes for which it is used. The value of a person's life, therefore, cannot be reduced to its role as a condition for realizing other goods of the person (Finnis 1993: 334). Consequently, the straightforward inference to the conclusion that continued life is of no benefit to patients in PVS is not valid.

If elements from the radical view according to which patients are not persons were admitted to the controversy at this point, then the straightforward inference might be shored up. But the further questions to which this view leads in this context make clear that it is a perspective foreign to the concerns which frame the controversy. If patients in PVS are not persons, then why should it be wrong intentionally to kill them? If these patients are not persons, then on what grounds are they to be treated differently from corpses? Questions like these might interest philosophers, but are not part of what puzzles those who are concerned practically with how to treat patients in PVS.

But there are other reasons for inferring that continued life is not a benefit to patients in PVS. One of these is the view that it is a necessary condition for something's being a benefit that the beneficiary experience it. This view is part of an account of the nature of benefits and does not appear to presuppose a dualistic distinction between the living human organism and the person. But this view is false. Surely one person can act to benefit another and succeed in providing the benefit without the other's ever knowing about the action or the benefit.

Perhaps the necessary condition for something's being a benefit can be restated to accommodate this possibility. A candidate would be the following: nothing can be a benefit to a person unless it contributes to some good in which the beneficiary consciously participates. But the restatement also seems false: Jones speaks well of Smith to Robinson, so as to improve Robinson's opinion of Smith. Jones succeeds, but Robinson does not act on this knowledge, and tells no one. Jones' action does not contribute to Smith's conscious interest in maintaining his reputation, but it is not obvious that there is no benefit to Smith. Another example: John is distracted by illness and fails to pay his bills. His friend Bill pays them, but before discovering this, John dies. While alive, John had an interest in paying his bills, although he was too sick to pay attention to it, and they were paid, but he did not discover this fact. He was the beneficiary of Bill's action, but never knew it.

Further difficulties in the view that benefits are essentially related to the experience of the beneficiary emerge by considering the fact that those incapable of experience can be harmed. This is acknowledged by all who address the issue of the care of patients in PVS from within the perspective of traditional medical ethics. Indeed, some who argue that withdrawing the means for providing food and water is permissible appeal to the harm involved in keeping them alive as a premise in their argument (Jennett 1993: 43).

Patients in PVS can be harmed by being killed, by being treated as spectacles or sex objects, by being used improperly for experimental purposes, and so on. Most of these and other potential harms to patients in PVS fall into the category of indignities, that is, of actions and omissions which harm by failing to respect the patient as a person. If indignities are harms to patients in PVS, then actions taken precisely to prevent or remove these indignities must be benefits to them. And so too must other actions taken precisely for the sake of respecting the personal dignity of these patients. The beneficial character of such actions appears to be acknowledged by some of those who do not believe that continued life support is a benefit to patients in PVS. For example, some of those who support the withdrawal of food and water also indicate the continuing need to maintain oral hygiene (Institute of Medical Ethics Working Party 1991: 97).

If maintaining oral hygiene can be a benefit to a patient in PVS, presumably because this kind of care shows respect for his or her personal dignity, then it is not clear why continuing the person's life, which can be done for this same reason, cannot also be a benefit. In short, a consideration of the nature of benefits, far from showing that the unconscious cannot receive them, strongly suggests that continuing their lives can be a benefit to them. This consideration is not meant to settle the moral issue in favour of continuing the provision of food and water, but to undermine one of the straightforward ways of showing that withdrawing this care is generally permissible.

However, this consideration indicates something further about the benefit of continuing to provide food and water to patients in PVS. The care of a person in need ordinarily includes an intention to maintain human solidarity with that person. That intention manifests love and respect for the person in need, and the benefit it anticipates is interpersonal, a good realized not only in the person cared for but within the community of patient and care givers. Frequently, this intention is not articulated as a distinct purpose for care, but included within the intention to restore functioning or alleviate suffering. But as the possibility of successfully doing either of these things diminishes, concerns for respecting and promoting the patient's dignity, including maintaining solidarity with him or her, come to the forefront. In the extreme case of patients in PVS, they are virtually the only considerations in play. It follows that providing food and water to patients in PVS does not have a purely symbolic significance, as if it were a kind of gesture. It is done to show respect for them as persons, and it does that in part by maintaining solidarity and refusing simply to leave them to their fate (Boyle 1992: 38–39).

In short, the claim that continuing life and the provision of food and water are not benefits to the patient cannot be sustained, and so the position that withdrawing these forms of care is permissible cannot be based on that claim. The argument must, therefore, be that these benefits, though real, are so small that they cannot justify the burdens of providing the care, that is, that the benefits are disproportionate to the burdens.

THE HARMS OR BURDENS OF CONTINUED TREATMENT

Many of the normal burdens to patients which justify the decision to forgo medical care are not present for patients in PVS. The pain, suffering and interference with the pursuit of valued activities which often provide reasons for discontinuing treatment are not possible for patients in PVS. Consequently, the burdens to the patient which might be relevant in determining that care is disproportionate to its benefits fall into two categories: the already discussed category of indignities and the category of actions that are harmful because they are against the patient's will.

To take the second category of harms first, a person's declaration that he or she does not want to be kept alive by being fed and hydrated through a nasogastric tube or gastrostomy is surely a morally relevant circumstance of his or her overall condition, and it is not unreasonable to think that ignoring such a declaration would be a harm to the patient. But most people in PVS have not made such declarations, and so this is not a general circumstance of patients in PVS. Some suggest that this fact is not important, because most people would reject such treatment if they had considered or were capable of considering the matter (Jennett 1993: 41, 43). However, guesses and inferences from surveys about public attitudes towards life in PVS do not provide evidence about what a given person decided or would have decided, and speculations about what reasonable people would prefer if in PVS presuppose certain controversial answers to questions at the heart of this dispute.

Of course, if providing food and water by gastrostomy or nasogastric tube were itself an indignity to the patient, then there would be reason, independent of the patient's will in the matter, for withdrawing these forms of care. But this condition is not fulfilled. These are forms of care routinely used for patients with a variety of ills, and are used in the care of patients in PVS precisely to show respect for their human dignity (Finnis 1993: 336).

The rejoinder to this claim is that continued life in PVS is itself an indignity, and so acting to continue it is a wrong. But here the indignity in question has shifted from actions or omissions which fail to respect the person to the condition of PVS itself. As already noted, this is a condition of grave disability which no one would desire for himself, herself or another. But when such a condition exists people can and morally must continue to act towards that person in ways which respect his or her inherent human dignity. The deprived and perhaps undignified condition of the person's life does not change that requirement, and would by itself justify withdrawal of treatment only if death were judged better for the person than such an existence. It is not clear how this comparative judgment could be known to be true, and how, if it were accepted as a practical judgment for deciding life and death questions, it would be limited so as not to justify killing patients in PVS, much less those whose lives are filled with pain and misery.

In short, the burdens or harms to patients in PVS of keeping them alive by providing food and water do not establish a general ground for thinking that withdrawing them is morally permissible. Consequently, if the burdens of treatment are to function as a reason for this judgment, the burdens in question must be those imposed on others. There are two kinds of such burdens: the suffering of family members and friends who must live with and experience the tragic condition of their loved one, and the overall costs of keeping these patients alive.

The suffering of family members of patients in PVS is in many cases a serious concern to which care givers must attend. But some family members at least appear to think that their suffering is justified by their effort to provide some level of care and contact with the patient, including the provision of food and water. So, this circumstance will not be a factor in all cases. Moreover, it is not clear how concerns for the welfare of family members should be factored into decisions about the care of patients in PVS. If the family is being ruined financially, or prevented from carrying on its essential business, say of work and raising children, then the concern about their welfare is part of the larger question of costs. But if family members are distraught primarily because of the permanently debilitated condition of the patient, and a decision is taken to withdraw care to deal with this concern, then the decision seems to be a decision to get things over with, perhaps to end the patient's life as a means to that, or at least a decision to end the care that binds them to the patient.

The specific costs of providing food and water by gastrostomy and nasogastric tube to patients in PVS are not high, particularly in comparison to the costs of other medical treatments. But the overall costs of caring for these patients, particularly over time, are high and could be higher still if they were treated aggressively (Boyle 1992: 40). It is the latter, overall costs which have figured in the discussion, and this raises the troubling question of whether withdrawing these forms of care is undertaken as perhaps the least objectionable way of withdrawing the patient from all care or of ending the patient's life as a way to avoid having further to care for him or her. Nevertheless, given the resource limitations of families and of health care systems in even the wealthy, Western societies in which the care for patients in PVS is a serious question, there is certainly a legitimate question as to whether the resources used for the maintenance of such patients should be better used (Finnis 1993: 335).

Still, families and societies differ in the level of support they can reasonably provide for patients in PVS, and since these patients do not require hospitalization, but can be cared for at home, avoiding much of the cost of caring for them is possible without withdrawing food and water and other forms of basic care. In other words, it does not follow from the fact that providing food and water by gastrostomy or nasogastric tube is initiated as part of medical care, ordinarily before the permanence of the vegetative condition is established, that they cannot also be part of the care appropriately given to people after specifically medical intervention is properly discontinued (Finnis 1993: 335).

In short, the arguments for the normative view that it is generally permissible to withhold food and water from patients in PVS, because of the condition itself or the general requirements for treating it, are not successful. These arguments do, however, suggest some of the factors, for example, the limited benefits of continued life and care, the patient's will in the matter, and the overall costs of the care, which appear to justify withdrawing food and water in some cases.

THE MORALLY RELEVANT CIRCUMSTANCES

The moral relevance of these factors is rejected by those who believe that withdrawing food and water from patients in PVS is necessarily wrong. This normative position has several foundations. One is the conviction that withdrawing these forms of care is morally equivalent to killing patients in PVS and another is the conviction that these are forms of elemental human care which are always required.

It seems clear that withdrawing life-sustaining treatments can be a way of killing people, particularly when they are deliberately withdrawn for the sake of ending the patient's life (Boyle 1992: 35–37). Some have denied this, but at the high price of attributing to the distinction between intentional actions and omissions with identical intentions a moral significance with no rational foundation (Finnis 1993: 331–333). There surely is a rational basis for distinguishing some decisions to withdraw life-sustaining treatments from actions (and omissions) chosen for the sake of ending life. But this does not justify attributing moral significance to the mere behavioural difference between actions and omissions, or between killing and letting die just as such (Grisez & Boyle 1979: 414–419).

The weakness of the position that withdrawing food and water from patients in PVS is inevitably intentionally killing them is that such conduct need not be undertaken with the intention of ending life. Perhaps that sometimes is the intent of those taking such a decision (Boyle 1992: 37), but such decisions can be taken because the limited benefits do not justify the costs involved. In such cases the patient's death is not intended, but is accepted as a side effect of a decision made for other reasons.

The argument that withdrawing food and water from patients in PVS is always wrong because these are obligatory forms of care also fails. There surely is an obligation to provide debilitated people with care that shows respect for their human dignity and maintains solidarity with them. But this general obligation does not settle the kind or level of care which must be provided. That must be determined by considering the capacities, resources and other responsibilities of those providing the care. The limitation of care based on these considerations does not involve a violation of the general obligation to care. For no moral obligation requires that people do what is strictly beyond their capacity to do, and this obligation does not require levels or kinds of care which can be provided only by setting aside other serious responsibilities. In short, the general obligation to provide care requires only that those responsible for providing it do what they can, and what people can do depends in part on their entire set of responsibilities. The generality applies to the case at hand: providing food and water by gastrostomy and nasogastric tube might sometimes be more than care providers can do for patients in PVS.

It follows, therefore, that circumstances of the particular case will be the decisive moral considerations in arriving at the moral judgment about the level of care to be provided to any patient in PVS. The condition itself and the essential requirements for caring for people who suffer from it are not sufficient to show either that withdrawing food and water is permissible or required or that continuing to provide them is required. As already suggested, the fact that a patient indicated prior to being in PVS that he or she did not want food and water artificially provided is one such circumstance. The cost of the care, in relation to the capacities, resources and other responsibilities of care givers is another.

The prior rejection of the artificial provision of food and water by the patient appears decisive, that is, it establishes a requirement to withdraw this form of care. The reason why prior refusal should be honoured is that continued care is significantly, if not completely, motivated by the intention to maintain solidarity with the patient and show respect for his or her human dignity. The decision to limit care drastically on the basis of the patient's refusal, therefore, has an altogether different human significance from withdrawing it without such direction. In the former case, care is withdrawn precisely out of respect for the patient, whose reasons for refusal need not be suicidal but can be based on the desire to remove from others the burdens of care. Respecting the generosity of a person's waiving his or her claims on others in no way shows disrespect for that person. In the latter case, the patient is removed from human care by the decisions of others, and generosity exercised for one who cannot speak for himself or herself is not, in fact, generosity but imposition. Thus, when not justified by other considerations, withdrawal of these forms of care can be abandonment of the patient and a refusal of the solidarity which respect for human dignity requires (Boyle 1992: 41–43; Grisez 1990: 33–34).

The factor of cost, in relation to the capacities, resources and other responsibilities of care givers, also can be morally decisive in some cases. Indeed, in one respect it has relevance to many, if not most, cases. For considerations of cost, broadly considered, ordinarily require that patients in PVS should not be maintained permanently by acute hospital care. There is little that expensive hospital care can do for these patients since they cannot be restored to good health and do not experience suffering. The resources of acute care hospitals are plausibly better used elsewhere. It follows that those who bear responsibility for these patients should take them home or provide some similar form of care for them. They should, of course, do what they can to provide care for these patients, and that might include continuing to provide food and water by way of a gastrostomy or nasogastric tube. But if a family, for example, could not, without expense and effort that would prevent the fulfilment of other serious responsibilities, continue to maintain the artificial means for providing food and water, then they could be rightly withdrawn. But a level of care which can be provided compatibly with other responsibilities is morally required. Thus, the relevant moral rule is that we must do what we can to care for patients in PVS, and to maintain the human ties with them which show our respect for their human dignity. But the application of this rule to the situation of different people with different resources and varying forms of social support must inevitably lead to different concrete moral judgments as to what it is right for them to do.

REFERENCES

Boyle, J. 1992. The American debate about artificial nutrition and hydration. In *The Dependent Elderly: Autonomy, Justice and Quality of Care*, ed. L. Gormally, pp. 38–46. Cambridge: Cambridge University Press.

Finnis, J. M. 1993. *Bland*: Crossing the Rubicon? *The Law Quarterly Review* 109: 329–337.

Grisez, G. 1990. Should nutrition and hydration be provided to permanently comatose and other mentally disabled persons? *Linacre Quarterly* 57(2): 30–43.

Grisez, G. and Boyle, J. 1979. *Life and Death with Liberty and Justice: A Contribution to the Euthanasia Debate*. Notre Dame: University of Notre Dame Press.

Institute of Medical Ethics Working Party on the Ethics of Prolonging Life and Assisting Death. 1991. Withdrawal of life-support from patients in a persistent vegetative state. *Lancet* 337: 96–98.

Jennett, B. 1993. The case for letting vegetative patients die. *Ethics & Medicine* 9(3): 40–44.

Plum, F. 1989. Artificial provision of nutrition: medical description of the levels of consciousness. In *Critical Issues in Contemporary Health Care*, ed. R. Smith, pp. 45–59. Braintree, MA: The Pope John Center.

14

Dilemmas at life's end: a comparative legal perspective

DIETER GIESEN[1]

INTRODUCTION

ISSUES OF DEATH and dying have become the focus of intense debate in recent times among theologians, ethicists, lawyers and the public at large.[2] This has to a significant extent been due to a number of controversial decisions of superior courts on these matters such as *Cruzan* v. *Director, Department of Health* in the United States,[3] *Airedale National Health Service Trust* v. *Bland* in the United Kingdom,[4] *Rodriguez* v. *British Columbia (Attorney General)* in Canada[5] and the *Wittig* and *Hackethal* cases in Germany.[6] There are two other reasons for this debate.[7] First, the dramatic advances in medical technology and pharmacology which have been made in the course of this century have made it possible to sustain the lives of terminally or otherwise hopelessly ill patients[8] for extended and often indefinite periods of time.[9] Ever greater power has been concentrated upon specialist medical practitioners, whose decisions to use, not to use or to discontinue life-sustaining treatment, have truly given them control over life and death. Secondly, as was stated by Mr Justice Stevens, of the United States Supreme Court, due to these 'advances, and the reorganization of medical care accompanying the new science and social conditions of death people are less likely to die at home, and are more likely to die in relatively public places, such as hospitals or nursing homes. Ultimately questions that might have been dealt with in intimacy by a family and its physician have now become the concern of institutions'.[10] Clearly, these treatment decisions are of the utmost moral and legal significance and it is therefore unsurprising that there have emerged a number of sharply conflicting ethical frameworks for the resolution of treatment dilemmas at life's end.[11]

A LEGAL AND ETHICAL FRAMEWORK

While a detailed and wide-ranging discussion of all the ethical and legal problems accompanying the provision of life-sustaining treatment is obviously beyond the scope of this chapter, it is possible to identify a number of basic principles which govern medical decision-making in Western society.[12] Furthermore, since the law is one of the chief means by which society translates its fundamental ethical concerns and central values into rules for the regulation of human conduct, these principles form the framework for the legal regulation of decisions on death and dying. As the German *Bundesverfassungsgericht* (Federal Constitutional Court) has put it, '[t]he ethical and the legal are conjoined in the medical matters to a much greater extent than in other social contexts'.[13]

The first of these principles is that of individual *autonomy*, which, in the medical context, means that a person has the right, in accordance with his own value commitments and beliefs, to determine whether and to what extent he shall submit himself to any recommended course of treatment. This principle, which is central to political morality in all democratic societies, is given legal expression in *the patient's right to self-determination*. Thus, the patient's valid consent is an essential prerequisite to the undertaking of medical procedures in all but the most exceptional circumstances.[14] This is also the case in relation to terminally and hopelessly ill patients and, accordingly, a patient has the right to refuse even life-sustaining treatment. A correlative of this right is the doctor's duty to respect his patient's decision as that of an autonomous legal subject.[15] As Professor Ian Kennedy has succinctly put it '[t]o abide by the refusal may be difficult for the doctor; but it is required by law, the principle of self-determination overruling any notion that the doctor knows best'.[16] Autonomy is not, however, without its limits.[17] First, the physician attending to the victim of a terminal illness may be required to engage in a rather more subtle appreciation of autonomy than simply acceding to a patient's request for active euthanasia, which is likely to be rooted in the fear and anxiety which inevitably accompany the dependency and helplessness of the terminally ill patient. Secondly, it has been emphasized in a series of important judgments in the United States that the patient's right to refuse medical treatment must be balanced against a number of legitimate state interests.[18]

Two further principles determine the legal and ethical duties which doctors owe their patients. According to the principle *neminem laedere* or non-maleficence a doctor ought not to inflict evil or harm or bring his patients into the risk of evil or harm.[19] The law closely reflects this position, imposing civil[20] and sometimes criminal sanctions[21] for failure to exercise due care in the performance of medical procedures and forbidding under the law of torts and the criminal law[22] unconsented-to intrusions upon the patient's bodily integrity. In relation to the law of murder and homicide there can be no exceptional category of reduced responsibility for the medical profession as such. Intentional homicide is a crime regardless of the professional status of the accused.[23]

The second principle, that of *beneficence*, is not as well reflected in the law as that of non-maleficence[24] and the Common Law has long been hesitant about imposing duties of affirmative action upon individuals. By contrast, the Civil Law jurisdictions, through the imposition of criminal law sanctions, have recognized the obligation of common humanity to rally to the aid of another human being in danger.[25] It is important to note that these basic principles are not only embodied in the various legal régimes governing the provision of health care, but are also central to traditional medical ethics as embodied in the Hippocratic Oath.[26]

Finally, as technological progress expands the possibilities for treating those who are terminally or hopelessly ill, fair and just criteria of access to life-sustaining treatment must be established. In guiding medical decision-making, a principle of *distributive justice* should be applied, whereby burdens and benefits are allocated according to ethically significant criteria, and *only* according to those criteria.[27]

COMPETENT HOPELESSLY ILL PATIENTS[28]

Active euthanasia

Active euthanasia may be defined as the (deliberate) administration of life-shortening substances with the intention to cause death in order to end pain and suffering.[29] This may be done in accordance with the wishes of the patient (voluntary euthanasia), without his consent (involuntary euthanasia) or where he is incapable of consenting (non-voluntary euthanasia).[30]

In spite of a number of legislative proposals, active euthanasia is forbidden by law, regardless of whether the patient has consented or not, and constitutes the crime of unlawful homicide (i.e. murder or manslaughter) in almost all major jurisdictions.[31] As Lord Goff summarized this prevailing position under English law, '[it] is not lawful for a doctor to administer a drug to his patient to bring about his death, even though that course is prompted by a humanitarian desire to end his suffering, however great that suffering may be . . . So to act is to cross the Rubicon which runs between on the one hand the care of the living patient and on the other hand euthanasia – actively causing his death to avoid suffering. Euthanasia is not lawful at common law'.[32] As Professor Glanville Williams put it: 'The law does not leave the issue in the hands of doctors; it treats euthanasia as murder'.[33]

In the Netherlands, however, very recent legislation has embodied the tendency of the highest Dutch courts[34] to tolerate active euthanasia by providing a defence in such cases. The new rather confused rules require that the patient's decision is voluntary, informed and certain and that the doctor concerned has consulted with colleagues and drawn up a detailed report of the decision-making process.[35] Compliance with these conditions will effectively entitle the doctor to exemption from prosecution under the Dutch Penal Code. These developments[36] will no doubt be welcomed by those commentators and campaigners who seek to legalize active euthanasia in their own jurisdictions. In their view the principle of individual autonomy entails a right to die and concomitant right on the part of the doctor to fulfil a patient's death wish and to practise active euthanasia.[37]

It is submitted, however, that this opinion represents a serious misinterpretation of the principles of autonomy, non-maleficence and beneficence.[38] As we have already pointed out, a person's autonomy is not without limits. The first is immanent in the concept itself. Self-determination is an inalienable right which is constitutionally protected in many countries.[39] It cannot, therefore, be renounced or conferred upon another person. 'Freedom does not stand naked. It is clothed by an "ought"; we are free to do what we ought to do . . . a freedom to do what one is obliged to do, not an entitlement to specific treatment by others'.[40] In short, to allow another person to decide about one's life is not an expression of autonomy but of heteronomy.[41] Furthermore, the patient who consults a physician may have already lost some of his most precious freedoms – for example, freedom to move about and freedom from the power of other persons. This position of heightened vulnerability and correspondingly increased dependency cannot be made the basis for eliminating his right to self-determination. Terminal illness is often accompanied by feelings of hopelessness and despair on the part of the patient, but it must not become the occasion for overbearing medical paternalism, however well intended.[42] What is most clearly required in such situations is a patient–physician relationship founded not on the outdated notion that 'doctor knows best', but upon complex layers of mutual loyalty, fidelity, respect, support and trust.[43] It is submitted that this vulnerable, arguably fiduciary relationship,[44] is seriously endangered by the advocacy and toleration, however partial, of active euthanasia. Patients will inevitably grow reluctant to entrust themselves to a profession which is perceived as sometimes curing and sometimes killing.[45] In the Netherlands, for example, the increasing laxity of legal controls and the ever louder rhetoric in favour of euthanasia have combined to discount the value of human life and have meant that 'a generation of doctors is being raised who learn that a doctor may treat a patient, or sometimes kill him'.[46]

Active euthanasia also poses a major threat to the principle of the *inviolability of life*, which, as the House of Lords, the Supreme Court of Canada, the United States Supreme Court and both the German *Bundesverfassungsgericht* (Federal Constitutional Court) and the *Bundesgerichtshof* (Federal Supreme Court) have recently held, the state has a legitimate interest in protecting.[47] Recent history shows us that once firm constraints against killing are removed, a general moral decline will result. The German experience of the Nazi euthanasia programme, during which *c.* 100 000 disabled persons were killed because they were classified as living 'lives not worth living', demonstrates the potential for perverse thinking and inhuman deeds once the first step upon the slippery slope is taken.[48] The principle of non-maleficence requires us to resist such steps.

Experience in the Netherlands to date suggests that, in practice, no sharp distinction can be drawn between voluntary and non-voluntary euthanasia. Instead, commentators have documented a continuum of killing, from the (quite rare) paradigm case of informed and rational choice to frequent instances of familial and medical pressure, to the elimination of defenceless newborns, adjudged to be a burden upon society and to the purging of old people's homes.[49] Indeed, a Dutch government report has stated that in 1990 over 1000 patients were put to death by their doctors without explicitly requesting active euthanasia.[50] With perhaps as many as 8% of all deaths in the Netherlands resulting from active euthanasia,[51] an atmosphere of fear and distrust has been created among the weakest and most vulnerable sections of that society.[52] Extension and acceptance of active euthanasia have meant that the right to life of individuals is no longer sacred and inviolable, but contingent upon the calculations of the state, endorsing the judgments of doctors as to whose lives are 'worthwhile' or not.

Admittedly, there may be very exceptional situations where society is reluctant to condemn an individual for taking the life of another. But statutory provisions allowing a court to mitigate an otherwise harsher penalty for murder or manslaughter[53] are sufficient to deal with such cases for what they are: isolated exceptions. Regardless of this very narrow sentencing discretion, courts must be firm, in such cases, in applying the substantive criminal law, unamended, by categorizing active euthanasia as unlawful homicide.[54] Given the importance of the state's commitment to the value of life and of the enforcement of those laws which clearly demonstrate this commitment, it is inappropriate to leave the decision as to mitigation to prosecuting authorities, much less, as is now the case in the Netherlands, to enable the doctor concerned to prevent both a proper investigation and criminal charges.[55]

Palliative care

Palliative care is the provision of therapy or drugs with the aim of relieving pain and making the patient comfortable until death occurs even if it may indirectly shorten the patient's life.[56] Such treatment is held to be ethically justifiable under the doctrine of 'double effect', provided that the alleviation of pain is the aim, that the patient (if competent) has given his consent, that death is imminent and that there is a favourable balance between the therapy and its results.[57] Clearly, there is, in many instances at the end of life, an apparent conflict between the principles of non-maleficence (not to kill) and beneficence (to relieve pain). The doctrine of double effect, which provides for the resolution of this dilemma while protecting the ethical integrity of the medical profession, is also reflected in the relevant jurisprudence.[58] It is submitted that this doctrine is useful in providing for a principled evaluation of conduct (and proposed conduct) and also that it corresponds with popular intuition in recognizing the significance of the *intentions* of the actor, here the attending doctor.[59] We cannot, with all due respect, share the more sceptical position of Ian Kennedy and Andrew Grubb on this matter.[60] We hold rather with Lord Devlin when, as Mr Justice Devlin, he instructed the jury in the case of *R* v. *Bodkin Adams*, that '[i]f the first purpose of medicine, the restoration of health, can no longer be achieved, there is still much for a doctor to do, and he is entitled to do all that is proper and necessary to relieve pain and suffering, even if the measures he takes may incidentally shorten life'.[61] A doctor in such situations must, however, proceed with great caution since his intention will be of primary importance in determining whether his conduct amounted to palliative care or to unlawful homicide, whether murder or manslaughter.[62]

Assisting suicide

The difference between active euthanasia and aiding in a terminally ill patient's suicide is essentially that between perpetrators and accessories. In the former case the doctor determines the eventual course of action, whereas in the latter he merely assists the patient to realize his autonomous decision to end his life. It must be emphasized, however, that while suicide may be looked upon as an act of self-determination and autonomy,[63] active euthanasia cannot. Thus, in almost all legal systems, while active euthanasia remains a punishable offence, suicide has generally been decriminalized,[64] although there remain strong ethical and public policy considerations against its permissibility.[65] The withdrawal of the criminal law from the area of attempted suicide involves a recognition that health and welfare measures may offer a more sensitive and successful means of dealing with what remains a personal tragedy and a serious social problem.[66] It cannot, however, be construed as a weakening of the fabric of the law which ensures the sanctity of life and thus in very many jurisdictions assisting suicide continues to be subject to criminal sanctions.[67]

Such criminal sanctions were held to be compatible with the Canadian Charter of Rights and Freedoms by the Supreme Court of that country in the recent case of *Rodriguez* v. *British Columbia (Attorney General)*.[68] In his majority judgment, Mr Justice Sopinka held that s. 241(b) Canadian Criminal Code, which makes it an offence to assist a suicide, fulfilled the state's aim of protecting the vulnerable and preventing a depreciation in the value of life without infringing the principle of proportionality embodied in the Charter. He added that Canada, like almost all other Western democracies, adhered to the fundamental conception of the sanctity of life and no consensus to depart from it in such cases could be identified.[69]

In short, the doctor is best advised not to comply with the patient's wish for a means to commit suicide.[70] Rather, he should try to help the patient to overcome his feelings of utter depression and despair and to strive to make the time remaining to the patient as comfortable as possible.[71]

Withholding or withdrawing treatment[72]

It must be stressed that the right to decline life-sustaining treatment is entailed by the individual's right to self-determination.[73] As Chief Justice Rehnquist put it in the majority decision of the United States Supreme Court in *Cruzan* v. *Director, Missouri Department of Health*, '[t]he logical corollary of the doctrine of informed consent is that the patient generally possesses the right not to consent, that is, to refuse treatment'.[74]

However, as we have noted previously, the principle of autonomy is not absolute, and courts in the United States, as well as in Canada[75] and Germany,[76] have recognized a number of important state interests which may qualify the patient's right to forego treatment in such cases.[77] These interests include the preservation of life, the prevention of suicide, the protection of third parties (for example children or other dependents) and the maintenance of the ethical integrity of the medical profession.[78] Such considerations are not, of course, decisive. Thus, where a patient has no vulnerable dependents, the state interest in the preservation of life will normally give way before the right of the patient to determine the course of his own life.[79] Neither does the ethical integrity of the medical profession come into question since the doctor's ethical and legal obligation shifts from a duty to save life to a duty to comfort and care for the patient and to ensure that he is able to die with dignity.[80]

There has, however, been much controversy as to exactly which medical treatment can be lawfully declined. Distinctions have been drawn, in this regard, between acts (unlawful) and omissions (lawful),[81] between withholding treatment (lawful) and withdrawing treatment (unlawful), and between discontinuing ordinary or life-saving treatment (unlawful) and discontinuing extraordinary treatment (lawful).[82] Unfortunately, none of these distinctions has proved very useful in determining the extent of legally permissible conduct in this field.[83] It is, therefore, more profitable to adopt a principled approach, taking the patient's right to self-determination and the doctor's correlative duties and responsibilities as the parameters of medical decision-making.[84]

INCOMPETENT TERMINALLY ILL PATIENTS

A number of factors may lead to an individual being held legally incompetent. Chief among these in the context of life-sustaining treatment are unconsciousness, as where the patient is said to be in a persistent vegetative state, mental illness and minority. As we shall see, each poses significant ethical and legal problems.[85] It must be made clear at the outset, however, that the right to refuse treatment, which we have already discussed, also extends to incompetent patients. Thus, a mentally ill person may still retain and a minor may gradually develop the natural capacity to give or refuse consent.[86] Furthermore, an adult person is presumed to be capable of consenting to medical procedures and therefore the onus of proving incompetence lies upon the doctor who seeks to avoid civil and criminal liability.[87] Each of these features reflects the central importance of the value of individual autonomy, a value the easy displacement of which courts in all jurisdictions will resist.[88]

Unconscious and mentally ill persons

In cases of incompetence the law is nonetheless vigilant to ensure that the autonomy and human dignity of the patient are respected and therefore the rules implementing the rights of competent patients also apply through the mechanism of substituted decision-making. The first important issue which arises in the context of patient incompetence is who should be allowed to exercise the rights of the patient.[89] There is little difficulty where the patient has, before the period of incompetency, authorized a surrogate or proxy to make decisions on his behalf. So far as such a substitute's consent or refusal of treatment is within the scope of the authority with which he has been invested, it must be respected by the attending medical staff and, where necessary, will generally be enforced by the courts.[90] In the absence of such a formally authorized proxy, the decision will have to be made by a court in the exercise of its wardship jurisdiction or by a court-appointed ward or guardian. It is important to note that, while courts may, and often do, appoint family members to this position, doctors who consult with the close relatives of the patient do not automatically forestall subsequent judicial scrutiny of their course of conduct. Thus, in *Re T (Adult: refusal of medical treatment)*[91] Master of the Rolls Lord Donaldson took the view that, while such consultation would be a desirable step, 'the next of kin has no legal right to consent or to refuse consent'.[92] Indeed, under recently introduced German legislation the guardian's decision must be confirmed by the wardship court where the incompetent patient is in danger of death or serious and lasting injury.[93] In a similar vein, the Supreme Court of Missouri has held that a guardian's decision to end life-sustaining treatment and thereby the life of the patient had to be balanced against the state's 'vital interest in preserving life'.[94]

The second important matter to be resolved in cases of incompetency is the *standard of decision-making* to which a surrogate must conform.[95] The alternatives are to decide ('objectively') in the patient's *best interests* or to attempt ('subjectively') to ascertain the decision which the patient himself would have made were he fully competent, by applying a substituted-judgment test.[96] Unfortunately, attempts to apply either test in isolation have led to conceptual confusion and therefore a different approach, embodying elements of both tests while emphasizing the patient's right to self-determination, has generally been preferred. Thus, the relevant German law provides that an incompetent's previously expressed wishes are to be respected as long as they do not interfere with his welfare.[97] The Supreme Court of New Jersey has developed similar though more detailed standards for decision-making in this context.[98] Depending on the availability of evidence as to the wishes of the patient a surrogate decision-maker is required to apply one of three tests:

(1) Where there is clear and convincing evidence that the patient would have refused the life-sustaining treatment it will be unlawful to proceed with these measures. The evidence required to comply with this subjective test would most obviously be constituted by a 'living will', an oral directive or a durable power of attorney. Although the patient's prior intentions may be also deduced from previous statements or from his religious beliefs, the United States Supreme Court has upheld the constitutionality of a requirement that such evidence be 'clear and convincing' as furthering the state's interest in the protection of life.[99]

(2) Where the evidence of the patient's wishes that such treatment be discontinued, although trustworthy, is not unequivocal,[100] a 'limited objective test' should be applied. In such cases treatment could be withheld if life with it would be more burdensome than beneficial to the patient.[101]

(3) Where there is no evidence at all of the patient's wishes, a fully objective test is applied. Accordingly, life-sustaining treatment may be withheld if it would cause such recurring and severe pain that its administration would be inhumane.

It must be added that where the patient was never competent in the sense of possessing the 'natural capacity' to consent outlined above, the subjective and limited objective tests can have no application. In such instances the state's *parens patriae* jurisdiction would include the power to authorize a surrogate decision-maker to end life-sustaining treatment where the burdens of continuing are clearly and markedly outweighed by the benefits of termination.[102]

In England it has been held that, since the *Mental Health Act*, 1959, came into force this *parens patriae* jurisdiction is no longer available to courts in cases involving incompetent adults. In *F* v. *West Berkshire Health Authority*,[103] the House of Lords was therefore only able to state that, in cases of sterilization and similarly controversial procedures, it would be highly advisable as opposed to obligatory for doctors concerned to seek the prior approval of the court.[104] Lord Goff held that a 'best interests' test should be applied in deciding whether to grant the declaratory relief sought in this manner and that the best interests of the incompetent patient were to be determined in accordance with the familiar *Bolam* test, by seeking to ascertain the views of a responsible body of medical practitioners.[105] In

Airedale National Health Service Trust v. *Bland*,[106] this approach was applied in relation to the termination of the tube-feeding of a patient in a persistent vegetative state.[107]

It is submitted that the *Bolam* test,[108] which has been overwhelmingly rejected outside England and Scotland,[109] and which leaves the last word to the (defendant) doctors, unjustifiably privileges the medical perspective in decision-making at the edges of life. It is indeed regrettable that British judges continue to endorse such medical paternalism which is untenable and outmoded and ultimately sets the patient's right to self-determination at nought.[110] As John Finnis has written in criticism of the *Bland* decision, even if the *Bolam* test had 'some appropriate sphere, its application or extension to the question who have or have not lives worth sustaining (and protecting against intentional termination) seems radically unsound . . . [The issue is one] of the true implications of principles and notions being put into practice by a group of citizens whose medical qualifications, experience and ethos confer no standing to settle for the whole community such issues of meaning, consistency, humanity and justice'.[111]

Incompetency due to minority

The primary decision-makers for minors are their parents, who are presumed to have their best interests at heart.[112] There is no clearly defined age at which a child is deemed by law to be capable of consenting to medical treatment. Instead the law regards the right of parents to make such decisions for their children as 'a dwindling right' which 'starts with a right of control and ends with little more than advice'.[113] It is important to note that these parental rights and correlative duties are only subject to limitation where substantial lack of concern for or neglect of the child's health and safety requires the state to intervene in exercise of its powers as *parens patriae*.[114] This reflects the importance of parental autonomy and the freedom of parents to raise their children in accordance with values and beliefs other than those held by the mainstream of society.[115] Only where the child is in an immediately life-threatening situation must the parent's right to refuse treatment yield to the right to life of their offspring. In such situations, as the United States Supreme Court put it, parents are not entitled to make martyrs of their children.[116]

The most problematic legal and ethical issues in the treatment of minors have arisen from the growth of neonatal intensive care.[117] Severely handicapped newborns who may benefit from this care, may be divided into two categories.[118] First, there are those who have a chance of survival in a handicapped state if treatment of complications other than the underlying defect is rendered (e.g. Down's syndrome children with an intestinal blockage).[119] Secondly, there are those who will not survive for long even if all available treatment is given (e.g. anencephalic newborns).[120] In either case it is of the utmost importance to emphasize that the life of each human person whether handicapped or not is protected from birth by law. Therefore, the (active) killing of severely handicapped newborns will constitute the crime of unlawful homicide, murder or manslaughter.[121]

Obviously neonates are not in a position to decide their fate for themselves and therefore it falls to their parents, as primary surrogate decision-makers, to act in their best interests.[122] In making such an assessment, however, it is important not to impose one's own value judgments upon the life of the newborn and to recall that the principle of *favor vitae* does not distinguish between handicapped and non-handicapped people.[123] It has therefore been accepted that a permanent handicap will only justify a decision to withdraw life-sustaining treatment when it is so severe that continued existence would not be a net benefit to the infant.[124] Courts faced with the dilemma of 'whether the life of this child is demonstrably going to be so awful that in effect the child must be condemned to die, or whether the life of this child is still so imponderable that it would be wrong for her [or him] to be condemned to die' must apply this test subjectively and determine the outcome from the infant's point of view.[125] If in doubt and to forestall the ascription of relative values to different human lives,[126] the court should decide in accordance with the principle of *favor vitae* and in favour of life-sustaining procedures.[127] Finally, where parents decide to submit their handicapped child to therapy considered futile by the general run of medical opinion, this decision should be respected so long as it would not cause the child substantial suffering.[128]

THE ALLOCATION OF SCARCE HEALTH CARE RESOURCES

As we noted at the outset, significant problems of access may be present in the context of medical treatment at life's end. At the level of micro-allocation of resources difficult choices may have to be made as to which patient or group of patients shall receive treatment when resources and facilities are limited.[129] Doctors and health care administrators therefore undoubtedly require clear ethical guidance in making such decisions, which may have life or death implications for their patients.

Two main approaches to these problems of distribution have been identified.[130] The first approach would require decision-makers to favour patients whose potential recovery would be of greatest benefit or utility to society. However, such a standard would be wholly unacceptable since it would involve leaving the decision as to which of two potential recipients is the more deserving of life-sustaining treatment to the medical profession, although such assessments are surely well outside the scope of medical expertise.[131] The principle of autonomy is also threatened, since those whose lifestyles deviate from the utilitarian norm would be forced to conform or to forego necessary health care.[132]

The alternative theory would employ 'a lottery or randomized approach which, in spite of the chance element it embodies, probably best serves the ethical integrity of the decision-making process'.[133] The most practicable and ethically acceptable approach, therefore, would be to adopt a system of waiting lists, based on the 'first come, first served' principle without favouritism for the powerful or the well-connected.[134] This approach respects the individual dignity and the autonomous choices of patients as to the lifestyles which they wish to pursue and the integrity of the doctor–patient relationship.

CONCLUSION

In each area discussed we have seen that the law seeks to give effect to the core ethical principles of individual autonomy, non-maleficence and beneficence. Each of these principles has shaped the legal response to active euthanasia, which remains a serious criminal offence in the overwhelming majority of jurisdictions. In the light of historical experience we found that these legal and ethical standards must be maintained to preserve the sanctity of human life and to prevent a slide into moral ambivalence. These concerns also require that cases of palliative treatments which shorten life be subjected to the utmost scrutiny. On the other hand it was recognized that respecting refusals of treatments which shorten life is ethically and legally permissible as an exercise of the patient's inalienable right to self-determination.

These principles apply with equal force in cases of incompetency. Thus, we saw that the decisions of a duly appointed proxy are respected by the law. In other cases the clearly expressed wishes of the patient will be implemented by the courts. In the case of minors, we found that the primary decision-makers are the parents and that the active killing of newborns constitutes active euthanasia and as such is subject to criminal sanctions. In general, treatment decisions on behalf of incompetents are subject to the presumption *in favorem vitae*, which guards against the imposition of the value judgments of others upon the vulnerable and incompetent patient. Finally, it was shown that access on a first-come-first-served basis represented the fairest and most acceptable approach to the allocation of such resources.

To conclude, then, it is necessary to reflect upon the future role of the law in this area. It has, on occasion, been claimed that courts are ill equipped to deal with the highly sensitive and personal questions which arise with regard to patient participation in medical decision-making,[135] especially in relation to treatment at life's end, and there have been judicial calls, most recently by the House of Lords in the *Bland* case,[136] for legislative intervention to provide decision-makers with clear and unequivocal guidance. The efficacy of statutory regulation is to be doubted, however, especially when it is considered that the courts would be required to use their discretion in applying such statutes to the inevitably diverse and unforeseeable range of cases which come before them. Regardless of the form which legal developments take, it is essential that they conform to the fundamental principles outlined in this discussion. Legislators and judges alike must, while seeking to give effect to the value of personal (here patient) autonomy and personality interests, ensure that the sanctity of human life and, thus, respect for human life is maintained against the tides of ethical relativism and moral decline.

NOTES

1 I gratefully acknowledge the valuable co-operation received from one of my Research Assistants at the Free University of Berlin, John Harrington, LL.B. (Dubl.), B.C.L. (Oxon.), in the course of the work for, and preparation of, this paper.

2 This interest has been spurred, in part by earlier important decisions from the United States: *In re Karen Quinlan*, 70 NJ 10, 355 A2d 647 (1976) and *Superintendent of Belchertown State School* v. *Saikewicz*, 373 Mass 728, 370 NE2d 417 (1977); further case law is referred to in the following notes. For a comparative law discussion cf. D. Giesen, 'Ethische und rechtliche Probleme am Ende des Lebens', JZ 1990, 929–943; D. Giesen, 'Euthanasie und Sterbehilfe aus juristischer Perspektive', 39 Zeitschrift für medizinische Ethik 151–171 (1993); also cf. *Hilfe zum Sterben? Hilfe beim Sterben!*, ed. by H. Hepp, with interdisciplinary contributions by Arno Anzenbacher, Dieter Birnbacher, Dieter Giesen, Johannes Gründel, Hermann Hepp, Eberhard Schockenhoff and Klaus Wilms. Vol. 147 of the *Schriftenreihe der Katholischen Akademie in Bayern* (Düsseldorf 1992) (refs.), and generally D. Giesen, *International Medical Malpractice Law* (Tübingen, Dordrecht, Boston & London 1988 [hereinafter cited: *International Medical Malpractice Law* (1988)]) paras 891–987 (refs.).

3 *Cruzan* v. *Director, Missouri Department of Health*, 497 US 261, 110 SCt 2841, 111 LEd2d 224, 58 USLW 4916 (1990); cf. J. Areen, P. A. King, S. Goldberg, A. M. Capron, *Law Science and Medicine* (Mineola [NY] 1984) 1063–1235; B. R.

Furrow, S. H. Johnson, T. S. Jost & R. L. Schwartz, *Health Law. Cases, Materials and Problems* (2nd ed St Paul [Minn.] 1991) 1061–1082; D. W. Louisell & H. Williams, *Medical Malpractice*, 4 vols. (New York 1993) 19B (for the fullest survey of recent American case law on death, and withholding and withdrawing life support).

4 *Airedale National Health Service Trust* v. *Bland* [1993] AC 789 (HL), [1993] 2 WLR 316, [1993] 1 All ER 821, (1993) 12 BMLR 64 (FamD, CA & HL).

5 *Rodriguez* v. *British Columbia (Attorney General)* (1993) 158 NR 1 (SCC).

6 BGH, 4 July 1984 3 StR 96/84 BGHSt 32, 367, JZ 1984, 893, NJW 1984, 2369 (Dr Wittig); OLG München, 31 July 1987 1 Ws 23/87 NJW 1987, 2940 (Dr Hackethal). Cf. generally D. Giesen, *International Medical Malpractice Law* (1988) paras 891–987.

7 For a comprehensive comparative survey, cf. D. Giesen, 'Law and Ethical Dilemmas at Life's End', in: *Council of Europe. Law and moral dilemmas affecting life and death. Proceedings of the 20th Colloquy on European Law*, Glasgow, 10–12 Sept 1990 (Strasbourg 1992) 82–110; cf. also, A. Laufs, *Arztrecht* (5th ed Munich 1993) paras 290 ff. (299).

8 'Terminally ill' is used to describe a patient whose illness is likely to cause death within a very short time, cf. United States President's Commission for the Study of Ethical Problems in Medicine and Biomedical and Behavioural Research: *Deciding to Forego Life-Sustaining Treatment* (Washington 1983) 1, 17–18 (hereinafter cited: DFLST) 26. The group of hopelessly ill patients is mainly comprised of those in a persistent vegetative state (PVS). This state has been held to describe 'a body which is functioning entirely in terms of its internal controls. It maintains temperature. It maintains heart-beat and pulmonary ventilation. It maintains digestive activity. It maintains reflex action of muscles and nerves for low level conditioned responses. But there is no behavioural evidence of either self-awareness or awareness of the surroundings in learned manner.' *Matter of Jobes*, 529 A2d 434, 438 (NJ 1987), quoting an expert witness.

9 It has been estimated that there are between 5000 and 10 000 patients in the United States who exist in the 'twilight world' of the persistent vegetative state, cf. D. D. Byrd, 'A Right to Die: Can a Massachusetts Physician Withdraw Artificial Nutrition and Hydration from a Persistently Vegetative Patient Following Cruzan v Director, Missouri Department of Health?' 26 New England LR 199–224, 199 (1991–92).

10 *Cruzan* v. *Director, Missouri Department of Health*, 497 US 261, 110 SCt 2841, 58 USLW 4916 (1990, per *Justice Stevens* at 2883).

11 DFLST 1, 17–18; A. M. Capron, 'Legal and Ethical Problems in Decisions for Death', 14 Law, Med & Health Care 141–144, 141 (1986); Paul Ramsey, *Ethics at the Edges of Life. Medical and Legal Intersections* (New Haven & London 1978); M. Phillips & J. Dawson, *Doctors' Dilemmas. Medical Ethics and Contemporary Science* (Brighton 1985) 21, 31–34, 52–55; J. Areen, P. A. King, S. Goldberg, A. M. Capron, *Law Science and Medicine* (Mineola [NY] 1984) 1077–1235; A. Kaufmann, 'Zur ethischen und strafrechtlichen Beurteilung der sogenannten Früheuthanasie', JZ 1982, 481–487, 481; A. Laufs, *Arztrecht* (5th ed Munich 1993) paras 290 ff.; M. von Lutterotti, 'Der Arzt und das Tötungsverbot', MedR 1992, 7–14.

12 Cf. T. L. Beauchamp & J. F. Childress, *Principles of Biomedical Ethics* (3rd ed New York & Oxford 1989), *in toto*; P. Ramsey, *Ethics at the Edges of Life. Medical and Legal Intersections* (New Haven & London 1978) 143–188; H. Schaefer, *Medizinische Ethik* (Heidelberg 1983) 195–217; F.J. Illhardt, *Medizinische Ethik* (Berlin, Heidelberg, New York & Tokyo 1985) 107–128; A. Laufs, *Arztrecht* (5th ed Munich 1993) paras 290 ff.; *Grundgesetzkommentar*, ed. Ingo von Münch & Philip Kunig (4th ed Munich 1992) para 36 to Article 1 GG (Sterbehilfe), paras 44 & 50 to Article 2 GG (P. Kunig).

13 BVerfG,. 25 July 1979 2 BvR 878/74

BVerfGE 52, 131 (170). This comment was endorsed by the Federal Supreme Court in the case of Dr Wittig, prosecuted for failing to render assistance to his patient whose suicide attempt had left her unconscious and grievously injured: BGH, 4 July 1984 3 StR 96/84 BGHSt 32, 367, JZ 1984, 893 (896), NJW 1984, 2369.

14 For a full comparative discussion of the right to self-determination in the health care context, cf. D. Giesen, *International Medical Malpractice Law* (1988) §§ 20–27. Also cf. J. Arras & R. Hunt, *Ethical Issues in Modern Medicine* (2nd ed Palo Alto [Cal.] 1983 [hereinafter cited: MM]) 64–84 (Bruce L. Miller & Gerald Dworkin); *Medical Ethics. A Clinical Textbook and Reference for the Health Professions*, ed. N. Abrams & M. D. Buckner (Cambridge [Mass.] & London 1983 [hereinafter cited: ME]) 3–12 (T.L. Beauchamp & J. Childress on autonomy).

15 W. J. Curran, M. A. Hall & D. H. Kaye, *Health Care Law, Forensic Science, and Public Policy* (4th ed Boston, Toronto & London 1990) 927–1013; D. Giesen, *International Medical Malpractice Law* (1988) para 495.

16 I. Kennedy, *Treat Me Right. Essays in Law, Medicine and Ethics* (Oxford 1988) 320.

17 E. Pellegrino & D. C. Thomasma, *For the Patient's Good. The Restoration of Beneficence in Health Care* (New York & Oxford 1988) 46–50.

18 Cf. *Cruzan* v. *Director, Missouri Department of Health*, 497 US 261, 110 SCt 2841, 58 USLW 4916, 111 LEd2d 224, 242 (1990); *Gray* v. *Romeo*, 697 FSupp 580, 588 (D RI 1988); *Superintendent of Belchertown State School* v. *Saikewicz*, 373 Mass 728, 370 NE2d 417, 425 (1977); *In re Conroy*, 98 NJ 321, 486 A2d 1209, 1223 (1985). It is submitted that these considerations are also applicable in other jurisdictions, cf. D. Giesen, *International Medical Malpractice Law* (1988) paras. 948–954; *Grundgesetzkommentar*, ed. Ingo von Münch & Philip Kunig (4th ed Munich 1992) para. 36 to Article 1 GG (Sterbehilfe), paras. 44 & 50 to Article 2 GG (P. Kunig).

19 T. L. Beauchamp & J. F. Childress, *Principles of Biomedical Ethics* (3rd ed New York & Oxford 1989) 120–193.

20 On standards of care in medical treatment cf. D. Giesen, *International Medical Malpractice Law* (1988) §§ 9–14.

21 At common law a doctor may be convicted of manslaughter where his gross negligence has led to the death of his patient, cf. *Akerele* v. *The King* [1943] AC 255, [1943] 1 All ER 367 (PC). In the same situation liability is imposed under § 222 StGB (German Criminal Code) for negligent killing.

22 J. G. Fleming, *The Law of Torts* (8th ed Sydney 1992) 24–26, 79–84 (on battery and consent); M. Brazier, 'Patient Autonomy and Consent to Treatment', (1987) 7 LS 169–193.

23 A. Laufs, *Arztrecht* (5th ed Munich 1993) paras 295–300 (refs.).

24 Cf. T. L. Beauchamp & J. F. Childress, *Principles of Biomedical Ethics* (3rd ed New York & Oxford 1989) 194–255; E. Pellegrino & D. C. Thomasma, *For the Patient's Good. The Restoration of Beneficence in Health Care* (New York & Oxford 1988); for an important survey, cf. B. R. Furrow, S. H. Johnson, T. S. Jost & R. L. Schwartz, *Health Law. Cases, Materials and Problems* (2nd ed St Paul [Minn.] 1991) 1056–1060 (on principles of autonomy and beneficence).

25 E.g., under § 323c StGB (German Criminal Code). It should be made clear that, although a doctor in a common law country is not legally obliged to go to the assistance of strangers, a patient who has submitted himself to the doctor's care is no longer considered a 'stranger' but a 'neighbour' within the sense of *Lord Atkin's* famous test in *Donoghue (or M'Allister)* v. *Stevenson* [1932] AC 562, [1932] All ER Rep 1 (HL). A doctor failing to treat such a patient will be liable in tort under the head of abandonment, cf. D.Giesen, *International Medical Malpractice Law* (1988) paras 713–729.

26 An English translation of the oath is printed

in full in D. Giesen, *Arzthaftungsrecht – Medical Malpractice Law* (Bielefeld 1981) 425.

27 T. L. Beauchamp & J. F. Childress, *Principles of Biomedical Ethics* (3rd ed New York & Oxford 1989) 256–306.

28 For a comparative review of the law governing the right of competent adult patients to forego medical treatment, cf. B. R. Furrow, S. H. Johnson, T. S. Jost & R. L. Schwartz, *Health Law. Cases, Materials and Problems* (2nd ed St Paul [Minn.] 1991) 1082–1103; D. Giesen, *International Medical Malpractice Law* (1988) paras 932–954 (refs.).

29 ME 38-45 (J. Rachels on active and passive euthanasia, L. C. Becker on killing and giving up); M. Brazier, *Medicine, Patients and the Law* (2nd ed Harmondsworth 1992) 444–445; British Medical Association, *Euthanasia. Report of the Working Party to Review the British Medical Association's Guidance on Euthanasia* (London 1988) 28–29; D. Giesen, *International Medical Malpractice Law* (1988) para 944.

30 J. K. Mason & R. A. McCall Smith, *Law and Medical Ethics* (4th ed London, Dublin & Edinburgh 1994) 315–317; S. McLean & G. Maher, *Medicine, Morals and the Law* (Aldershot 1983) 42–60.

31 I. Kennedy, *Treat Me Right. Essays in Law, Medicine and Ethics* (Oxford 1988) 321; Art 20 French Code of Medical Deontology, 28 Jun 1979; BGH, 4 July 1984 3 StR 96/84 BGHSt 32, 367, JZ 1984, 893, NJW 1984, 2639; A. Laufs, *Arztrecht* (5th ed Munich 1993) paras 295–300 (refs.); *Handbuch des Arztrechts*, ed. A. Laufs & W. Uhlenbruck (Munich 1992) § 132 n4 (at 780).

32 *Airedale National Health Service Trust* v. *Bland* [1993] AC 789 (HL), [1993] 2 WLR 316, [1993] 1 All ER 821, (1993) 12 BMLR 64 (FamD, CA & HL, *Lord Goff* at 867c–d).

33 G. Williams, *Textbook of Criminal Law* (2nd ed London 1983) 580; also cf. J. K. Mason & R. A. McCall Smith, *Law and Medical Ethics* (4th ed London, Dublin & Edinburgh 1994) 318.

34 Hoge Raad der Nederlanden, 27 Nov 1984 NJ 1985, 451 no. 106; 21 Oct 1986 EuGRZ 1987, 282. For a short review of these judicial developments, cf. J. Stapel, 'Die Sterbhilfediskussion in den Niederlanden' ZRP 1986, 318–322; *M. von Lutterotti*, 'Der Arzt und das Tötungsverbot', MedR 1992, 7–14 (refs.).

35 The Independent, No. 1969 of 10 Feb 1993 at 1; The New York Times, No. 49 237 of 9 Feb 1993 at A1, A7, No. 49 238 of 10 Feb 1993 at A5.

36 J. K. M. Gevers, 'Legislation on euthanasia: recent developments in the Netherlands', (1992) 18 JME 138–141.

37 Cf. for example, H. Kuhse, 'The Case for Active Voluntary Euthanasia', 14 Law, Med & Health Care 145–148 (1986); P. Singer, 'Taking Life: Euthanasia', MM 210–215; P. Singer & H. Kuhse, 'Resolving arguments about the sanctity of life', (1988) 14 JME 198–199; cf. T. A. Long, 'Two philosophers in search of a contradiction: a response to Singer and Kuhse', (1990) 16 JME 95–96; for a critical assessment of Kuhse's and Singer's utilitarian approach cf. *Hilfe zum Sterben? Hilfe beim Sterben!*, ed. H. Hepp, with interdisciplinary contributions by Arno Anzenbacher, Dieter Birnbacher, Dieter Giesen, Johannes Gründel, Hermann Hepp, Eberhard Schockenhoff and Klaus Wilms. Vol. 147 of the *Schriftenreihe der Katholischen Akademie in Bayern* (Düsseldorf 1992) (refs.).

38 E. Pellegrino & D. C. Thomasma, *For the Patient's Good. The Restoration of Beneficence in Health Care* (New York & Oxford 1988) 44ff. *Hilfe zum Sterben? Hilfe beim Sterben!*, ed. H. Hepp, with interdisciplinary contributions by Arno Anzenbacher, Dieter Birnbacher, Dieter Giesen, Johannes Gründel, Hermann Hepp, Eberhard Schockenhoff and Klaus Wilms. Vol. 147 of the *Schriftenreihe der Katholischen Akademie in Bayern* (Düsseldorf 1992) (refs.).

39 In England: *Airedale National Health Service Trust* v. *Bland* [1993] AC 789 (HL); [1993] 2 WLR 316, [1993] 1 All ER 821, (1993) 12 BMLR 64 (FamD, CA & HL, *Lord Goff* at 866b–d); *Sidaway* v. *Bethlem Royal Hospital Governors* [1985] AC 871,

[1985] 1 All ER 643 (CA, per *Lord Scarman* at 649g–h); in the United States: *Schloendorff* v. *Society of New York Hospital*, 211 NY 125, 105 NE 92 (1914) (NY CA, per *Justice Cardozo* at 93); in Germany: BGH, 9 Dec 1958 VIZR 203/57 BGHZ 29, 46 (54), LM § 276 [Ca] BGB No 8, NJW 1959, 811.

40 E. Pellegrino & D. C. Thomasma, *For the Patient's Good. The Restoration of Beneficence in Health Care* (New York & Oxford 1988) 45.

41 A. Eser, 'Neues Recht des Sterbens? Einige grundsätzliche Betrachtungen', in A. Eser. (ed.), *Suizid und Euthanasie* (Stuttgart 1976) 392–407 (400).

42 On medical paternalism generally, cf. D. Giesen, *International Medical Malpractice Law* (1988) §§ 20, 51.

43 R. M. Veatch, *A Theory of Medical Ethics* (New York 1981) 214–226; also cf. E. Pellegrino & D. C. Thomasma, *For the Patient's Good. The Restoration of Beneficence in Health Care* (New York & Oxford 1988) 109–110.

44 The existence of such a special fiduciary relationship between doctor and patient was recognized both in Australia and in Canada, cf. *Kondis* v. *State Transport Authority* (1984) CLR 672, (1984) 55 ALR 225, (1984) ALJR 531, (1984) Aust Torts Reps § 80–311 (HC of A), and *McInerney* v. *MacDonald* (1992) 137 NR 35, [1992] 2 SCR 138, 93 DLR4th 415, (1993) 12 CCLT2d 225 (SCC); *Norberg* v. *Wynrib* [1992] 2SCR 318 (additional reasons to:) [1992] 2 SCR 226, [1992] 4 WWR 577, (1992) 68 BCLR2d 29, (1992) 138 NR 81, (1992) 92 DLR4th 449, (1992) 12 CCLT2d 1 (SCC, per *Justice McLachlin* at 35); for an ethical view cf. E. Pellegrino & D. C. Thomasma, *For the Patient's Good. The Restoration of Beneficence in Health Care* (New York & Oxford 1988). By contrast, in *Sidaway* v. *Bethlem Royal Hospital Governors* [1985] AC 871, [1985] 2 WLR 480, [1985] 1 All ER 643, 1 BMLR 132 (HL), the House of Lords rejected the contention that the doctor–patient relationship is of fiduciary character (per *Lord Scarman* at 651a–b).

45 'For him [a doctor] to . . . become a professional killer or assistant in suicide by direct action, would, I believe, change profoundly his role in society, to the severe detriment first of trust and thence of good medicine', G. R. Dunstan, 'The presumption in favour of life', in *New Prospects of Medicine*, ed. J. M. Austyn (Oxford, New York & Tokyo 1986) 71–83 (82).

46 R. Fenigsen, 'A Case Against Dutch Euthanasia', 19/5 Hastings Center Report (Special Supplement: 'Mercy, Murder and Morality. Perspectives on Euthanasia') 22–30 [30 first column] (1989).

47 *Airedale National Health Service Trust* v. *Bland* [1993] AC 789 (HL), [1993] 2 WLR 316, [1993] 1 All ER 821, (1993) 12 BMLR 64 (FamD, CA & HL, per *Lord Goff* at 865h–j); *Rodriguez* v. *British Columbia (Attorney General)* (1993) 158 NR 1 (SCC, per *Justice Sopinka* at 40); also cf. *Re T (Adult: refusal of medical treatment)* [1992] 3 WLR 782, [1992] 4 All ER 649, (1992) 9 BMLR 46, [1992] 2 FLR 458 (CA, per *Master of the Rolls Lord Donaldson* at 661e–f); *Cruzan* v. *Director, Missouri Department of Health*, 497 US 261, 110 SCt 2841, 58 USLW 4916, 111 LEd2d 224, 242 (1990, per *Chief Justice Rehnquist* at 242); BVerfG, 25.2.1975 1 BvF 1–6/74 BVerfGE 39, 1, JZ 1975, 205 (G. Kriele), NJW 1975, 573; 28.5.1993 2 BvF 2/90, 2 BvF 4/92, 2 BvF 5/92 JZ 1993 (Sonderheft) 1–51; BGH, 18.1.1983 VI ZR 114/81 BGHZ 86, 240 (252–253); BGH, 4 July 1984 3 StR 96/84 BGHSt 32, 367, JZ 1984, 893, NJW 1984, 2369 (Dr Wittig).

48 R. J. Lifton, *The Nazi Doctors. Medical Killing and the Psychology of Genocide* (New York 1986); G. A. Annas, 'Mengele's Birthmark: the Nuremberg Code in United States Courts', 7 Jnl of Contemporary Health Law & Policy 17–45 (1991); T. L. Beauchamp & J. F. Childress, *Principles of Biomedical Ethics* (3rd ed New York & Oxford 1989) 141; cf. also, Hans Jonas, *Technik, Medizin und Ethik. Zur Praxis des Prinzips Verantwortung* (Frankfurt/M. 1985) 219 ff., 242 ff. For an impressive statement of the legal position under Ger-

man law today, cf. *Handbuch des Arztrechts*, ed. A. Laufs & W. Uhlenbruck (Munich 1992) § 132 (pp. 776–789 with ample refs.) (W. Uhlenbruck).

49 R. Fenigsen, 'A Case Against Dutch Euthanasia', 19/1 Hastings Center Report (Special Supplement) 22–30 [24, on newborns, and 30 on familial pressure and old people] (1989).

50 The Remmelink Report, cf. The Independent, 17 Feb 1993 at 8.

51 The Independent, 17 Feb 1993 at 8.

52 R. Fenigsen, 'A Case Against Dutch Euthanasia', 19/1 Hastings Center Report (Special Supplement) 22–30 [26]; cf. also, criticisms of Fenigsen's article and his response thereto in 19/6 Hastings Center Report 47–51 (1989). Indeed, in its highly significant decision in *Rodriguez* v. *British Columbia (Attorney General)* (1993) 158 NR 1 (SCC), the Supreme Court of Canada noted the 'worrisome' increase in involuntary active euthanasia which has followed the relaxation of Dutch law on this matter (per *Justice Sopinka* at 35).

53 For example: § 216 StGB (German Criminal Code); Art 114 Swiss Criminal Code; § 77 Austrian Criminal Code.

54 A. Laufs, *Arztrecht* (5th ed Munich 1993) paras 295–300 (refs.).

55 As Henk Ten Have, Professor of Medical Ethics at Nijmegen University, put it, it would be farcical to suggest that a doctor who has illegally killed a patient will then volunteer that information to the relevant authorities, cf. The Independent, 17 Feb 1993 at 8.

56 L. A. Lacewell, 'A Comparative View of the Roles of Motive and Consent in the Response of the Criminal Justice System to Active Euthanasia', (1987) 6 Med Law 449–463, 450.

57 Sacred Congregation for the Doctrine of the Faith, Declaration on Euthanasia, *Acta Apostolicae Sedis* (AAS) LXXII (1980) 542–552 (in the Latin original), published in English by the Catholic Truth Society, London 1980; *A New Dictionary of Christian Ethics*, ed. J. Macquarrie & J. Childress (London 1986) 162–163 (R. A. McCormick SJ on the principle of double effect), 210–212 (T. Wood on euthanasia), 353–354 (T. Wood on the sacredness of life). Cf. also M. Brazier, *Medicine Patients and the Law* (2nd ed Harmondsworth 1992) 446–449; T. L. Beauchamp & J. F. Childress, *Principles of Biomedical Ethics* (3rd ed New York & Oxford 1989) 127–134; J. K. Mason & R. A. McCall Smith, *Law and Medical Ethics* (4th ed London, Dublin & Edinburgh 1994) 329–330; 56. Deutscher Juristentag Berlin 1986, Strafrechtliche Abteilung, Beschluss I.3, NJW 1986, 3073.

58 I. Kennedy & A. Grubb, *Medical Law: Text with Materials* (2nd ed London 1994) 1205–1207; A. Laufs, *Arztrecht* (5th ed Munich 1993) paras 290–303 (refs.).

59 Cf. Lord Goff of Chieveley, 'The Mental Element in the Crime of Murder', (1988) 104 LQR 30–59.

60 I. Kennedy & A. Grubb, *Medical Law: Text with Materials* (2nd ed London 1994) 1205–1207.

61 *R* v. *Bodkin Adams* [1957] CrimLR 365 (per *Mr Justice Devlin* at 375); on the function of medicine in these circumstances, cf. E. J. Cassell, 'The Function of Medicine', MM 238–242; M.A. Somerville 'The Song of Death: The Lyrics of Euthanasia', 9 Jnl of Contemporary Health Law & Policy 1–76 (1993).

62 British Medical Association, *Euthanasia. Report of the Working Party to Review the British Medical Association's Guidance on Euthanasia* (London 1988) 69; A. Laufs, *Arztrecht* (5th ed Munich 1993) para. 292.

63 S. McLean & G. Maher, *Medicine, Morals and the Law* (Aldershot 1983) 45–46. However, Immanuel Kant rejected the notion that suicide involves an exercise of individual autonomy as incoherent: I. Kant, *Metaphysische Anfangsgründe der Tugendlehre* (Königsberg 1797) § 6; for English translations of relevant Kantian maxims cf. MPM 434–437 (Immanuel Kant on duties towards the body in regard to life and on suicide).

64 D. Giesen, *International Medical Malpractice Law* (1988) paras 227 n 36, 706–712, 941, 949 (refs.).

65 Cf. *Hyde* v. *Thameside Area Health Authority* (1981) 282 BMJ 1716, [1981] CLY 1854, (1981) The Times, 16 April, (1986) 2 PN 26 (CA, per *Master of the Rolls Lord Denning*; *Satz* v. *Perlmutter*, 362 So2d 160 (Fla App 1978), affd 379 So2d 359 (Fla 1980); BGH, 10 Mar 1954 GSSt 4/53 BGHSt 6, 147, LM § 330c [now § 323c] StGB No 7, JZ 1954, 639, NJW 1954, 1049.

66 *Rodriguez* v. *British Columbia (Attorney General)* (1993) 158 NR 1 (SCC, per *Justice Sopinka* at 27).

67 *Suicide Act*, 1961 (9 & 10 Eliz II c 60) ss 1–2; Art 580 Italian Criminal Code § 78 Austrian Criminal Code; Art 294 Dutch Criminal Code. It is submitted that this position is preferable to that obtaining in Scotland whereby an unsustainable distinction is drawn between administering and merely supplying a lethal drug to a terminally ill patient, cf. S. McLean & G. Maher, *Medicine, Morals and the Law* (Aldershot 1983) 46 n 46. In German law it is not a crime for a doctor to assist a patient to commit suicide as long as the patient has full control over the course of events and is not incompetent. However, if the patient passes over into a state of unconsciousness and is in danger of dying the doctor will be guilty of a criminal offence if he fails to take steps to save the patient's life under §§ 212, 13 or § 323c StGB (German Criminal Code), cf. BGH, 4 July 1984 3 StR 96/84 BGHSt 32, 367, JZ 1984, 893, NJW 1984 2369 (Dr Wittig).

68 *Rodriguez* v. *British Columbia (Attorney General)* (1993) 158 NR 1 (SCC, per *Justice Sopinka* at 27).

69 *Rodriguez* v. *British Columbia (Attorney General)* (1993) 158 NR 1 (SCC, per *Justice Sopinka* at 33–37).

70 P. D. G. Skegg, *Law, Ethics and Medicine* (Oxford 1984) 112.

71 G. Gillett, 'Euthanasia, letting die and the pause', (1988) 14 JME 61–68.

72 Cf. British Medical Association, *Euthanasia. Report of the Working Party to Review the British Medical Association's Guidance on Euthanasia* (London 1988) 23–24; K. C. Calman, 'Ethical Implications of Terminal Care', in: *Medicine, Ethics and Law. Current Legal Problems*, ed. M. D. A. Freeman (London 1988) 112; *Moral Problems in Medicine*, ed. S. Gorovitz, R. Macklin, A. L. Jameton, J. M. O'Connor & S. Sherwin (Englewood Cliffs [NJ] 1983 [hereinafter cited: MPM]), 277–295 (T. Goodrich on killing and letting die, J. Rachels on active and passive euthanasia, B. Steinbock on the intentional termination of life).

73 DFLST 40. In a recent decision of the English Court of Appeal, *Butler-Sloss* LJ reaffirmed that '[a] man or woman of full age and sound understanding may choose to reject medical advice and medical or surgical treatment either partially or in its entirety. A decision to refuse medical treatment by a patient capable of making the decision does not have to be sensible, rational or well considered.' *Re T (Adult: refusal of medical treatment)* [1992] 3 WLR 782, [1992] 4 All ER 649, (1992) 9 BMLR 46, [1992] 2 FLR 458 (CA, per *Lord Justice Butler-Sloss* at 664j). Cf. also *Malette* v. *Shulman* (1990) 72 OR2d 417, (1990) 67 DLR4th 321, (1990) 2 CCLT2d 1 (CA).

74 *Cruzan* v. *Director, Missouri Department of Health*, 497 US 261, 110 SCt 2841, 58 USLW 4916, 111 LEd2d 224, 242 (1990, per *Chief Justice Rehnquist* at 236).

75 *Rodriguez* v. *British Columbia (Attorney General)* (1993) 158 NR 1 (SCC, per *Justice Sopinka* at 40).

76 BGH, 4 July 1984 3 StR 96/84 BGHSt 32, 367 (Dr Wittig).

77 *Cruzan* v. *Director, Missouri Department of Health*, 497 US 261, 110 SCt 2841, 58 USLW 4916, 111 LEd2d 224, 242 (1990); *Gray* v. *Romeo*, 697 FSupp 580, 588 (D RI 1988); *Superintendent of Belchertown State School* v. *Saikewicz*, 373 Mass 728, 370 NE2d 417, 425 (1977); *In re Conroy*, 98 NJ 321, 486 A2d 1209, 1223 (1985).

78 It is submitted that these considerations are also applicable in other jurisdictions, cf. D. Giesen, *International Medical Malpractice Law* (1988) paras 948–954 (refs.); also cf. *Grundgesetzkommentar*, ed. Ingo von Münch & Philip Kunig (4th ed Munich 1992) para 36 to Article 1 GG (Sterbehilfe),

paras 44 & 50 to Article 2 GG (P. Kunig).

79 *Cruzan* v. *Director, Missouri Department of Health*, 497 US 261, 110 SCt 2841, 58 USLW 4916, 111 LEd2d 224, 242 (1990), per *Justice Brennan* at 262–263); W. J. Curran, M. A. Hall & D. H. Kaye, *Health Care Law, Forensic Science, and Public Policy* (4th ed Boston, Toronto & London 1990) 934–966.

80 Indeed, as it was put by the Supreme Court of Massachusetts, 'the value of life . . . is lessened not by a decision to refuse treatment, but by the failure to allow a competent human being the right of choice', *Superintendent of Belchertown State School* v. *Saikewicz*, 373 Mass 728, 370 NE2d 417, 425 (1977).

81 Indeed, although it forms a cornerstone of his and the rest of their Lordships' ruling in *Airedale National Health Service Trust* v. *Bland* [1993] AC 789 (HL), [1993] 2 WLR 316, [1993] 1 All ER 821, (1993) 12 BMLR 64 (HL), *Lord Mustill* (at 895a) refers to 'the morally and intellectually dubious distinction between acts and omissions'.

82 On the related question of the moral significance and practical viability of the distinction between the provision of nutrition and medical treatment, cf. *Airedale National Health Service Trust* v. *Bland* [1993] AC 789 (HL), [1993] 2 WLR 316, [1993] 1 All ER 821, (1993) 12 BMLR 64 (FamD, CA & HL, per *Lord Keith* at 861d–f); cf. also I. Kennedy & A. Grubb, 'Withdrawal of Artificial Hydration and Nutrition: Incompetent Adult. Airedale NHS Trust v. Bland', (1993) 1 Med L Rev 359–370 on the one hand and, on the other, J. Finnis, '*Bland*: Crossing the Rubicon?', (1993) 109 LQR 329–337.

83 Thus, for example, in *Cruzan* v. *Director, Missouri Department of Health*, 497 US 261, 110 SCt 2841, 58 USLW 4916, 111 LEd2d 224, 242 (1990), *O'Connor* J. (concurring), rejected as untenable the distinction sometimes drawn in this regard, between artificial feeding and other forms of life-sustaining treatment (at 248).

84 *In re Conroy*, 98 NJ 321, 486 A 2d 1209 at 1223 (1985); cf. generally, D. Giesen, *International Medical Malpractice Law* (1988) paras 948–950 (refs.).

85 United States President's Commission for the Study of Ethical Problems in Medicine and Biomedical and Behavioral Research: Making Health Care Decisions, 3 vols. (Washington 1982 [hereinafter cited: MHCD]) i.167 ff.; W. J. Curran, M. A. Hall & D. H. Kaye, *Health Care Law, Forensic Science, and Public Policy* (4th ed Boston, Toronto & London 1990) 1014–1024. For a detailed comparative survey of the legal and ethical aspects of incompetency, cf. D. Giesen, *International Medical Malpractice Law* (1988) paras 955–987 (refs.). For a thorough survey of the problems engendered by incompetence see *Decision-Making and Problems of Incompetence*, ed. A. Grubb (Chichester, New York, Brisbane, Toronto & Singapore 1994).

86 In England: *Hewer* v. *Bryant* [1970] 1 QB 357, [1969] 3 WLR 425, [1969] 3 All ER 578 (CA, per *Master of the Rolls Lord Denning* at 528e); *Gillick* v. *West Norfolk and Wisbech Area Health Authority and the DHSS* [1986] AC 112, [1985] 3 WLR 413, [1985] 3 All ER 402 (HL, per *Lord Scarman* at 423b). In Germany: BGH, 5 Dec 1958 VI ZR 266/57 BGHZ 29, 33, LM § 107 BGB No 3, NJW 1959, 811; 28 June 1988 VI ZR 288/87 BGHZ 105, 45 (47–48). In Austria: OGH, 19 Dec 1984 3 Ob 562/84 SZ 57 (1984) 1036 (No 207), JBl 1985, 548 (550). Also cf. B. R. Furrow, S. H. Johnson, T. S. Jost & R. L. Schwartz, *Health Law. Cases, Materials and Problems* (2nd ed St Paul [Minn.] 1991) 1104–1159; D. Giesen, *International Medical Malpractice Law* (1988) paras 917–931, 975–987 (comparative) and D. Giesen, 'Decision-Making and Problems of Incompetence: Comparative Legal Developments', in: *Decision-Making and Problems of Incompetence*, ed. Andrew Grubb (Chichester, New York, Brisbane, Toronto & Singapore 1994) 7–26 (refs.).

87 *R* v. *Hallstrom* [1986] QB 1090, [1986] 2 WLR 883, [1986] 2 All ER 306 *Justice McCullough* at 314f–g), MHCD i.171; cf. also D. Giesen, *International Medical*

Malpractice Law (1988) para 919 (refs.).

88 Cf. *Kirby* v. *Leather* [1965] QB 367, [1965] 2 WLR 1318, [1965] 2 All ER 441 (CA); BGH, 4 July 1984 3 StR 96/84 BGHSt 32, 367 (Dr Wittig); OLG München, 31 July 1987 1 Ws 23/87 NJW 1987, 2940 (Dr Hackethal).

89 MHCD i.177 ff.

90 In *Cruzan* v. *Director, Missouri Department of Health*, 497 US 261, 110 SCt 2841, 58 USLW 4916, 111 LEd2d 224, 242 (1990) *Justice O'Connor* held (at 250) that, although it was not necessary for the decision at hand, state courts might well be constitutionally required to give effect to the decisions of such a surrogate decision maker, so as to protect the patient's liberty interests; on proxy consent for adult incompetents, cf. R. M. Veatch, 'The Case of Karen Quinlan', MM 270–273; P. Ramsey, 'The Saikewicz Precedent: What's Good for an Incompetent Patient?', MM 274–281; also cf. G.J. Annas, 'Quinlan, Saikewicz, and Now Brother Fox', ME 337–340. In England under s. 3(1) *Enduring Powers of Attorney Act* 1985 the incompetent person's wishes must only be respected in relation to his 'property and affairs'.

91 *Re T (Adult: refusal of medical treatment)* [1992] 3 WLR 782, [1992] 4 All ER 649, (1992) 9 BMLR 46, [1992] 2 FLR 458 (CA).

92 *Re T (Adult: refusal of medical treatment)* [1992] 3 WLR 782, [1992] 4 All ER 649, (1992) 9 BMLR 46, [1992] 2 FLR 458 (CA, per *Master of the Rolls Lord Donaldson* at 653f). This is also the position in German law, cf. BGH, 9 Dec 1958 VI ZR 203/57 BGHZ 29, 46, LM § 276 [Ca] BGB No 8, NJW 1959, 811.

93 § 1904 BGB (German Civil Code); cf. M. Coester, 'Von anonymer Verwaltung zu persönlicher Betreuung – Zur Reform des Vormund- und Pflegschaftsrechts für Volljährige', Jura 1991, 4–9.

94 *Cruzan* v. *Harmon*, 760 SW2d 408, 425–426 (Mo 1988).

95 MHCDi.180–181.

96 DFLST 132, 135; MHCDi.178–179. Cf. also D. Giesen, *International Medical Malpractice Law* (1988) paras 980–987 (refs.).

97 § 1901 Abs 1 and 2 BGB (German Civil Code).

98 *In re Conroy*, 98 NJ 321, 486 A2d 1209 (1985).

99 *Cruzan* v. *Director, Missouri Department of Health*, 497 US 261, 110 SCt 2841, 58 USLW 4916, 111 LEd2d 224, 242, (1990, per *Chief Justice Rehnquist* at 234–247).

100 W. J. Curran, M. A. Hall & D. H. Kaye, *Health Care Law, Forensic Science, and Public Policy* (4th ed Boston, Toronto & London 1990) 966–1006 (on patients without clearly expressed wishes, discussing cases from *Karen Ann Quinlan* to *Cruzan*).

101 'By this we mean that the patient is suffering, and will continue to suffer throughout the expected duration of his life, unavoidable pain, and that the net burdens of his prolonged life . . . markedly outweigh any physical pleasure, emotional enjoyment, or intellectual satisfaction that the patient may still be able to derive from life' *In re Conroy*, 98 NJ 321, 486 A2d 1209 (per *Justice Schreiber* at 1232).

102 D. Giesen, *International Medical Malpractice Law* (1988) para 987 (refs.).

103 *F* v. *West Berkshire Health Authority, sub nom F, Re* [1990] 2 AC 1, [1989] 2 WLR 1025, [1989] 2 All ER 545, (1989) 4 BMLR 1 (HL).

104 Cf. also *Frenchay Healthcare National Health Service Trust* v. *S* [1994] 2 All ER 403 (CA).

105 *F* v. *West Berkshire Health Authority, sub nom F, Re* [1990] 2 AC 1, [1989] 2 WLR 1025, [1989] 2 All ER 545, (1989) 4 BMLR 1 (HL, per *Lord Goff* at 567f–h). A 'best interests' test has also been endorsed in New Zealand, cf. *Auckland Area Health Board* v. *Attorney General* [1993] 1 NZLR 235 (HC).

106 *Airedale National Health Service Trust* v. *Bland* [1993] AC 789 (HL), [1993] 2 WLR 316, [1993] 1 All ER 821, (1993) 12 BMLR 64 (FamD, CA & HL). Cf. also, I. Kennedy & A Grubb, 'Withdrawal of Artificial Hydration and Nutrition: Incompetent Adult. Airedale NHS Trust v Bland', (1993) 1 Med L Rev 359–370.

107 *Lord Keith, Lord Goff, Lord Lowry* and *Lord Browne-Wilkinson* endorsed the *Bolam* test in this context. *Lord Mustill* raised doubts about applying a principle of civil liability 'in a field dominated by the criminal law' and stated that there was no reason in logic why on such a decision the opinions of the doctors should be decisive: *Airedale National Health Service Trust* v. *Bland* [1993] AC 789 (HL), [1993] 2 WLR 316, [1993] 1 All ER 821, (1993) 12 BMLR 64 (HL, per *Lord Mustill* at 895g–i).

108 *Bolam* v. *Friern Hospital Management Committee* [1957] 1 WLR 582, [1957] 2 All ER 118, 1 BMLR 1 (QBD, per *McNair* J). The essence of the test is that '[a] doctor is not guilty of negligence if he has acted in accordance with a practice accepted as proper by a responsible body of medical men skilled in that particular art' (per *Justice McNair* at 122).

109 For a comparative survey of other common law jurisdictions, cf. D. Giesen, 'From Paternalism to Self-determination to Shared Decision-making', in: Acta Juridica (Cape Town) 1988, 107–127; D. Giesen & John Hayes, 'The Patient's Right to Know – A Comparative View', (1992) 21 Anglo-Am LR 101–122; D. Giesen, 'Vindicating the Patient's Rights: A Comparative Perspective', 9 Journal of Contemporary Health Law and Policy 273–309 (1993). More recent Common Law decisions are *Rogers* v. *Whitaker* (1992) 175 CLR 479, (1992) 67 ALJR 47, (1992) 109 ALR 625, (1992) Aust Torts Reps § 81–189 (HC of A) and now also *Daphne Castell* v. *Andrew de Greef* (Case # 976/92 [not yet published]), where the Supreme Court of South Africa (Cape Town Division) in February 1994 expressly decided to discard the *Bolam* test in consent cases and to adopt in its stead the aforementioned *Rogers* decision from Australia, also stating its agreement with established case law of the German *Bundesgerichtshof* (Federal Supreme Court) which also applies a (subjective) patient-oriented test (per *Justice Ackermann, Judge-President Friedman & Justice Farlam*). The *Rogers* decision is now approvingly commented upon by J. Keown, 'Burying *Bolam*: Informed Consent Down Under', [1994] CLJ 16–19. Also cf. the following footnote.

110 The fact that the decision in *Bland* whether to continue life-sustaining treatment is based on the *Bolam* test means that justification cannot be found for the decision by calling in aid the concept of self-determination. There is never any justification for the medical profession, on its own terms, to decide the ethically charged question whether life-sustaining treatment should be halted. The decision in *Bland* might have been rationally defensible if it had been based, as suggested in this chapter, on the will of the patient regarding further treatment. In cases such as this where the patient is unconscious this determination must, of course, be made by someone else. The basis for the decision in this case, however, is not the personal opinion of the decision-maker, but still the will of the patient. This may, as outlined earlier, be determined according to a subjective or a more objective test, depending on the evidence available as to the will of the patient. Where the test is objective there must, clearly, be a strong presumption in favour of the value and the sanctity of life.

Indeed, the *Bolam* test, both in its content and in its application, is also inadequate to determining ordinary treatment and disclosure malpractice, cf. D. Giesen, 'Medical Malpractice and the Judicial Function in Comparative Perspective', (1993) 1 Medical Law International 3–16; D. Giesen, 'Legal Accountability for the Provision of Medical Care: A Comparative View', (1993) 86 Journal of the Royal Society of Medicine 648–652; for a broad comparative law perspective, cf. D. Giesen, *International Medical Malpractice Law* (1988) paras 561–563, 566, 573, 580–581, 591, 649–650, 678, 680–681, 729, 777–778, 786, 789, 790, 799, 845, 903–910, et passim, on medical paternalism endorsed by judicial paternalism.

111 J. Finnis, '*Bland*: Crossing the Rubicon?', (1993) 109 LQR 329–337 (334). The German Federal Supreme Court is also on record as holding a similar opinion, BGH, 18 Jan 1983 VI ZR 114/81 BGHZ 86, 240 (252–253) (wrongful life case). Also cf. Hans Jonas, *Technik, Medizin und Ethik. Zur Praxis des Prinzips Verantwortung* (Frankfurt/M. 1985); Paul Ramsey, *Ethics at the Edges of Life. Medical and Legal Intersections* (New Haven & London 1978); M. Phillips & J. Dawson, *Doctors' Dilemmas. Medical Ethics and Contemporary Science* (Brighton 1985) 21, 31–34, 52–55.

112 D. Giesen, *International Medical Malpractice Law* (1988) para 955 (refs.); A.R. Holder, 'The Duty to Prolong Life', ME 378–381 (381).

113 *Hewer* v. *Bryant* [1970] 1 QB 357, [1969] 3 WLR 425, [1969] 3 All ER 578 (CA, per *Lord Denning* MR at 528e). This formulation was approved by the House of Lords in *Gillick* v. *West Norfolk and Wisbech Area Health Authority and the DHSS*)1986] AC 112, [1985] 3 WLR 413, [1985] 3 All ER 402 (HL, per *Lord Scarman* at 423b).

114 *Re P (A Minor)* (1982) 12 FamL 88, [1982] CLY 2082 (CA). Cf. also German Federal Constitution (Grundgesetz) Art 6 II 2.

115 D. Giesen, Kindesmisshandlung? Zur Kinder- und Familienfeindloichkeit in der Bundesrepublik Deutschland (Paderborn, Munich, Vienna & Zurich 1979) 69, 107, 111, 124: J. Goldstein, 'Medical Care for the Child At Risk: On State Supervention of Parental Autonomy', Yale Law Journal 86, 645–670 (1977).

116 *Prince* v. *Massachusetts*. 321 US 158 (1944).

117 Cf. D. Giesen, *International Medical Malpractice Law* (1988) paras 965–968; DFLST 197–229 (refs.).

118 For relevant American case law, cf. W. J. Curran, M. A. Hall & D. H. Kaye, *Health Care Law, Forensic Science, and Public Policy* (4th ed Boston, Toronto & London 1990) 1007–1013; also cf. B. F. Brooks, 'Ethical Dilemmas in the Treatment of Critically Ill Newborns', 1 Journal of Contemporary Health Law & Policy 133–141 (1985).

119 *Re B (A Minor) (Wardship: Medical Treatment)* [1981] 1 WLR 1421 (CA).

120 *Re C (A Minor) (Wardship: Medical Treatment)* [1990] Fam 26, [1989] 3 WLR 240, [1989] 2 All ER 782 (CA).

121 R v. *Arthur* (1981) 12 BMLR 1 (*Mr Justice Farquharson*), cf. also I. Kennedy & A. Grubb, *Medical Law: Text with Materials* (2nd ed London 1994) 1247–1249.

122 *Re C (A Minor) (Wardship: Medical Treatment)* [1990] Fam 26, [1989] 3 WLR 240, [1989] 2 All ER 782 (CA, per *Master of the Rolls Lord Donaldson* at 787g).

123 G. R. Dunstan, 'The presumption in favour of life', in *New Prospects of Medicine*, ed. J. M. Austyn (Oxford, New York & Tokyo 1986) 71–83.

124 DFLST 218–219.

125 *Re B (A Minor) (Wardship: Medical Treatment)* [1981] 1 WLR 1421 (CA, per *Lord Justice Templeman* at 1424B); also cf. *Re J (A Minor) (Wardship: Medical Treatment)* [1991] Fam 33, [1991] 2 WLR 140, [1990] 3 All ER 930, (1992) 9 BMLR 10 (CA).

126 It is a matter of concern that recent decisions of the English Courts have ignored the principle of the sanctity of human life in favour of an unmodified 'best interests' test, cf. *Re J (A Minor) (Wardship: Medical Treatment)* [1991] Fam 33, [1991] 2 WLR 140, [1991] 3 All ER 903, (1992) 9 BMLR 10 (CA); *Re B (A Minor) (Wardship: Medical Treatment)* (1980) [1981] WLR 1421, [1990] 3 All ER 927 (CA).

127 D. Giesen, *International Medical Malpractice Law* (1988) para 966 (refs.).

128 DFLST 219–220.

129 C. C. Havighurst, *Health Care Law and Policy. Readings, Notes, and Questions* (Westbury & New York 1988 with 1992 Supplement) 919–1064 (on cost containment regulations in general and cost controls in government programmes).

130 D. Giesen, *International Medical Malpractice Law* (1988) para 1336 (refs.).

131 D. Giesen, *International Medical Malpractice Law* (1988) para 1336.
132 J. E. Giles, *Medical Ethics* (Cambridge [Mass] 1983) 185.
133 J. E. Giles, *Medical Ethics* (Cambridge [Mass] 1983) 184.
134 'The equal right of every human to live, and not relative personal or social worth, should be the ruling principle. When not all can be saved and all need to die, this ruling principle can be applied only or best by random choice among equals.' P. Ramsey, *A Human Lottery? Ethical Issues in Modern Medicine*, ed. J. Arras & R. Hunt (2nd ed Palo Alto [Cal] 1983) 480 ff (470).
135 MHCD i.175. Cf. generally, B. Bromberger, 'Patient Participation in Medical Decision-Making: Are the Courts the Answer?', (1983) 6 UNSWLJ 1–23; but cf. J. G. Fleming, 'Is There a Future for Tort?', (1984) 58 ALR 131–142, who predicts that in the future courts could well make up lost ground in expanding areas, 'as in the United States, in the civilised mission of furthering civil rights, privacy and other personality interests' (142).
136 *Airedale National Health Service Trust* v. *Bland* [1993] AC 789 (HL), [1993] 2 WLR 316, [1993] 1 All ER 821, (1993) 12 BMLR 64 (HL, per *Lord Browne-Wilkinson* at 879j).

15

Physician-assisted suicide: the last bridge to active voluntary euthanasia

YALE KAMISAR

SOME 30 YEARS AGO an eminent constitutional law scholar, Charles L. Black, Jr, spoke of 'toiling uphill against that heaviest of all argumental weights – the weight of a slogan.'[1] I am reminded of that observation when I confront the slogan the 'right to die.'

THE 'RIGHT TO DIE'

Few rallying cries or slogans are more appealing and seductive than the 'right to die.' But few are more fuzzy, more misleading, or more misunderstood. The phrase has been used loosely by many people to embrace at least four different rights:

1 the right to reject or to terminate unwanted medical procedures, including life-saving treatment;
2 the right to commit suicide or, as some call it, the right to 'rational' suicide;
3 the right to assisted suicide, that is, the right to obtain another's help in committing suicide; and
4 the right to active voluntary euthanasia, that is, the right to authorize another to kill you intentionally and directly.

Each of these four 'rights' should be kept separate and distinct. Unfortunately, many times they are not.

First of all, neither the 1976 *Quinlan* case[2] nor the 1990 *Cruzan* case[3] (the only case involving death, dying and the 'right to privacy' ever decided by the US Supreme Court) establishes an absolute or general right to die – a right to end one's life in any manner one sees fit. The only right or liberty that the *Quinlan* Court established and the *Cruzan* Court recognized is the right under certain circumstances to refuse or to reject life-sustaining medical treatment or, as many have called it, the right to die *a natural death*.

Indeed, the *Quinlan* case explicitly distinguished between letting die on the one hand, and both direct killing and assisted suicide on the other.[4] No less prominent an advocate of assisted suicide and active voluntary euthanasia than the Hemlock Society's Derek Humphry recognizes that the *Quinlan* case 'is significant,' *inter alia*, for 'distinguishing between suicide and the passive withdrawal of life supports.'[5]

As did *Quinlan*, the *Cruzan* case, the one 'right to die' case that rivals *Quinlan* for prominence, involved the right to end artificial life support.[6] *Cruzan*, too, provides small comfort to proponents of a constitutional right to assisted suicide.

In *Cruzan*, a 5–4 majority, *per* Chief Justice Rehnquist, 'assumed for purposes of this case' that a competent person has 'a constitutionally protected right to refuse lifesaving hydration and nutrition.'[7] But the Court declined to call the liberty a 'fundamental right,' a characterization that requires a state to provide a compelling justification before restricting it. Instead, the Court called the right 'a Fourteenth Amendment liberty interest.'[8]

By avoiding 'fundamental right' language, the Court, it seems, would permit a state to restrict the 'liberty interest' in terminating unwanted life-sustaining medical treatment upon a lesser showing of need than would have been required if the interest had been deemed 'fundamental.' 'Any reasonable state interest' might suffice.[9] In any event the *Cruzan* Court did not assume or even suggest that one has so much as a 'Fourteenth Amendment liberty interest' in *assisted suicide*. Quite the contrary. The Court asserted that a state has an undeniable interest 'in the protection and preservation of human life' and supported this assertion by noting:

> [T]he majority of States in this country have laws imposing criminal penalties on one who assists another to commit suicide. We do not think a State is required to remain neutral in the face of an informed and voluntary decision by a physically able adult to starve to death.[10]

I share the view that the language quoted above amounts to an endorsement of laws prohibiting assisted suicide (and laws permitting state intervention to prevent suicide).[11]

Cruzan is not the only Supreme Court case on which proponents of a right to assisted suicide rely. They also find support for their views in the Court's abortion cases.[12] In *Roe* v. *Wade*,[13] the Court informed us that 'a right of privacy, or a guarantee of certain areas or zones of privacy,' which had earlier been invoked to invalidate restrictions on the use of contraceptives, 'is broad enough to encompass a woman's decision whether or not to terminate her pregnancy.'[14] The Court cleared the way for its ultimate holding by rejecting the state's argument that 'a fetus is a person' within the meaning of the Constitution – 'the word "person," as used in the Fourteenth Amendment, does not include the unborn.'[15]

Although *Roe* did not concern the termination of a human life, as the Court perceived the matter, the case has been read very broadly to support a 'right' or 'liberty' to commit suicide and to enlist the assistance of others in doing so.[16] So far as I am aware, however, no one who has read *Roe* this broadly has taken into account that later in the same Term the Court rejected the notion that 'our Constitution incorporates the proposition that conduct involving consenting adults only is always beyond state regulation.'[17] It is noted at this point that '[t]he state statute books are replete with constitutionally unchallenged laws against prostitution, suicide . . . and duels, although these crimes may only directly involve "consenting adults."'[18]

The Court must have meant *assisted* suicide, not suicide, for two reasons: (1) suicide itself does not involve consenting adults; and (2) at the time the Court made this observation there were no state laws against suicide, but there were many criminalizing *assisted* suicide.

A plausible argument may be made that the 'right of privacy' which protects a woman's right to terminate her pregnancy, at least in its early stages, includes the 'right' or 'liberty' of a person, at least one terminally ill, to make the choice whether to continue to live until death comes naturally or to hasten death by the use of 'physician-prescribed medications.'[19] But a much more persuasive argument may be made, I believe, that the 'right of privacy' invoked in *Roe* encompasses the autonomy of sexual activity and relationships.

As Justice Blackmun wrote in a much-publicized consensual sodomy case, '[s]exual intimacy is "a sensitive, key relationship of human existence, central to . . . the development of human personality"'; 'individuals define themselves in a significant way through their intimate sexual relationships with others' and 'much of the richness of a relationship will come from the freedom an individual has to *choose* the form and nature of these intensely personal bonds.'[20] But Justice Blackmun wrote in dissent.

A majority of the Court in that case, *Bowers* v. *Hardwick*, upheld the challenged ban against consensual sodomy as applied to homosexuals even though the activity took place in private. *Roe* and other 'right of privacy' cases were explained away on the ground that they involved family, marriage, procreation, contraception and abortion. '[A]ny claim that these cases . . . stand for the proposition that any kind of private sexual conduct between consenting adults is constitutionally insulated from state proscription is unsupportable.'[21]

Robert Sedler, a well-known law professor and one of the lawyers challenging the constitutionality of Michigan's prohibition against assisted suicide, maintains that 'the essence of the "liberty" protected by the due process clause is *personal autonomy*' which, he contends, encompasses a person's right 'to control his or her own body, and to define his or her own existence' (which, he claims, includes the right to end one's existence in accordance with one's principles).[22] How does or can Professor Sedler reconcile his views with *Bowers* v. *Hardwick*, which rejected a similar argument in the context of sexual activities and relationships? A sphere of conduct like that at issue in *Hardwick* seems much closer to marriage, procreation, the use of contraceptives and abortion than the right to assisted suicide. Sedler does not attempt to reconcile his views with *Bowers* v. *Hardwick*. He ignores the case entirely.

COMPARING AND CONTRASTING SUICIDE, ASSISTED SUICIDE AND ACTIVE EUTHANASIA

The right to active voluntary euthanasia

In recent decades we have witnessed a good deal of change in attitudes toward death and dying, especially 'letting die.' But it is no less true today than it ever was that *active* voluntary euthanasia (sometimes called 'consensual homicide') is murder. Although there has long been a high incidence of failures to indict and jury nullification in these cases,[23] the law on the books in every state is clear: If one intentionally and actively kills another, neither the fact that he did so at the deceased's request nor the fact that the defendant was motivated by 'mercy' excuses the homicide. One cannot waive one's right not to be killed.[24]

To be sure, some commentators have forcefully argued that one should be able to waive one's right not to be killed, at least where the person is competent and makes an 'informed' decision that continued existence is no longer desirable or sensible under the circumstances.[25] But to date no American legislature nor any American court has accepted this argument in the context of active voluntary euthanasia.

The right to assisted suicide

Assisted suicide falls somewhere between the termination of life support and active voluntary euthanasia. (More about just where it falls later.) Active voluntary euthanasia occurs when a person other than the one who dies performs the last act – the one that actually brings about death. Assisted suicide takes place when another person provides assistance but the suicidant commits the last act herself. Although the two practices differ with respect to who performs the 'last act,' they are similar in that each involves the active intervention of another person to promote or to bring about death.

As the *Cruzan* Court noted, assisted suicide (although less widely condemned than active voluntary euthanasia) is a crime in a majority of American states. Most of the states that prohibit assisted suicide do so by specific legislation, while some treat it as a form of murder or manslaughter.[26]

Suicide, attempted suicide and assisted suicide

It is often said that since there is a 'right' to commit suicide it follows that there is a right to assisted suicide as well. But I do not think if fitting or proper to speak of *a right* to commit suicide.

Although one usually has the *capacity* to commit suicide, one does not have the *right* to do so. The fact that we no longer punish suicide or attempted suicide does not mean that we *approve* of these acts or that we *recognize* that an individual's right to 'self-determination' or 'personal autonomy' extends this far.

The decriminalization of both suicide and attempted suicide did not come about because suicide was deemed a 'human right' or even because it was no longer considered objectionable. Rather, it occurred because punishment was seen as unfair to innocent relatives of the suicide and because those who committed or attempted to commit the act were thought to be prompted by mental illness.[27] However, the judgment that there is no form of criminal punishment that is acceptable for a completed suicide and that criminal punishment is singularly inefficacious to deter attempts to commit suicide does not mean that there is a 'right' to commit the act. Much less does it mean that one has a justifiable claim to assistance in committing the act.[28]

That criminal punishment was thought to have no deterrent effect on would-be suicides does not mean it would be ineffective in the case of someone considering *assisting another* to commit suicide. And there is good reason to invoke the criminal law in the latter case: '[T]he interests in the sanctity of life' represented by the prohibition against criminal homicide would seem to be 'threatened by one who expresses a willingness to participate in taking the life of another, even though the act may be accomplished with the consent, or at the request of, the suicide victim.'[29]

This, at least, was the judgment of the eminent scholars who drafted the American Law Institute's *Model Penal Code* (hereinafter the Code) in the 1950s and 1960s. The Code is considered 'the principal text in criminal law teaching, the point of departure for criminal law scholarship, and the greatest single influence on the many new state codes that have followed in its wake.'[30]

Although it criminalizes neither suicide nor attempted suicide, it does make *aiding or soliciting another* to commit suicide a felony.[31]

The Code's reporters considered the argument that in certain cases the criminality of assisted suicide should turn upon 'the presence of a selfish motive' – a position advanced by one of its special consultants, Glanville Williams, a renowned British commentator and a leading proponent of assisted suicide and voluntary euthanasia. In the end, however, the reporters concluded that 'the wiser course' in these cases 'is to maintain the prohibition and rely on mitigation in the sentence when the ground for it appears.'[32]

Recently, a proponent of physician-assisted suicide asked: 'How should the law respond when a physician or other person helps an individual do something that is legal in every state, when that legal activity is suicide?'[33] It may be good advocacy to frame the question this way, but to do so strikes me as quite misleading.

As already pointed out, the reasons that led to the decriminalization of suicide and attempted suicide do not apply when one person 'helps' *another* to commit suicide. Although there may be 'a certain moral extravagance in imposing criminal punishment on a person who has sought his own self-destruction [and] who more properly requires medical or psychiatric attention,'[34] self-destruction 'is still a harm to be avoided, not a right to be encouraged.'[35] That is why, despite the fact that suicide itself is no longer a crime, 'helping' *another* commit suicide – if 'help' means 'intentionally providing the physical means' or 'intentionally participat[ing] in a physical act' by which that other person dies by suicide[36] – remains a crime in most states.

WOULD A NARROW EXCEPTION TO CURRENT CRIMINAL PROHIBITIONS REMAIN A NARROW EXCEPTION FOR VERY LONG?

Assisted suicide versus active voluntary euthanasia

Consider the following cases: A competent patient who has clearly made known her wish to die accomplishes her purpose by swallowing a lethal dose of medication which her physician has (*a*) placed under her pillow or on the night table next to her bed; (*b*) placed in her hand; (*c*) put in her mouth. How should we characterize these cases?

It is fairly clear that (*a*) constitutes assisted suicide, but what of cases (*b*) and (*c*)? I would say that (*b*) is also a case of assisted suicide because the lethal process has not yet become irreversible. The patient still has a choice – she could change her mind before putting the medication in her mouth and swallowing it. I think case (*c*) is a very close call, but even here one could argue that this, too, is an act of assisted suicide – if the patient is able to remove the substance from her mouth or spit it out, but instead chooses to swallow it. If so, then even here, one could argue, the patient still retains the final choice.

Lawrence Gostin, the Editor-in-Chief of the *Journal of Law, Medicine and Ethics*, would disagree with me. He would say that both (*b*) and (*c*) should be classified as active euthanasia because in both cases the physician did not merely take part in the events leading up to the commission of the suicide but 'active[ly] participat[ed] in an overt act directly causing death.'[37] (But if this can be said of the physician who puts a lethal dose of medication in a patient's hand, why can it not also be said of the doctor who places the medication within a patient's easy reach?)

Whether one agrees with Gostin or me does not matter very much. What does matter, I think, is that the distinctions among these closely related acts are so fine that reasonable people (if I may include myself in that group) cannot agree on which side they fall.[38]

If so, how can these distinctions be defended on principle or maintained in practice? Once we cross the line between the termination of life support and the active intervention of another to promote or to bring about death, how can we – and why should we – stop short of active voluntary euthanasia?

One who turns to the literature on the law and morality of assisted dying soon discovers that the line between assisted suicide and voluntary euthanasia is often blurred and sometimes completely obliterated. Voluntary euthanasia 'has been variously described as "assisted suicide"' and suicide has sometimes been called 'self-administered euthanasia.'[39] According to one leading writer on the subject, active voluntary euthanasia is 'a form of suicide' and the case for voluntary euthanasia 'depends upon the case for the righteousness of suicide.'[40] Another commentator similarly maintains that 'the permissibility of euthanasia follows from the permissibility of suicide.'[41] Still another considers voluntary euthanasia 'essentially a form of suicide involving the assistance of others.'[42]

The fine distinction between assisted suicide and voluntary euthanasia – who performs the 'last act' – was badly smudged by the hard-fought campaigns in the states of Washington (1991) and California (1992) to legalize physician 'aid-in-dying' – a label covering *both* assisted suicide *and* active voluntary euthanasia.[43] I followed both campaigns very closely and came away with the impression that many members of the media and general public *either* did not understand the distinction between the two practices *or* did not accept it.

Derek Humphry, the founder of the Hemlock Society, has probably written more about the general subject than anyone else, and his books have undoubtedly been read by more people than any others in the field. He uses the terms suicide, assisted suicide, euthanasia and self-deliverance quite loosely and almost interchangeably.

In a recent book, *Dying with Dignity*, Humphry tells his readers that he had 'no knowledge or interest in euthanasia' until he helped his first wife die by furnishing her 'a lethal potion of drugs with which she could end her life at a time chosen by her.'[44] Thirty pages later he describes this incident as a personal 'euthanasia experience.'[45] At another point he tells us that 'justifiable suicide' is 'rational and planned self-deliverance' or 'autoeuthanasia.'[46] Some ninety pages later he recalls that before the advent of Hemlock 'active voluntary euthanasia (also known as self-deliverance and autoeuthanasia) was a taboo subject in America.'[47] In a chapter on 'Euthanasia for the Elite,' he maintains that '*euthanasia* is already widely available to the elite,' because '[w]ell off or well connected people often have medical friends who, in secret, *will pass out lethal drugs* or actually make the injection.'[48]

Some, no doubt, would dismiss Derek Humphry as a 'popularizer.' But then they must deal with the eminent lawyer-philosopher, Ronald Dworkin. On the opening page of his new book, *Life's Dominion*, Professor Dworkin observes:

> The argument over *euthanasia* has suddenly exploded into front-page news. Doctors are now beginning openly to admit what the profession once kept secret: that doctors sometimes kill patients who ask to die, *or help such patients to kill themselves*.[49]

Then, to illustrate his point that *euthanasia* 'has provoked intense controversy' not only in the Netherlands but in America and elsewhere, Dworkin discusses two cases. The first involves a New York physician who 'prescribed lethal drugs for a leukemia patient and told her how many she should take to die.' The second involves a British doctor who 'injected potassium chloride [a drug that has no analgesic effect] into a rheumatoid arthritis patient . . . begging to be killed.'[50] Some 180 pages later, Professor Dworkin discusses the British case again. He then turns to what he calls 'a similar case' – the aforementioned New York case.[51] I think it fair to say that the fact that the British doctor performed active euthanasia and that the American doctor only helped his patient commit suicide (and, arguably, provided a relatively low level of assistance at that)[52] does not interest Dworkin. What does seem to bother him is that the British doctor was convicted of attempted murder while the American doctor, who was involved in 'a similar case,' was not even prosecuted.

Even if one believes (as Dworkin, Humphry and others evidently do not) that there is an important distinction between assisted suicide and active voluntary euthanasia in principle, it will be extremely difficult to contain that principle in any subsequent litigation or to adhere to the distinction in practice.

If a patient's inability to commit suicide 'for either physiological or psychological reasons' entitles her under certain circumstances to the active intervention of another person in order to bring about her death,[53] why should not a patient's inability – *despite* preliminary assistance – to perform the last death-causing act, for either physiological or psychological reasons, entitle her to active voluntary euthanasia? If assisted suicide is appropriate when patients 'need more help from the physician than merely abating treatment, but less help than would be required if they were asking the physician to kill them,'[54] why is not active voluntary euthanasia appropriate when less help than 'killing them' would *not* suffice, when patients are unable to perform the ultimate act and thus nothing less than 'killing them' *is* required to 'help' them die an 'easy' death?

Suppose a patient is unable to swallow the pills that will bring about her death or is otherwise too weak to perform the last act that will fulfill her persistent wish to die. If there is or ought to be a right to assisted suicide, how can it be denied to such a person simply because she lacks the physical capacity to perform the final act by herself?

Dr Timothy Quill, who helped a long-standing patient die by suicide, does believe in drawing a line between assisted suicide and voluntary euthanasia,[55] but even he has a difficult time adhering to that line. Quill tells, approvingly, a 'moving story' about a physician who prescribed barbiturates to a patient in an advanced stage of AIDS but who did not 'abandon his patient' when this help proved inadequate:

> The patient wanted to take the barbiturates he had saved for an overdose, but was too weak to feed them to himself. Faced with this moment of truth, the doctor helped his patient swallow the pills.[56]

Can (should) the right to assisted suicide be confined to the terminally ill? To those suffering unbearable pain?

One can understand an argument without accepting it. I understand the basic argument for assisted suicide (and perhaps active voluntary euthanasia as well): Life has value only so long as it has meaning for the person whose life it is and respect for 'self-determination' and 'personal autonomy' should entitle a competent person to decide for herself whether, when and how she chooses to end her life. If this argument is convincing, however, I have great difficulty understanding why the 'right' or 'liberty' to assisted suicide should be limited to the 'terminally ill' and/or those suffering unbearable pain.

If one is trying to establish a right to assisted suicide it is good tactics to frame the issue narrowly – to speak, for example, only of a right to assisted suicide *for the terminally ill*. Thus, lawyers for the American Civil Liberties Union (ACLU) have challenged the constitutionality of Michigan's ban on assisted suicide *insofar as it prohibits terminally ill patients* from committing suicide by making use of physician-prescribed medications.[57] But is there any principled way to so limit the right? If either autonomy or the merciful termination of an unendurable existence is the basis for this right, why limit it to the terminally ill?

First of all, 'there is, in fact, no consensus on what is a "terminal condition."'[58] For example, although many states still define such a condition as one that will shortly result in death *regardless* of the utilization of available medical treatment, several states have recently adopted provisions defining the condition as one that will soon cause death in *the absence* of medical intervention.[59] Even if we could all agree on a definition of 'terminal condition,' however, 'under a variety of circumstances life may be unendurable to a reasonable person, even though he does not face the prospect of immediate and painful death.'[60]

Timothy Quill, one of the most eloquent proponents of physician-assisted suicide, would limit the right in various ways, but he would not confine it to the terminally ill. The patient must have a condition, he tells us, 'that is incurable and *associated* with severe, unrelenting suffering.'[61] Dr Quill does 'not want to *arbitrarily* exclude persons with incurable, but not imminently terminal progressive illness, such as ALS (motoneurone disease) or multiple sclerosis.'[62] But is it any less arbitrary to exclude the quadriplegic? The victim of a paralytic stroke? A person afflicted with severe arthritis?

If personal autonomy and the termination of suffering are the key factors fueling the right to assisted suicide, why exclude those with non-terminal illnesses or disabilities who might have to endure greater 'unbearable suffering' for much longer periods of time than those who are likely to die in the near future? Why does not a person who must continue to live what she considers an unendurable existence for ten or twenty more years have an equal – or even greater – claim on the liberty interest in assisted suicide than those with terminal conditions?[63]

In an effort to distinguish the terminally ill from all others who might seek death by suicide, Professor Sedler maintains that 'the state cannot assert any valid interest' in requiring a terminally ill person to wait until death comes naturally because '*there can be no valid interest in "preserving life" when there is no "life left to preserve."*'[64] I really do not understand this argument.

Surely, Sedler is not saying that one who is terminally ill is no longer a 'person' or a 'human being'? Such a person may have a number of months to live (a common definition of terminal illness is six months or less to live) and her mental powers can hardly be substantially impaired if she 'chooses' to die by suicide. For the present, at ieast, Sedler and his confrères are not contending that persons who are *no longer competent* should have a right to assisted suicide. Thus, if they prevail, and their ground rules are adopted, assisted suicide could take place only if the person seeking such a death retains sufficient decision-making capacity to exercise a voluntary, competent choice. How can it be said that such a person has 'no "life left to preserve"'?

Of course, such a person may *feel* or honestly *believe* that her life is not a 'life' worth preserving. But so too may many others who suffer from debilitating illnesses or severe disabilities, but who are not terminally ill.

As I understand the position of those advocating a constitutional right to assisted suicide, one should have the same right to enlist the aid of others in dying by suicide as one presently has to refuse or to withdraw life-sustaining medical treatment.[65] If so, it is fairly clear that once established the right to assisted suicide would not be restricted to the terminally ill. For, as demonstrated by the *Elizabeth Bouvia* case and other decisions involving quadriplegics who apparently had long life expectancies, the right to refuse or to reject medical treatment has not been so limited.[66] (Nor, for that matter, has it been limited to the presently competent.)

Another restriction often placed on the right to assisted suicide is that the person asserting this right must be experiencing 'intractable pain' or undergoing 'unbearable suffering.' At first blush this appears to be a small, easily identifiable group. But a closer look reveals this is not so.

First of all, although 'pain' and 'suffering' are often lumped together, the two classifications are not identical. 'Not all pain leads to suffering (the pain of the victorious distance runner leads to pleasure), nor does suffering require the presence of physical pain (the anguish of knowing one has Alzheimer's disease).'[67]

If 'pain and suffering' means or includes physical pain, experts in the field maintain that, although pain is admittedly notoriously undertreated in America,[68] 'almost all terminally ill patients can experience adequate relief with currently available treatment.'[69] Thus a renowned pain control expert, the Memorial Sloan-Kettering Cancer Center's Kathleen Foley, reports:

> We frequently see patients referred to our Pain Clinic who have considered suicide as an option, or who request physician-assisted suicide because of uncontrolled pain. We commonly see such ideation and request dissolve with adequate control of pain and other symptoms, using combinations of pharmacologic, neurosurgical, anesthetic or psychological approaches.[70]

To be sure, '[d]ying patients often undergo substantial psychological suffering that is not fully or even principally the result of physical pain.'[71] But suffering 'has no objective correlation with a patient's (medical) condition'[72] – it is 'variable from person to person' and 'externally unverifiable.'[73]

If a right to assisted suicide were established, how could this right be denied an otherwise qualified candidate who *says* her pain or suffering is 'unbearable'? As a practical matter, would we not defer to the patient's own assessment of her pain or suffering? As a matter of principle, shouldn't we?

So long as a person is competent and her desire to enlist the aid of others in dying by suicide is firm and persistent, why should her 'right' to end her life in the manner she chooses (if such a right exists) be denied because her condition does not satisfy someone else's standard of suffering?

Once a right to assisted suicide is established, any requirement that the patient experience intolerable suffering will probably turn on the patient's own view of her suffering – or drop out entirely. In a sense, the requirement has *already* dropped out. The Washington and California proposals to legalize 'physician aid-in-dying' required only that a 'qualified patient' be afflicted with a terminal illness and express an enduring request for physician intervention. Of course, such a patient need not be suffering from a *painful* terminal illness or, if she is, might be receiving analgesic medications that, even by the patient's own admission, adequately relieve her physical pain.

As ethicist Albert Jonsen recently observed, the language of legislative proposals, such as those defeated in Washington and in California, is strong evidence that 'fear of uncontrolled pain' (and, I would add, 'unbearable suffering')

> is no longer a major feature of the justifying arguments [for 'aid-in-dying']. Autonomy, not pain or its merciful alleviation, is the principal and even sole justifying argument offered by modern proponents. Opponents who argue, as in the Washington and California campaigns, that modern methods of pain control can virtually eliminate the category of 'intractable' pain are correct enough, but they miss the mark: the right to choose death, not the presence of pain, is now the issue.[74]

THE NEED FOR A COURT TO CONSIDER THE BROAD IMPLICATIONS OF A 'NARROW' RIGHT TO ASSISTED SUICIDE FOR THE TERMINALLY ILL

Professor Sedler tells us that the constitutional challenge he and his ACLU colleagues have mounted against Michigan's anti-assisted suicide law is 'specific and narrow' – whether the law is invalid *insofar as* it prohibits the terminally ill from obtaining medications from physicians that will enable them to commit suicide – and that the courts should address only this particular issue.[75] Indeed, he goes so far as to say that the kind of 'slippery slope' arguments I have made have 'no place' in constitutional litigation and cannot be utilized 'to avoid' facing and confronting the specific question he and his colleague have framed.[76]

I could not disagree with him more. I do not believe a court can *responsibly* face and confront the 'narrow' issue presented *without* considering the general implications of the asserted right – without taking into account the 'slippery slope' arguments I have made (if one wants to call them that).

I have contended that drawing a line between the terminally ill and other seriously ill or disabled persons (who may have to endure more pain and suffering for a much longer period of time) is neither sensible nor principled. I have maintained, too, that the same may be said for drawing a line between assisted suicide (for those who need some assistance from a physician) and active voluntary euthanasia (for those who need a physician to perform the last, death-causing act). Is a judge supposed to put on blinders and forge straight ahead without thinking about the consequences and ramifications of her 'narrow' and 'specific' holding? Is this the way we are supposed to go about resolving constitutional issues?

As the three justices who played the decisive role in reaffirming *Roe* v. *Wade* observed:

> Consistent with other constitutional norms, legislatures may draw lines which appear arbitrary without the necessity of offering a justification. But courts may not. We must justify the lines we draw.[77]

An eminent constitutional law professor, Herbert Wechsler, has felicitously spelled out this important point:

> [T]he main constituent of the judicial process is precisely that it must be genuinely principled, resting with respect to every step that is involved in reaching judgment on analysis and reasons quite transcending the immediate result that is achieved. To be sure, the courts decide, or should decide, only the case they have before them. But must they not decide on grounds of adequate neutrality and generality, tested not only by the instant application but by others that the principles imply?[78]

Professor Sedler is unable to find any 'principled difference' in the applicable constitutional doctrine between 'the right of *a terminally ill* person' to withhold or to withdraw life-sustaining medical treatment and the right of such a person to enlist the aid of a physician in committing suicide.[79] It is now fairly clear, however, that the fact that a person may be kept alive for many years (for example, a respirator-dependent quadriplegic whose mental powers are unimpaired) is not a sufficient reason to deny her the right or liberty to terminate life support.[80] Why, then, if a right to assisted suicide exists for the terminally ill, should it be denied to those who may be kept alive for many years? Whatever the answer, is it not appropriate for a judge to consider this question *before* deciding whether there is a right to assisted suicide for the terminally ill?

In arguing that there is a right to personal autonomy that encompasses the right to assisted suicide, Professor Sedler and his colleagues rely very heavily on the US Supreme Court's abortion cases. Physician-assisted suicide was not, of course, the issue before the Court in any of those cases. If it is appropriate to transcend the 'narrow' and 'specific' issue presented in a case *once* it is decided, and to dwell instead – and to build on – its broad implications, why is it improper to *anticipate* the implications of a *soon-to-be decided* case and to call the court's attention to them?

That a proponent of the right to assisted suicide would speak only of – and wish the courts to think only about – such a right *for the terminally ill* is quite understandable. Such a narrowly circumscribed claim causes less alarm and commands more general support than does a broader right to assisted suicide. And, as Justice Frankfurter once observed, 'the function of an advocate is to seduce.'[81]

But the function of a court is to resist seduction, to rest its judgment on a principle of general significance that may be consistently applied, and to produce an intellectually coherent reason for a result which in *like cases* will produce *a like result*. If so, how can a conscientious judge *avoid* considering what *other* fact situations not presently before the court are (or are not) like cases? If I may quote Justice Frankfurter a second time:

> I am aware that we must decide the case before us and not some other case. But that does not mean that a case is dissociated from the past and unrelated to the future. We must decide this case with due regard for what went before and no less regard for what may come after.[82]

Robert Sedler is part constitutional law commentator and part constitutional litigator. In his first article on the subject Sedler-the-litigator appeared to dominate – he refused to consider whether a right to assisted suicide would or should extend beyond terminally ill persons. But in a more recent article, Sedler-the-commentator seems to have come to the fore – this time Professor Sedler does address the issue. He concludes that the right would and should be available not only to those who have 'no life left to preserve' (his characterization of the terminally ill), but to some who do have 'life left to preserve' (for example, the person debilitated by multiple sclerosis who may live for several additional years).[83] Comments Sedler:

> The claim of the multiple sclerosis victim that for him life has become unendurable, like the claim of the terminally ill person seeking to hasten inevitable death, is objectively reasonable . . . [S]ince the multiple sclerosis victim is helpless to bring about his own death, a ban on physician assistance to enable him to die so is obviously an undue burden on his right to end an unendurable life.[84]

Is Sedler's claim that there is or ought to be a right to assisted suicide for the terminally ill at bottom only one aspect of a claim that there is or ought to be such a right for any competent adult whose wish to die by suicide is 'objectively reasonable'? If so, why stop with the victim of multiple sclerosis? As already pointed out, there are all sorts of reasons why life may seem intolerable to a *reasonable* person.[85] 'To argue that suicide is rational to escape physical pain [or, I would add, to end a physically debilitated life], but not suicide for any other reason, is to show oneself out of touch with the depth and complexity of human motives.'[86] Moreover, all sorts of seriously ill or severely disabled persons may have an 'objectively reasonable' wish to die, though they may be physically or psychologically unable to bring about their own deaths. They, too, may need someone else to perform the 'last act.'

How do we go about determining whether a competent person's firm conclusion that life has become 'intolerable' is 'objectively reasonable'? Do we turn to the writings of philosophers (many of whom are in disagreement on this point)? Do we conduct opinion polls?

Moreover, if self-determination or personal autonomy is the major force driving the right to assisted suicide, why should a competent person's firm conclusion that life has become unendurable for her *have to be* 'objectively reasonable'? Why should not a competent person's *own evaluation* of her situation suffice?

I think it noteworthy that when a Michigan trial judge recently held that there is a constitutional right to assisted suicide – so far as I am aware, the first American court squarely ever to do so – he drew a line *neither* (*a*) between terminally ill people seeking to die by suicide and others wishing to do so *nor* (*b*) between those experiencing severe 'pain and suffering' and others whose pain and suffering was, or could be brought, under control. It is to this decision that I now turn.

THE MICHIGAN EXPERIENCE

In February 1993, shortly after the number of people Jack Kevorkian had helped to commit suicide had risen to fifteen, the Michigan legislature passed a law making assisted suicide a felony, punishable by up to four years in prison. The new law prohibits one with knowledge that another person intends to commit suicide from 'intentionally providing the physical means' by which that other person does so or from 'intentionally participat[ing] in a physical act' by which she does so.[87]

The law contains a number of exceptions. It recognizes the right to reject unwanted medical treatment, even life-sustaining procedures, by specifically excluding 'withholding or withdrawing medical treatment' from its coverage. It also recognizes the principle of 'double effect' – that there is a significant distinction between the intended effects of one's actions and the unintended though foreseen effects. It does so by exempting 'prescribing, dispensing or administering' medication or treatment designed 'to relieve pain or discomfort and not to cause death, even if the medication or procedure may hasten or increase the risk of death.' (Of course, if the medication administered *were* designed to cause death, at the patient's request, it would be a case of active voluntary euthanasia.)

These provisions led a prominent authority on legal issues in medicine, George Annas, to say that, given its exceptions, the Michigan law was likely to withstand constitutional challenge.[88] I would have put it even more strongly. But before the year was out, in *People* v. *Kevorkian*, Wayne County Circuit Judge Richard Kaufman ruled that the law violated the constitutionally protected 'right' or 'liberty' to assisted suicide.[89]

According to Judge Kaufman, (*a*) under certain conditions a competent adult has a right to commit 'rational' suicide and (*b*) a total ban against assisted suicide 'unduly burdens' this right.[90] Although the right is limited, it is not confined to the 'terminally ill.' Nor does it require unendurable 'pain and suffering.' Indeed, Judge Kaufman made no effort to distinguish between those experiencing intolerable pain and suffering and those whose pain or suffering was, or could be brought, under control.

The key factor, according to Judge Kaufman, is the presence or absence of 'an objective medical condition' that is 'extremely unlikely to improve.' If a person's quality of life is significantly impaired by such a medical condition, even though it is not a life-threatening condition (presumably blindness, the loss of a hand or permanent paralysis of a part of the body), and her decision is made without undue influence, she may avail herself of the newly discovered right. But if a person's quality of life is significantly diminished for any other reason (for example, disgrace, financial ruin, the loss of one's entire family in an airplane crash), she may not invoke the right – no matter how competent she is or how firm and persistent her desire to die.

Many in the media reported that Judge Kaufman had drawn a line between 'rational' assisted suicide (which a state cannot prohibit) and the 'irrational' kind (which a state may prevent). But this is not quite accurate. At one point in his opinion, Judge Kaufman did express the view that 'if an adequate, meaningful line can be drawn between rational and irrational suicide, the liberty provision of the Due Process Clause protects a person's decision to commit rational suicide.'[91] But the line he ultimately drew is *not* a line between 'rational' and 'irrational' suicide. Rather, it is a line between *one category* of 'rational' suicide – would-be suicides whose lives are significantly impaired by irreversible medical conditions – and *other* categories of 'rational' suicide.

Judge Kaufman did not say that a suicide by one whose life is substantially impaired by a medical condition constitutes the only form of 'rational' suicide. He concluded, however, that such suicides are the only ones that may *safely* be afforded constitutional protection.

This is the line that must be drawn, Judge Kaufman told us, 'since any form of *rational* suicide that did not include the presence of an objective medical condition would be *too close* to irrational suicide.'[92] If constitutional protection were extended to *all* persons who have a rational wish to die 'the possibility that irrational suicide would increase is too great.'[93] Thus, the state may prohibit not only 'irrational' suicide and assisted suicide, but some classes of 'rational' suicide and assisted suicide as well – those 'where no objective medical condition is present.'

In his extensive discussion of the 'rationality' of suicide, Judge Kaufman relied heavily on the writings of Alfred Alvarez (an historian of attitudes toward suicide) and Richard Brandt (a prominent American philosopher). So far as I can tell, however, neither commentator would draw the line where Judge Kaufman did. For example, in a passage that Judge Kaufman quotes with apparent approval, Professor Brandt observes:

> If we look over a list of the problems that bother people, and some of which various writers have regarded as good and sufficient reasons for ending life, one finds (in addition to serious illness) things like the following: some event which has made one feel ashamed or has cost one loss of prestige and status; reduction to poverty as compared with former affluence; the loss of a limb or physical beauty; the loss of sexual capacity; some event which makes it seem impossible that one will achieve things by which one sets store; loss of a loved one; disappointment in love; the infirmities of increasing age. It is not to be denied that such things can be serious blows to one's prospects of happiness.[94]

After discussing the views of the ancient Greeks and Romans, the Old Testament and early Christian doctrine, Judge Kaufman concludes that 'there is significant support in our traditions and history for the view approving suicide or attempted suicide.'[95] If Judge Kaufman is right about this (though I doubt that he is), his own opinion makes plain that such historical support was not limited to suicide by those whose quality of life was significantly impaired by an objective medical condition. Thus, in a passage that Judge Kaufman quotes, Alfred Alvarez observes:

> According to Justinian's *Digest* suicide of a private citizen [during Roman times] was not punishable if it was caused by 'impatience of pain or sickness, *or by another cause*,' or by *weariness of life* . . . lunacy, or *fear of dishonor*. Since this covered *every rational cause*, all that was left was the utterly irrational suicide 'without cause,' and that was punishable . . . [96]

In the course of his opinion, Judge Kaufman sets forth and rejects an argument I made in a recent article – that the social sanctioning of 'rational' suicide and assisted suicide is likely to lead to an increase in 'irrational' (or coerced or 'manipulated') suicide and assisted suicide.[97] He dismisses this argument on the ground that I did not provide any support for it. 'Couldn't one as effectively claim,' asks Kaufman, 'that by drawing a clear legal line between rational suicide and irrational suicide, the stigma of committing irrational suicide would increase?'[98]

Is this line of reasoning persuasive? Does it find any support in our recent experience with the 'right to die'? Until the recent legal assault on laws prohibiting assisted suicide, many of us thought we *had* drawn a fairly clear legal line – between the refusal or rejection of life-sustaining medical treatment and the active intervention of another to promote or to bring about death. So far as I know, however, nobody has suggested that drawing such a line has *increased the stigma* of assisted suicide or active voluntary euthanasia. Quite the contrary. At this very moment the firmly established right to refuse or to withdraw medical treatment is being used as a lever – as an argument for expanding the 'right to die' to include assisted suicide and active voluntary euthanasia as well.[99]

Does Judge Kaufman (or anybody else for that matter) really believe that affording constitutional protection to one form of 'rational' suicide and assisted suicide will *increase the stigma* attaching to 'irrational' suicide? (Or the stigma associated with other forms of 'rational' suicide?)

In writing the article Judge Kaufman quotes from, I relied heavily on the studies of geriatric psychiatrists (who work with suicidal people every day) and suicidologists (who perform 'psychological autopsies' of people who commit suicide). They report that a suicide rarely occurs in the absence of a major psychiatric disorder and that this observation is equally true in suicides among the elderly.[100] More significant for our purposes, these experts underscore the inability of depressed persons to recognize the severity of their own symptoms and the failure of primary physicians to detect major depression, especially in elderly patients.[101]

'Ageism' – the prejudices and stereotypes applied to the elderly solely on the basis of their age – may manifest itself in a failure to recognize treatable depression, the view that an elderly person's desire to commit suicide is more 'rational' than a younger person's would be, or, more generally, the attitude that the elder has every reason to be depressed.[102] As one authority has pointed out: 'Although we shrink from the idea of elderly suicide and euthanasia, we encourage it by our neglect and indifference.'[103] As another commentator has observed:

> Suicidal persons are succumbing to what they experience as an overpowering and unrelenting coercion in their environment to cease living. This sense of coercion takes many familiar forms: fear, isolation, abuse, uselessness, and so on.[104]

Is it not fair to assume, as I do, that these pressures will intensify in a society that sanctions assisted suicide (and thereby suicide as well)? Is it not fair to assume that once assisted suicide is a lawful alternative and people are 'doing it' and free to talk about it, more people, especially the sick and the old and the vulnerable, will see this as the unselfish course to take – a tempting way to spare both oneself and one's family the burdens of serious illness and/or advanced age?

Of course, I cannot *prove* that in a suicide-permissive society a substantial number of people who otherwise would not have pursued this route will be encouraged or pressured or 'manipulated' into choosing death by suicide or assisted suicide.[105] But then Judge Kaufman offers no support for his view that if a line were not drawn 'requir[ing] the presence of objective medical findings, the possibility that irrational suicide would increase is too great.'[106]

If a judge can deny constitutional protection to *some* forms of 'rational' assisted suicide out of concern that if he did not do so 'irrational' assisted suicide might get out of hand, why can a legislature not prohibit *all* forms of 'rational' assisted suicide on the same ground? If a judge may give weight to the writings of philosophers in arriving at his conclusions about the 'rationality' of suicide (Judge Kaufman quotes philosopher Richard Brandt six times, three times at considerable length), why can a legislature not rely on the studies and published findings of suicidologists and geriatric psychiatrists to reach a different conclusion?

After all, as one commentator said (and I am happy to report that he is a philosopher):

> If philosophers have something to say to the law, so also has the law something to say to philosophers. Attention to the working, or the possible working, of any institution or principle may well give us insight into weaknesses which remain concealed so long as it is posed in sufficiently abstract terms.[107]

SOME FINAL THOUGHTS

When I first wrote about this subject, thirty-six years ago, the chance that any state would legalize active voluntary euthanasia seemed minuscule and the possibility that any court would find the right of active voluntary euthanasia protected by the Due Process Clause seemed so remote as to be almost inconceivable. Not any more.

Before this decade ends I believe there is (*a*) a strong probability that at least several states will decriminalize active voluntary euthanasia (no doubt under the euphemistic label 'aid-in-dying'); and (*b*) a distinct possibility that at least several appellate courts will announce a state or federal constitutional right to active voluntary euthanasia. I continue to believe the US Supreme Court will not discover or recognize such a right, but the possibility that it may can no longer be disregarded.

What we cannot do in one step – perhaps even think about doing – we can often do in two or three or four. The modern history of our activities and beliefs about the law and ethics of death and dying is a good illustration – it is 'a history of lost distinctions of former significance'[108] (e.g. 'extraordinary means' versus 'ordinary means,' the respirator versus the feeding tube).

My colleague Carl Schneider has called this step-by-step process 'a psychological aspect of slippery slopes': They work partly by 'domesticating one idea' (say, disconnecting the respirator) and thus making its nearest neighbor (terminating 'artificial' feeding) 'seem less extreme and unthinkable.'[109]

What many used to call 'negative' or 'passive' euthanasia has become a *fait accompli* in modern medicine. The next sequence of events is likely to be physician-assisted suicide for (*a*) the terminally ill, (*b*) those with an 'objective medical condition' that significantly diminishes the quality of life, and (*c*) those whose wish to die is 'objectively reasonable.' If so, as this progression unfolds, active voluntary euthanasia will become more thinkable, more tenable and more supportable.

Proponents of an expansive 'right to die' have had considerable success in overcoming resistance step by step, blotting out one distinction after another. And there is no reason to think that this process will come to a halt. One important distinction remains – and it is *not* the distinction between assisted suicide and active voluntary euthanasia. As I have tried to show, this distinction is too thin to endure for very long. Indeed, even now, it is a distinction that the media, the public and even many commentators on the subject are either unable or unwilling to take seriously.

The one formidable distinction that remains is the one that is presently under attack – 'the historic divide'[110] between the termination of medical treatment and the active intervention of another to promote or to bring about death. If opponents of active voluntary euthanasia are unable to defend the bridge spanning this divide, they will have lost the war. For if this bridge falls, the flimsy bridge between assisted suicide and active voluntary euthanasia seems sure to follow.

AFTERWORD

In April 1994 I finished my chapter and sent it to the editor of this collection for publication. But the next 20 months turned out to be an extraordinarily eventful time for those interested in the law, politics and ethics of assisted suicide.

In May 1994, the Chief Judge of the US District Court in Seattle, Washington, Barbara Rothstein, became the first federal judge to strike down a statute outlawing assisted suicide on Fourteenth Amendment due process grounds. In *Compassion in Dying v. Washington*,[111] she invalidated a Washington state law prohibiting assisted suicide in so far as it placed an undue burden on competent, terminally ill adults who seek physician-assisted suicide. From a constitutional perspective, concluded Judge Rothstein, there is no meaningful distinction between the right to refuse or to withdraw medical treatment – a course of action that results in death – and the right of a competent, terminally ill person to achieve the same end by using drugs prescribed or provided by a physician.

Until Judge Rothstein's ruling only one other American court, a Michigan trial court, had ever held that there is a constitutional right to assisted suicide.[112] But seven months later, in *People v. Kevorkian*[113] a 5–2 majority of the Michigan Supreme Court held that there was no constitutional right to, or liberty interest in, assisted suicide, explicitly rejecting the analysis utilized in *Compassion in Dying*.[114] The fact that within the space of seven months a federal district court and a state supreme court reached opposite conclusions as to whether one has a constitutionally protected 'right' or 'liberty' to obtain a physician's assistance in committing suicide indicated that American courts would disagree about the issue until the US Supreme Court resolved it. But two events occurred in 1994 that may have a significant impact on how the constitutional issue is ultimately resolved:

The New York State Task Force Report

On 25 May 1994, the 24-member New York State Task Force on Life and the Law issued a 181-page report unanimously rejecting proposals to legalize assisted suicide and active voluntary euthanasia.[115] 'In light of the pervasive failure of our health care system to treat pain and diagnose and treat depression,' concluded the Task Force, 'legalizing assisted suicide and euthanasia would be profoundly dangerous for many individuals who are ill and vulnerable.'[116] The risks would be greatest, continued the Task Force, 'for those who are elderly, poor, socially disadvantaged, or without access to good medical care.'[117]

Although some of the Task Force members were of the view that assisted suicide and euthanasia are inherently wrong, others were not.[118] But even members of this second group concluded that legalizing assisted suicide 'would be unwise and dangerous public policy.'[119] They regarded 'the consequences of quietly tolerating assisted suicide as a private act of agreement between two individuals in extreme cases as profoundly different from the consequences of legalizing the practice.'[120]

The US Supreme Court is likely to be influenced significantly by the Task Force's thoughtful discussion of the 'state of vulnerability' produced by serious illness; the uncertainty in estimating a patient's life expectancy and the fallibility of medical practice generally; the severe shortcomings of current pain relief practices and palliative care; the very small number of individuals who make an informed, competent choice to die by suicide (particularly if appropriate pain relief and supportive care are provided) and cannot achieve their goal without another person's assistance; and the recognition that assisted suicide and euthanasia 'will be practiced through the prism of social inequality and prejudice that characterizes the delivery of services in all segments of society, including health care.'[121]

To be sure, any American legislature remains free to reject the Task Force report as a matter of public policy.[122] But how can it be said that a legislature that is impressed by the same *non*religious arguments against assisted suicide that influenced the Task Force and reaches the same conclusions the Task Force did has acted *unconstitutionally*?

Oregon legalizes physician-assisted suicide

After losing two hard-fought campaigns in the states of Washington (1991) and California (1992),[123] proponents of assisted suicide achieved some success in Oregon. In November 1994 Oregon voters approved a measure

(Ballot Measure 16) permitting physicians, under certain conditions, to prescribe lethal medication for competent, terminally ill patients, who request it.[124]

Although the Oregon vote was a victory for advocates of physician-assisted suicide, this development may cut *against* the establishment of a constitutional right or liberty to assisted suicide. For one thing, the vote demonstrates again that when American voters actually cast their ballots, they are closely divided on the issue: The more extensive Washington and California proposals failed by a 54–46% vote; the more limited Oregon proposal barely passed by a 51–49% margin. Moreover, the fact that proponents of assisted suicide finally gained a victory in one state might lead a Justice who *favors* some form of physician-assisted suicide as a matter of public policy to *decline* to constitutionalize the area. He or she might do so on the ground that judicial intervention at this time might halt a political process that is viewed as moving in the right direction and might increase divisiveness and defer stable settlement of the issue.[125]

As one leading *proponent* of physician-assisted suicide recently observed:

> Legalizing of physician-assisted suicide should be understood not as a matter of recognizing rights but as a policy aimed at making available a compassionate option of last resort for competent, terminally ill patients. Since we do not know whether such a policy will produce more good than harm, it should be viewed as an experiment . . .
>
> . . . Regardless of the ultimate judicial outcome, the Oregon referendum legalizing physician-assisted suicide is virtually certain to be implemented. One or more states will likely follow suit. With competent evaluate research we will be in a position to deliberate whether this policy experiment proves to be a success.[126]

Although 1994 seemed to be a most eventful year for those interest in the law and ethics governing death and dying, the events of that year were dwarfed by the momentous occurrences of 1996.

Until 1996, no American appellate court, state or federal, had ever held that there was a constitutional right to assisted suicide (no matter how narrow the circumstances or stringent the conditions). But in the spring of 1996 – within the span of a single month – two federal courts of appeals so held – an 8–3 majority of the Ninth Circuit (sitting *en banc*) in *Compassion in Dying v. Washington*[127] and a three-judge panel of the Second Circuit in *Quill v. Vacco*.[128] In October 1996 the US Supreme Court announced that it would review both cases.[129] (Oral arguments were presented in January 1997 and a decision is expected by June.)

Compassion in Dying v. Washington

The *Compassion in Dying* majority concluded first that 'there is a constitutionally-protected liberty interest in determining the time and manner of one's own death.'[130] After weighing this individual interest against the state's countervailing interests (such as the state's general interest in preserving life, its more specific interest in preventing suicide, and its interest in protecting the integrity of the medical profession), the court arrived at its next conclusion: Insofar as a Washington statute totally banning assisted suicide 'prohibited physicians from prescribing life-ending medication for use by terminally ill, competent adults who wish to hasten their own deaths, [the statue] violates the Due Process Clause.'[131]

The Ninth Circuit could see 'no ethical or constitutionally cognizable difference between a doctor's pulling the plug on a respirator and his prescribing drugs which will permit a terminally ill person to end his own life.'[132] Thus, the court found 'the state's interests in preventing suicide do not make its interests substantially stronger here than in cases involving other forms of death-hastening medical intervention.'[133]

I think the Ninth Circuit went awry by lumping together two different kinds of 'rights to die.'[134] It failed to realize that the right to forgo unwanted medical treatment and the right to enlist the assistance of a physician in committing suicide are not merely *sub*categories of *the same* broad right or liberty interest – controlling the time and manner of one's death.[135]

Until the ruling in *Compassion in Dying*, the so-called 'right to die' meant only a 'right against intrusion,'[136] a right to resist 'a direct invasion of bodily integrity, and in some cases, the use of physical restraints, both of which are flatly inconsistent with society's basic conception of personal dignity.'[137] To be sure, a total prohibition against assisted suicide does close an 'avenue of escape,' but, unlike a refusal to honor a competent patient's request to terminate life-sustaining treatment, it does not force one into 'a particular, all-consuming, totally dependent, and indeed rigidly standardized life: the life of one confined to a hospital bed, attached to medical machinery, and tended to by medical professionals.'[138]

Not only would a prohibition against rejecting life-sustaining treatment impose a more onerous burden on persons affected than does a ban against assisted suicide, it would also impair the autonomy of a great many more people. More than three-fourths of the two million people who die in this country every year do so in hospitals and long-term care institutions and most of these individuals die 'after a decision to forgo life-sustaining treatment has been made.'[139] If life-sustaining treatment could not be rejected, vast numbers of patients would be 'at the mercy of every technological advance.'[140]

Moreover, if patients could refuse potentially lifesaving treatment at the outset but not discontinue the treatment once it went into effect, many patients probably would not seek such treatment in the first place.[141]

In short, allowing a patient to die at some point is a practical condition upon the successful operation of medicine. The same can hardly be said of physician-assisted suicide or physician-administered active voluntary euthanasia.

Quill v. Vacco

Although the Second Circuit, which decided *Quill v. Vacco*, summarily rejected the Ninth Circuit's due process analysis,[142] it, too, found a constitutional right to, or liberty interest in, assisted suicide by invoking another provision of the Fourteenth Amendment – the Equal Protection Clause.

The *Quill* court was no more impressed than the *Compassion* court had been with the 'action-inaction distinction' or, more specifically, the difference between 'allowing nature to take its course, even in the most severe situations, and intentionally using an artificial death-producing device.'[143] Indeed, the *Quill* court went a step further. What it considered to be the moral and legal identity of these two means of hastening death became the crux of its equal protection analysis.

The Equal Protection Clause, the *Quill* court reminded us, 'directs that "all persons similarly circumstanced shall be treated alike," '[144] but New York had not done so: terminally ill persons on life support systems 'are allowed to hasten their death by directing the removal of such systems,' but persons off life support who are 'similarly situated' except for being attached to life-saving equipment 'are not allowed to hasten death by self-administering prescribed drugs.'[145]

The *Quill* court would have us believe that, much like the person who had been speaking prose all his life without knowing it, many physicians and other health professionals have been helping people commit suicide almost every day of their professional lives without realizing it:

> The ending of life [by the withdrawal of life support] *is nothing more nor less than assisted suicide*. It simply cannot be said that those mentally competent, terminally-ill persons who seek to hasten death but whose treatment does not include life support are treated equally.[146]

As noted earlier,[147] most of the two million people who die every year in this country do so after refusing some form of medical intervention. 'Under the [*Quill*] court's logic,' observes George Annas, 'there is an epidemic of suicide and homicide in the nation's hospitals.'[148]

With all deference, I find it hard to believe that the *Quill* court thought through where its rationale would lead and whether it was prepared to go there.[149] As I have spelled out elsewhere,[150] what the *Quill* Court did in effect was to lubricate the 'slippery slope' with the Equal Protection Clause.

As I understand the *Quill* analysis, and as I apply that analysis, it leads to the following conclusions: (a) mentally competent *non*-terminally ill people who are *not* attached to life-sustaining equipment have a right to determine the time and manner of their deaths because *if they were on life support* they would be able to do so by directing removal of such support; (b) mentally competent terminally ill people (and if I am right about part (a), *non*-terminally ill people as well) who are *unable* to perform the last, death-causing act themselves, and thus need a physician to do it for them (e.g., administer a lethal injection), are entitled to physician-administered voluntary euthanasia because, except for the arbitrary fact that they lack the capacity to perform the death-producing act themselves, they are 'similarly situated' to other mentally competent persons who wish to 'hasten their deaths' and *are* able to perform the 'last act' themselves.

Although one would not know this from the *Quill* opinion, the right to forgo life-saving medical treatment has not been limited to the terminally ill.[151] If, as the *Quill* court insists, there is no legally cognizable distinction between competent, *terminally* ill persons off life-support who wish to 'hasten their deaths' but cannot do so and 'similarly situated persons who *are on* life support, and thus *able* to control the time and manner of their deaths, then the same reasoning leads to the conclusion that competent, *non*-terminally ill persons who are *off* life support, and for that reason alone unable to control the timing of their deaths, are being treated 'unequally'.

The *Quill* court's equal protection analysis also has a bearing on the viability of the distinction between physician-assisted suicide (where the suicidant herself performs the last, death-causing act) and physician-assisted active voluntary euthanasia (where the physician does not merely provide assistance but performs the act that actually brings about death). Unlike the *Compassion* majority, whose position on this issue appears rather tentative,[152] the *Quill* court seems quite willing to honor the distinction between assisted suicide and active voluntary euthanasia.[153] But it is highly unlikely that this distinction could survive the kind of equal protection analysis the Second Circuit utilized in *Quill*.

If the only reason a person cannot avail herself of physician-assisted suicide is her inability to perform the last, death-causing act herself, that situation seems no less arbitrary and no more relevant than the fact that a person does not happen to be dependent on a life-support system. If a person otherwise 'eligible' for physician-assisted suicide, and determined to end her life by the active intervention of another, needs someone else to administer the lethal medicine, how can she be denied this right or liberty (assuming it *is* a right or liberty) *simply because* she cannot perform the last, death-causing act herself?

As Holmes once observed, although 'all rights tend to declare themselves absolute to their logical extreme,' all are 'limited by the neighborhood of principles of policy other than those on which the particular right is founded, and which become strong enough to hold their own when a certain point is reached.'[154] The right to refuse treatment has come to mean the right to remove the feeding tube as well as the respirator and the right to direct the removal of life support for an incompetent relative as well as for oneself. But surely when the right to refuse treatment becomes the basis for an alleged right to the active intervention of a physician to promote or to bring about death, the anti-suicide tradition is, to use Holmes' phrase, 'strong enough to hold [its] own'.

I need not argue that a legislature must arrive at this conclusion.[155] I need only maintain that if a legislature *does* do so, its judgment should not be overturned by the courts.

NOTES

I am indebted to University of Michigan law student Marc Spindelman for valuable research assistance and for helpful comments.

1 Charles Black, *The People and the Court* 88 (1960).

2 *In re*: Quinlan, 70 N.J. 10, 355 A. 2d 647 (1976).

3 *Cruzan* v. *Director, Missouri Department of Health*, 497 U.S. 261 (1980).

4 See *Quinlan*, 355 A. 2d at 665, 670 & n. 9. 'The assertion that rejection of life-saving medical treatment by competent patients constitutes suicide,' observes Norman Cantor, *The Permanently Unconscious Patient, Non-Feeding and Euthanasia*, 15 Am. J. Law & Med. 381, 433 (1989), 'has been uniformly rejected – usually based on a distinction between letting nature take its course and initiating external death-causing agents.'

5 Derek Humphry & Ann Wickett, *The Right to Die* 242 (First Hemlock Society ed. 1990).

6 In *Quinlan* the state court permitted an unconscious patient to be removed from a respirator, as her family desired; in *Cruzan*, the Supreme Court upheld the state's power to keep an unconscious patient on a feeding tube, over her family's objection, because the patient had not left clear instructions for ending life-sustaining treatment.

7 497 U.S. at 279.

8 *Id.* at 279 n. 7.

9 See John Robertson, *Cruzan and the Constitutional Status of Nontreatment Decisions for Incompetent Patients*, 25 Ga. L. Rev. 1139, 1174–75 & n. 132 (1991).

10 497 U.S. at 280.

11 See Louis Michael Seidman, *Confusion at the Border: Cruzan, 'The Right to Die,' and the Public/Private Distinction*, 1991 Sup. Ct. Rev. 47, 53, 62.

12 See, e.g., Robert Sedler, *The Constitution and Hastening Inevitable Death*, Hastings Center Rep., 23 no. 5 (1993), at 20. Professor Sedler is one of the lawyers challenging the constitutionality of a Michigan law which makes assisted suicide a felony.

13 410 U.S. 113 (1973).

14 *Id.* at 152–53. But the right is not absolute. Thus, the state's compelling interest in

protecting life *after* viability enables it to proscribe abortion during that period except when necessary to protect the mother's life or health.

15 *Id.* at 157–58.

16 See, e.g., Sedler, *supra* note 12.

17 *Paris Adult Theatre* v. *Slaton*, 413 U.S. 49, 68 (1973) (a well-known obscenity case).

18 *Id.* at 68 n. 15.

19 See, e.g., Sedler, *supra* note 12, at 24.

20 *Bowers* v. *Hardwick*, 478 U.S. 186, 205 (1986) (dissenting opinion).

21 *Id.* at 191.

22 Sedler, *supra* note 12, at 23. This view seems very close to the attitude of the Romans, who, we are told, looked on suicide 'as a carefully considered and chosen validation of the way they had lived and the principles they had lived by,' Alfred Alvarez, *The Background*, in Suicide: The Philosophical Issues 7, 22 (M. Battin & D. Mayo eds. 1980).

In formulating his argument, Professor Sedler uses snippets from the Court's long opinion in *Planned Parenthood* v. *Casey*, 112 S. Ct. 2791 (1992), such as '[a]t the heart of liberty is the right to define one's concept of existence, of meaning, of the universe, and of the mystery of human life.' *Id.* at 2807. *Casey* did reaffirm *Roe*, but so far as I am aware nobody has suggested that it overruled *Bowers* v. *Hardwick*.

Moreover, in reaffirming the 1973 abortion cases the *Casey* majority relied heavily on '[t]he obligation to follow precedent' and the 'indispensable' nature of 'a respect for precedent.' *Id.* at 2808. Three of the Justices who voted to reaffirm *Roe* (none of whom was on the Court when *Roe* was decided) observed that '[w]e do not need to say whether each of us, had we been Members of the Court [when *Roe* was decided], would have concluded, as the *Roe* Court did, that [the weight of the State's interest in protecting the potentiality of life] is insufficient to justify a ban on abortions prior to viability . . . The matter is not before us in the first instance . . . ' *Id.* at 2817 (O'Connor, Kennedy and Souter, JJ.).

23 See Yale Kamisar, *Some Non-Religious Views Against Proposed 'Mercy-Killing' Legislation*, 42 Minn. L. Rev. 969, 971–73 (1958).

24 See e.g. Wayne LaFave & Austin Scott, 1 *Substantive Criminal Law* 330 (2d ed. 1986); Alan Meisel, *The Right to Die* 61–62 (1989); Lawrence Gostin, *Drawing a Line between Killing and Letting Die: The Law, and Law Reform, on Medically Assisted Dying*, 21 J. L. Med. & Ethics 94, 96 (1993); Sanford Kadish, *Letting Patients Die: Legal and Moral Reflections*, 80 Cal. L. Rev. 857, 858 (1992).

25 See, e.g., Dan Brock, *Voluntary Active Euthanasia*, Hastings Center Rep., 22 no. 2 (1992) at 10, 14.

26 According to Thomas Marzen, '*Out, Out Brief Candle: Constitutionally Prescripted Suicide for the Terminally Ill*', 21 Hastings Con. L. Q. 799, 804 (1994), 'assisted suicide is separately punishable by statute in thirty states.' Marzen lists the 30 specific criminal code provisions in a long footnote, *id.* at 804, n. 21. The same 30 states are listed in Alan Meisel, *The Right to Die: 1994 Cum. Supp. No. 1* at 60–61.

According to Timothy Quill, a well-known proponent of physician-assisted suicide, 36 states prohibit the practice. See Quill, *Death and Dignity*, 141 (1993). Quill is probably including those states which ban the practice under their general criminal homicide laws as well as those that do so by specific legislation. In some states which do not have specific statutes on the subject it is unclear whether assisted suicide is treated as a type of murder or manslaughter. Until recently this ambiguity reigned in the state of Michigan. It was only after several trial courts dismissed murder indictments against Jack Kevorkian for assisting in suicides on the ground that such an act was not covered by the general homicide laws of the state that the legislature enacted specific legislation on the subject.

27 See Thomas Marzen, *et al.*, *Suicide: A Constitutional Right*?, 24 Duq. L. Rev. 1, 68–100 (1985).

28 See Leon Kass, *Is There a Right to Die*?,

Hastings Center Rep. 23, no. 1 (1993) at 34, 35.

29 American Law Institute, *Model Penal Code and Commentaries, Part 1*, § 210.5 (1985) at p. 100.

30 Sanford Kadish, *The Model Penal Code's Historical Antecedents*, Rutgers L. J. 521 (1988).

31 American Law Institute, *Model Penal Code*, Part II, § 210.5 (Official Draft, 1962).

32 See Model Penal Code (Tentative Draft No. 9, 1959) at pp. 56–57.

33 Robert Weir, *The Morality of Physician-Assisted Suicide*, 17 Law, Med. & Health Care 116, 125 (1992).

34 American Law Institute, Model Penal Code and Commentaries, Part I, § 210.5 (1985) at p. 94.

35 Thomas Marzen, *supra* note 26, at 804. As Marzen notes, *id.* at n. 20, every American state provides for the involuntary commitment of persons who are a danger to themselves.

36 At this point, I am quoting from the language of Michigan's 1993 law against assisted suicide. See generally George Annas, *Physician-Assisted Suicide – Michigan's Temporary Solution*, 328 N. Eng. J. Med. 1573 (1993). See also the discussion in note 38 *infra*. 'Providing the means of suicide appears to be the act against which the assistance statutes are primarily directed.' Note, *Criminal Liability for Assisting Suicide*, 86 Colum. L. Rev 348, 360 (1986).

37 Gostin, *supra* note 24, at 96.

38 As pointed out in David Watts & Timothy Howell, *Assisted Suicide Is Not Voluntary Euthanasia*, 40 J. Am. Geriatr. Soc. 1043 (1992), assisted suicide involves various levels of assistance. According to the authors, they include *supplying information*; writing *prescriptions* for lethal medication that a patient might use to kill herself; providing the *physical means*, i.e., the lethal dose of medication or poison itself; and 'supervising or directly aiding' the suicide, the type of involvement characterizing the activities of Jack Kevorkian. But see Glenn Graber, *Assisted Suicide Is Not Voluntary Active Euthanasia, But It's Awfully Close*, 41 J. Am. Geriatr. Soc. 88 (1993) (editorial).

Not surprisingly, those who favor assisted suicide but balk at active voluntary euthanasia, try to put as much distance as possible between the two concepts by comparing and contrasting relatively *low levels* of assistance with active euthanasia. When they speak of assisted suicide they usually talk about supplying Hemlock Society material or other information, providing a prescription or discussing required doses – but not supervising the suicide or intentionally furnishing the physical means by which a person dies by suicide. See e.g. Weir, *supra* note 33, at 118 (emphasis added):

> If a physician is involved, the difference [between assisted suicide and active euthanasia] in personal involvement is between providing a suicidal patient with a prescription that would be lethal if taken by the patient in certain amounts, compared with the physician personally administering a lethal injection to the patient at the patient's request . . . A physician who responds to a patient's request for assistance in committing suicide cannot be certain, *merely by providing a prescription or discussing dosage*, either that the patient will follow through with the attempt at self-destruction or that the attempt at causing his or her death will actually work.

I very much doubt that supplying information about suicide is or should be viewed as 'assisted suicide' at all. I do not think any American prosecutor would try to convict someone for providing a friend or relative *information* that might prove useful in committing suicide – even if it could be established (and this would be extremely hard to do) that the defendant's intent was to cause death.

There is plenty of information about how to commit suicide in Derek Humphry's best-selling book, *Final Exit: The Practicalities of Self-Deliverance and Assisted Suicide for the Dying* (1991). Indeed, as the author makes plain in his Introduction, the book 'is aimed at helping the public and the health professional achieve death with dignity for those who desire to plan for it.' *Id.* at 18. Hundreds of thousands of copies of this book have been sold and no doubt many have been given or lent to friends and relatives. So far as I know, no prosecutions have been brought for such acts. If a prosecutor were foolhardy enough to try to convict someone of assisted suicide for lending a sick friend or relative a copy of *Final Exit* I think he would soon run afoul of the First Amendment.

I have not studied the other twenty-nine state laws banning assisted suicide, but I am familiar with the Michigan statute. It does not cover *supplying information* about suicide at all. Nor do I believe, although this is less clear, that it prohibits a physician from prescribing drugs for a sick patient who might use them to kill herself – not at least if it is a prescription for drugs that have a legitimate medical use. The statute prohibits one 'who has knowledge that another person intends [to] commit suicide' from 'intentionally' 'participat[ing] in a physical act' or 'provid[ing] the physical means' by which the other person commits suicide. I share the view that 'physicians who write prescriptions do not provide the 'physical means' to commit suicide, any more than someone who gives a person money to fill the prescription or a car to get it would provide the physical means.' Annas, *supra* note 36, at 1574.

39 George Smith, *All's Well that Ends Well: Toward a Policy of Assisted Rational Suicide or Merely Enlightened Self-Determination*, 22 U. C. Davis L. Rev. 275, 279–80 (1989).

40 Joseph Fletcher, *Morals and Medicine* 176 (1954). Fletcher was a famous medical ethicist and a prolific writer who advocated active euthanasia for some fifty years.

41 James Rachels, *The End of Life: Euthanasia and Morality* 86–87 (1986).

42 Raanan Gillon, *Suicide and Voluntary Euthanasia* in Euthanasia and the Right to Death 173–74 (A. B. Downing ed. 1969).

43 See generally Alexander Morgan Capron, *Proposition 161: What Is at Stake?*, Commonweal, Sept. 1992 (Special Supp.) at 2; Rob Carson, *Washington's I-119*, Hastings Center Rep. 22, no. 2 (1992) at 7. Both the Washington state proposal to legalize 'aid in dying' (Initiative 119) and the California proposal to do the same (Proposition 161) failed by a 54 percent to 46 percent margin. See Alexander Morgan Capron, *Even in Defeat, Proposition 161 Sounds a Warning*, Hastings Center Rep. no. 1 (1993) at 32.

44 Derek Humphry, *Dying with Dignity: Understanding Euthanasia* 70 (1992).

45 *Id.* at 102.

46 *Id.* at 79.

47 *Id.* at 171.

48 *Id.* at 159. (Emphasis added.)

49 Ronald Dworkin, *Life's Dominion: An Argument about Abortion, Euthanasia, and Individual Freedom* 3 (1993). (Emphasis added.)

50 See *id.* at 3–4. The American case involved Dr Timothy Quill, who was not prosecuted for assisted suicide, a felony in his state; the British case involved Dr Nigel Cox, who was convicted of attempted murder. See *id.* at 184–86.

51 See *id.* at 184–85.

52 See the discussion in note 38 *supra*.

53 Weir, *supra* note 33, at 118.

54 *Id.*

55 See Timothy Quill, *Death and Dignity: Making Choices and Taking Charge* 157–60 (1993).

56 *Id.* at 137.

57 See Sedler, *supra* note 12, at 20.

58 Marzen, *supra* note 26, at 814.

59 See Yale Kamisar, *When is There a Constitutional 'Right to Die'? When is There* No *Constitutional 'Right to Live'?*, 25 Ga. L. Rev. 1203, 1210–11 (1991) and authorities collected therein. Moreover 'terminal' is variously defined as occurring in 'a relatively short time,' 'imminent,' when treatment only 'postpones the moment of death,' when the patient is 'incurable' and/or her condition 'hopeless.' See *id.*; Marzen, *supra* note 26, at 814 & n. 54.

60 Alan Sullivan, *A Constitutional Right to Suicide*, in Suicide: The Philosophical Issues 229, 241 (M. Battin & D. Mayo eds. 1980).

61 Quill, *supra* note 26, at 162. (Emphasis added.)

62 *Id.* (Emphasis added.)

63 See Marzen, *supra* note 26, at 800. See also Robert Wennberg, *Terminal Choices* 99 (1989).

64 Sedler, *supra* note 12, at 24. (Emphasis in the original.)

65 See *id.* at 23–24.

66 See *Bouvia* v. *Superior Court* (Glenchar), 225 Cal. Rep. 297 (Ct. App. 1986). Elizabeth Bouvia was not terminally ill, unconscious, or mentally retarded. Indeed, she was 'intelligent, very mentally competent' and 'alert.' *Id.* at 300, 305. Nevertheless, the California Court of Appeal granted the relief she sought – removal of the nasogastric tube keeping her alive against her will. To the same effect are *McKay* v. *Bergstedt*, 801 P. 2d 617 (Nev. 1990) and *State* v. *McAfee*, 385 S.E. 2d 651 (Ga. 1989). Both cases involved respirator-dependent quadriplegics who apparently had long life expectancies.

To be sure, none of these cases were decided by the US Supreme Court, but they have been well received by lawyers, physicians, bioethicists and medico-legal commentators. Thus Professor Alan Meisel recently called the view that a patient must be terminally ill for life support to be stopped one of the 'myths' about terminating medical treatment that should be dispelled. See Meisel, *Legal Myths about Terminating Life Support*, 109 Archives Int. Med. 1497, 1498–99 (1991).

Moreover, in the *Cruzan* case, the Supreme Court failed to attach any significance to the fact that Nancy Cruzan was not dying or terminally ill, as these terms are usually defined. No doubt many thought that she 'might as well be dead' or that she was 'better off dead,' but if her feeding tube had not been removed (after the case was remanded and additional evidence was presented that she would have wanted to die under the circumstances), she might have been kept alive another twenty or thirty years.

67 Daniel Callahan, *The Troubled Dream of Life: Living with Mortality* 95 (1993).

68 Judith Ahronheim & Doron Weber, *Final Passages* 99–114 (1992). The authors note that '[t]he majority of clinicians – including cancer specialists – receive very inadequate training in pain assessment and pain management,' *id.* at 99, and that important information about pain control for the terminally ill and other patients has only 'started to enter the curriculum of medical schools.' *Id.* at 112.

69 *Id.* at 102.

70 Kathleen Foley, *The Relationship of Pain and Symptom Management to Patient Requests for Physician-Assisted Suicide*, J. Pain & Sym. Management 1991; 6: 289,290. Adds Dr Foley, *id.* at 292: 'The high cost of pumps, drugs, and home care supervision on a 24-hour basis makes [pain control] only available to a limited number of patients who have appropriate health care coverage. By rationing pain management on a financial basis, patients are being forced to consider death as their only option.'

71 Dan Brock, *Voluntary Active Euthanasia*, Hastings Center Rep. 22, no. 2 (1992), at 10, 16.

72 Maurice A. M. deWachter, *Euthanasia in the Netherlands*, Hastings Center Rep. 22, no. 2 (1992), at 23, 25.

73 Callahan, *supra* note 67, at 102.

74 Albert Jonsen, *To Help the Dying Die – A New Duty for Anesthesiologists?* (Editorial), Anesthesiology 78: 225, 227 (1993).

75 See Sedler, *supra* note 12, at 22–24.

76 *Id.* at 23.

77 *Planned Parenthood* v. *Casey*, 112 S. Ct. 2791, 2817 (1992) (O'Connor, Kennedy & Souter, JJ.) (plurality opinion).

78 Herbert Wechsler, *Toward Neutral Principles of Constitutional Law*, 73 Harv. L. Rev. 1, 15 (1959). I think it fair to say that the present Supreme Court would readily agree. As the majority observed in the recent *Casey* case, *supra* note 77, at 2814: 'The Court must take care to speak and act in ways that allow people to accept its decisions on the terms the Court claims for them, as grounded truly in principle, not as compromises with social and political pressures having, as such, no bearing on the principled choices that the Court is obliged to make.'

79 See Sedler, *supra* note 12, at 24. (Emphasis added.)

80 See text at note 66 *supra* and accompanying footnote. Although I suspect that nowadays almost everyone would agree that there is a

right or liberty to terminate either futile or excessively burdensome 'medical treatment,' sometimes the distinction between this right and the right to commit suicide (or to seek assistance in order to achieve this end) becomes exceedingly thin. By overlooking this distinction, some courts, perhaps inadvertently, may have provided support for a right to physician-assisted suicide. Consider in this regard the interesting – and troublesome – case of *McKay* v. *Bergstedt*, note 66 *supra*.

At the age of ten, as the result of a swimming accident, Kenneth Bergstedt became a quadriplegic. He lived for the next twenty-one years with the aid of a respirator. Then, faced with the imminent death of his ill father, Bergstedt decided, as the majority put it, 801 P. 2d at 620, that 'he wanted to be released from a life of paralysis held intact by the life-sustaining properties of a respirator . . . He despaired over the prospect of life without the attentive care, companionship and love of his father.'

At this point, Bergstedt petitioned the district court for an order permitting the removal of his respirator by a person who could also administer a sedative, thereby relieving the pain that would otherwise precede his demise. In addition, he sought an order granting this person immunity from civil or criminal liability. The district court granted the relief sought.

Although Bergstedt did not survive the date of the state supreme court's opinion in his case, the court confirmed his right to remove his life support system. It rejected the view that Bergstedt's petition constituted an attempt to commit suicide or seek suicide assistance, viewing his request as simply the exercise of his right to decline medical treatment – his 'right to allow the natural consequences of his condition to occur – unimpeded by artificial barriers.' *Id.* at 632.

Justice Springer dissented, arguing forcefully (and, I think, persuasively) that although the court would not recognize a right to suicide or suicidal assistance if a person were able to do the deed himself, the majority had in essence done just that in this case because of Bergstedt's disabled condition (*id.* at 635):

> [Bergstedt's] request to forgo mechanical respirator has been made in a context suggesting that his intent may be suicidal . . . [He] had been living steadily for over [twenty] years, breathing with the aid of a ventilator, until he reached a time in his life when he decided to die because, like most other suicides, life had become, temporarily at least, intolerable for him.

Relying heavily on an *amicus* brief filed by Thomas Marzen, a leading authority on the law of assisted suicide and the general counsel for the National Legal Center for the Medically Dependent and Disabled, the dissent maintained that although Bergstedt's breathing device had been introduced during a medical emergency by medical personnel, it had become something more than mere medical *treatment*. The machine had become an 'integral part' or a 'real extension' of Bergstedt's person and could no longer be regarded mere 'treatment.' See *id.* at 635.

81 Felix Frankfurter, *Mr Justice Jackson*, in Felix Frankfurter on the Supreme Court 509, 511 (P. Kurland ed. 1970).

82 *West Virginia State Board* v. *Barnette*, 319 U.S. 624, 660–61 (1943) (dissenting opinion).

83 See Robert Sedler, *Constitutional Challenges to Bans on 'Assisted Suicide': The View from Without and Within*, 21 Hastings Con. L. Q. 777, 792 (1994) (forthcoming).

84 *Id.* at 792–93.

85 See text at note 60 *supra*. See also the text at notes 94 and 96 *infra*.

86 Philip Devine, *The Ethics of Homicide* 199 (1978).

87 Actually, the Michigan law criminalizes assisted suicide only temporarily. It establishes a commission on death and dying which is given fifteen months to develop and submit recommendations as to legislation 'concerning the voluntary self-termination of life.' The ban against assisted suicide is automatically repealed six months after the commission makes its recommendations. For a careful, detailed analysis of the Michigan law, see Annas, *supra* note 36.

88 *Id.* at 1574.

89 *People* v. *Kevorkian*, No. 93-11482 (Mich. Cir. Ct. Wayne County Dec. 13, 1993). Professor Sedler and his ACLU colleagues were not directly involved in this case. The ACLU and Jack Kevorkian 'have kept at some considerable distance from each other,' Sedler, *supra* note 12, at 21. In another case brought by Sedler and his colleagues, a case also on appeal, Wayne County Circuit Judge Cynthia Stephens struck down the law on technical grounds under the state constitution, but indicated that had she not been able to invalidate the law on such grounds she would have blocked its enforcement on the basis of what she called a due process right to assisted suicide. See *Hobbins* v. *Attorney General*, No. 93-306-178 CZ (Mich. Cir. Ct. Wayne County May 20, 1993), *appeal docketed*, No. 164963 (Mich. App. Aug. 13, 1993). For criticism of Judge Stephens' opinion see Yale Kamisar, *'Right to Die' Can't Be the Last Word*, Legal Times, June 14, 1993, at 29–30.

90 As Thomas Marzen has observed, *supra* note 26, at 808:

> Any claim that the Constitution ought properly to recognize a right to assisted suicide necessarily assumes a recognized liberty to suicide itself. Yet paradoxically, suicide is now nowhere a crime and, in this sense, the state imposes no 'burden' of any kind on completion of the act. The plea for recognition of a right to assisted suicide thus amounts to a plea for suicide of a *special sort*: suicide that is done with expert aid and instruction to assure its painless and certain completion.

91 *People* v. *Kevorkian*, slip op. at 33.

92 *Id.* at 34. (Emphasis added.)

93 *Id.*

94 *Id.* at 31–32, quoting Richard Brandt, *The Rationality of Suicide*, in Suicide: The Philosophical Issues 117, 123 (M. Battin & D. Mayo eds. 1980).

95 Slip op. at 24.

96 *Id.* at 21, quoting Alfred Alvarez, *The Background*, in Suicide: The Philosophical Issues 7, 22 (M. Battin & D. Mayo eds. 1980). (Emphasis added.) On the same page of his opinion, Judge Kaufman notes that '[t]he idea that *one's honor* or one's quality of life would allow society to recognize the act of suicide as not contrary to societal norms has great historical support.' (Emphasis added.)

97 Slip op. at 28–29, quoting Yale Kamisar, *Are Laws against Assisted Suicide Unconstitutional?* Hastings Center Rep., 23, no. 3 (1993), at 32, 37.

98 Slip op. at 29.

99 See text at notes 65 and 79 *supra*.

100 See James Brown, *et al.*, *Is It Normal for Terminally Ill Patients to Desire Death?*, 143 Am. J. Psych. 208, 210 (Feb. 1986); Yeates Conwell & Eric Caine, *Rational Suicide and the Right to Die*, 325 New Eng. J. Med. 1100, 1101 (Oct. 1991); Herbert Hendin & Gerald Klerman, *Physician-Assisted Suicide: The Dangers of Legalization*, 150 Am. J. Psychiatry 1434 (1993); Roberta Richardson, *et al.*, *Coping with the Suicidal Elderly: A Physician's Guide*, 44 Geriatrics 43–44 (Sept 1989).

101 See David Clark, *'Rational' Suicide and People with Terminal Conditions or Disabilities*, 8 Issues in Law & Med. 147, 155, 162 (1992); Conwell & Caine, *supra* note 100, at 1101.

102 See George Colt, *The Enigma of Suicide* 392–95 (1991); Clark, *supra* note 101, at 163; Conwell & Caine, *supra* note 100, at 1102; Richardson, *supra* note 100, at 47.

103 Colt, *supra* note 102, at 394.

104 Sociologist Menno Boldt, quoted in Colt, *supra*, at 342.

105 For a discussion of 'circumstantial' and 'societal' manipulation in the context of suicide, see Margaret Pabst Battin, *Manipulated Suicide*, in Suicide: The Philosophical Issues 169 (M. Battin & D. Mayo eds. 1980).

106 Slip op. at 34.

107 Devine, *supra* note 86, at 188.

108 Thomas Mayo, *Constitutionalizing the 'Right to Die'*, 49 Maryland L. Rev. 103, 144 (1990).

109 Carl Schneider, *Rights Discourse and Neonatal Euthanasia*, 76 Calif. L. Rev., 151, 168 (1988). Although Karen Ann Quinlan's parents obtained permission to remove their daughter from the respirator, they did not request permission to remove

the feeding tube that was to keep her alive for another nine years. They probably declined to do so because they viewed feeding as 'natural' or 'basic' or 'ordinary' care. If the Quinlans had sought permission to remove their daughter's feeding tube, they would have run into strong resistance and most probably would have been rebuffed. For in the 1970s the distinction between the feeding tube and other forms of life support was quite formidable. If such a case arose today, of course, the feeding tube would be removed without any fanfare. See the discussion in Kamisar, *supra* note 59, at 1220–24.

110 Albert Alschuler, *Reflection*, in Active Euthanasia, Religion, and the Public Debate 105, 108 (The Park Ridge Center, 1991).

111 850 F. Supp. 1454 (UDC, WD Wash., 1994). For the subsequent history of this case, see note 127 *infra*.

112 This decision, by Wayne County Circuit Judge Richard Kaufman, is discussed at considerable length in the text at notes 89–107 *supra*.

113 527 NW 2d 714 (Mich. 1994) (consolidated with Hobbins v. Attorney General).

114 The Michigan court denied that those who choose to discontinue life-sustaining medical treatment are, in effect, committing suicide: 'There is a difference between choosing a natural death summoned by an uninvited illness or calamity, and deliberately seeking to terminate one's life by resorting to death-inducing measures unrelated to the natural process of dying. *Id.* at 728–29.

115 The New York State Task Force on Life and the Law, *When Death Is Sought: Assisted Suicide and Euthanasia in the Medical Context* (1994). The Task Force included eight medical doctors (two of whom were deans of medical schools), two bioethicists who were not medical doctors, four lawyers, six clergymen (one of whom was also a law professor), the state commissioner of health, the state commissioner on the quality of care for the mentally disabled and a member of the New York Civil Liberties Union. In addition, a nurse and three medical doctors served as consultants to the task force.

116 *Id.* at ix (Executive Summary).

117 *Id.*

118 See *id.* at 138–40.

119 See *id.* at 140. See also John Arras, *News from the Circuit Courts: How Not to Think About Physician-Assisted Suicide*, 2 BioLaw S: 171, S: 175, S: 184–85 (Special Section, July–Aug., 1996) (views of one Task Force member who believed assisted suicide or active voluntary euthanasia might be appropriate in certain rare instances, but balked at legalizing these practices for fear of the social consequences of decriminalization). Consider, too, Yale Kamisar, *The Reasons So Many People Support Physician-Assisted suicide – And Why These Reasons Are Not Convincing*, 12 Issues in Law & Med. 113, 116–18 (1996).

120 New York State Task Force Report, *supra* note 115, at 140–41. 'In addition to regulating and restraining behavior,' observed the Task Force, 'our laws also serve a highly symbolic function.' It continued, *id.* at 141:

> The legal prohibition, while not uniformly honored, preserves the gravity of conduct to assist suicide and prevents abuse . . ..
>
> . . . While not a tidy or perfect resolution, [the total ban] serves the interests of patients far better than legalizing the practice. By curtailing the autonomy of patients in a very small number of cases when assisted suicide is a compelling and justifiable response, it preserves the autonomy and well-being of many others. It also prevents the widespread abuses that would be likely to occur if assisted suicide were legalized.

121 See *id.* at 72, 121, 125, 131–33, 145, 147.

122 Thus, essentially for the reasons set forth in Charles Baron *et al.*, *A Model State Act to Authorize and Regulate Physician-Assisted Suicide*, 33 Harv. J. Leg. 1, 14–16 (1996), I disagree with Judge Michael Hogan, who ruled in Lee v. Oregon, 891 F. Supp. 1429 (D. Or. 1995), that the Oregon Act permitting and regulating physician-assisted suicide for the terminally

ill discriminates against the terminally ill as a class in violation of the Equal Protection Clause.

123 See note 43 *supra*.

124 See Michael Betzold, *Oregon Gives Approval; Renewed Ban Likely in Michigan*, *Detroit Free Press*, Nov. 10, 1994, p. 5B; William Crum, *Doctors Split on Oregon's Legalization of Assisted Suicide*, *Ann Arbor News*, Nov. 11, 1994, p. A7; Timothy Egan, *Suicide Law Placing Oregon on Several Uncharted Paths*, *NY Times*, Nov. 25, 1994, p. 1.

Unlike the proposals which failed earlier, the Oregon measure requires that medication prescribed under the Act be self-administered. According to the campaign director of Oregon Right to Die, the Oregon measure was adopted for this reason and because the state medical association dediced to remain neutral, breaking with the National Office of the American Medical Association (which opposed physician-assisted suicide). See Betzold, *supra*; Egan, *supra*. Moreover, as discussed earlier (see note 38 *supra*), writing a prescription for a lethal medication that a patient might take to end her life constitutes a relatively low level of assistance.

125 Cf. Ruth Bader Ginsburg, *Speaking in a Judicial Voice*, NYUL Rev. 1185, 1208 (1992): '*Roe* [v. *Wade*] . . . halted a political process that was moving in a reform direction and thereby, I believe, prolonged divisiveness and deferred stable settlement of the issue.' This was the last article Judge Ginsburg wrote before being appointed to the US Supreme Court.

126 Franklin G. Miller, *Legalizing Physician-Assisted Suicide by Judicial Decision: A Critical Appraisal*, 2 BioLaw S: 136, S: 144 (Special Section, July–Aug., 1996).

127 79 F. 3d 790 (9th Cir. 1996) (Reinhardt, J.), *cert. granted sub nom.*, Washington v. Glucksberg, 65 USLW 3085 (US Oct. 1, 1996) (No. 96-110). Judge Rothstein's decision had been reversed by a three-judge panel of the Ninth Circuit, 49 F. 3d 586 (9th Cir., 1995) (2–1, per Noonan, J.). But the following year a majority of the Ninth Circuit, sitting *en banc*, vacated the panel decision and affirmed Judge Rothstein's ruling.

128 80 F. 3d 716 (2d Cir. 1996) (Miner, J.), *cert. granted sub nom.* Dennis v. Vacco, 64 USLW 3795 (US Oct. 1, 1996) (No. 95-1858).

129 See notes 127–28 *supra*.

130 Compassion in Dying, 79 F. 3d at 793.

131 *Id.*

132 *Id.* at 824.

133 *Id.*

134 See the discussion in text at notes 1–11 *supra*.

135 See the discussion in Alexander Morgan Capron, *Liberty, Equality Death!*, Hastings Center Rep., May/June, 1996, pp. 23–24.

136 New York State Task Force Report, *supra* note 115, at 71.

137 *Id.*

138 Jed Rubenfeld, *The Right to Privacy*, 102 Harv. L. Rev. 737, 794 (1989). See also Arras, *supra* note 119, at S: 182; Miller, *supra* note 126, at S: 142.

139 See *Cruzan*, 497 US at 302–3 (Brennan, J., dissenting).

140 New York State Task Force Report Report, *supra* note 115, at 75. See Also Daniel Callahan, The Troubled Dream of Life 77–81 (1993).

141 See Giles R. Scofield, *Exposing Some Myths About Physician-Assisted Suicide*, 18 Seattle UL Rev. 473, 481 (1995).

142 '[T]he right contended for here,' noted the Second Circuit, 80 F. 3d at 724, 'cannot be considered so implicit in our understanding of ordered liberty that neither justice nor liberty would exist if it were sacrificed. Nor can it be said that [the claimed right] is deeply rooted in the nation's traditions and history. Indeed, the very opposite is true.'

143 *Quill*, 80 F. 3d at 729 (quoting the district court, which had found such a distinction significant).

144 *Id.* at 725.

145 *Id.* at 729. 'A finding of unequal treatment,' added the court, *id.*, 'does not, of course, end the inquiry, unless it is determined that the inequality is not rationally related to some legitimate state interest.' The court then concluded that to the extent

that the statute prohibited a physician from assisting a mentally competent, terminally-ill person to die by suicide, it was 'not rationally related to any legitimate state interest.' *Id.* at 731.

146 *Id.* at 729. (Emphasis added.) Actually, if one shares the *Quill* court's view that the action–inaction distinction is irrelevant and takes the *Quill* court's argument where it logically leads, ending a person's life by removing her life support would be *more than* assisted suicide – it would be voluntary euthanasia. Assisted suicide occurs when another person renders assistance (e.g. provides the lethal drugs), but *the suicidant herself* commits the last act – the one that brings about death. However, that is *not* an accurate description of what happens when a physician terminates life support. In such a case, according to the *Quill* court, it is the physician herself who is performing the last act, the death-causing act, and this constitutes euthanasia, not assisted suicide. See the discussion in the text at notes 23–56 *supra*. I have made plain my view that there is a significant distinction between the termination of life support and active intervention to promote or to bring about death. However, assuming arguendo that the distinction is neither legally nor morally significant (the position taken by both the *Compassion* and *Quill* courts), the 'active' counterpart to forgoing life-sustaining treatment would not be assisted suicide but active voluntary euthanasia (considered murder everywhere in the United States).

147 See text *supra* at note 139.

148 George J. Annas, *The 'Right to Die' in America: Sloganeering from Quinlan and Cruzan to Quill and Kevorkian*, 34 Duquesne L. Rev. 875, 896 (1996). 'Homicide' is an ugly word, but if one takes the *Quill* court's analysis seriously, an 'epidemic' of 'homicide' is not mere hyperbole. For the reasons discussed in note 146 supra, the *Quill* court's logic does lead to the conclusion that what has been going on in the nation's hospitals for many years is technically 'homicide', not 'suicide' or 'assisted suicide.'

149 Cf. Louis Henkin, *Foreword: On Drawing Lines*, 82 Harv. L. Rev. 63, 65–66 (1968): 'To avoid difficult questions, to support a result dictated by intuition or sympathy, perhaps to achieve a majority for that result, the Justices [sometimes] seize a rationale that comes to mind, without asking where it leads and whether they are prepared to go there.'

150 See Yale Kamisar, *The Right to Die: On Drawing (and Erasing) Lines*, 35 Duq. L. Rev. 481, 487–89 (1996).

151 See note 66 supra and accompanying text. See also 1 ALAN MEISEL, THE RIGHT TO DIE 470 (2nd ed. 1995).

152 Although it noted that whether there was a constitutional right to, or liberty interest in, active voluntary euthanasia (as well as physician-assisted suicide) was a question that had to be answered in a future case, the Ninth Circuit could not resist suggesting how it would resolve the question in a future case, 79 F. 3d at 831–32: 'We would be less than candid, however, if we did not acknowledge that . . . we view the critical line in right-to-die cases as the one between the voluntary and involuntary termination of an individual's life . . .. We consider it less important who administers the medication than who determines whether the terminally ill person's life shall end.' Of course, in voluntary euthanasia, *as well as* in assisted suicide, the patient *herself* determines whether her life shall end.

153 In response to the argument that the state had an interest in 'preventing the sort of abuse that "has occurred in the Netherlands . . .,"' the *Quill* court pointed out that the relief sought by the plaintiffs would not lead to such abuse because they 'do not argue for euthanasia at all,' only for assisted suicide for terminally ill patients 'who would self-administer the drugs.' See 80 F. 3d at 730–31. Moreover, the court noted that 'euthanasia falls within the definition of murder.' *Id.* at 730 n. 3.

154 Hudson County Water Co. v. McCarter, 209 US 349, 355 (1908) (Holmes, J.).

155 See text at note 122 *supra* and accompanying footnote.

16

Euthanasia in the Netherlands: sliding down the slippery slope?

JOHN KEOWN

INTRODUCTION

THERE IS ONLY one country in which euthanasia is officially condoned and widely practised: the Netherlands. Although euthanasia is proscribed by the Dutch Penal Code, the Dutch Supreme Court held in 1984 that a doctor who kills a patient may in certain circumstances successfully invoke the defence of necessity, also contained in the Code, to justify the killing. In the same year, the Royal Dutch Medical Association (KNMG) issued its members with guidelines for euthanasia. Since that time the lives of thousands of Dutch patients have been intentionally shortened by their doctors.

A requirement central to both the legal and medical guidelines has been the free and explicit request of the patient. Defenders of the guidelines have claimed that they permit voluntary euthanasia but not euthanasia without request; that they are sufficiently strict and precise to prevent any slide down a 'slippery slope' to euthanasia without request, and that there has been no evidence of any such slide in the Netherlands.

The question addressed in this chapter can be simply put: Does the Dutch experience of euthanasia lend any support to the claims of supporters of voluntary euthanasia that acceptance of voluntary euthanasia does not lead to acceptance of non-voluntary euthanasia or does it, rather, tend to support the claims of opponents of voluntary euthanasia that voluntary euthanasia leads down a 'slippery slope' to euthanasia without request?

The 'slippery slope' argument is often thought of as one argument but it is more accurately understood as comprising two independent yet related forms: the 'logical' and the 'empirical'. In its logical form, the argument runs that acceptance of voluntary euthanasia leads to acceptance of at least non-voluntary euthanasia (that is, the killing of patients incapable of requesting euthanasia such as newborns or those with advanced senile dementia) because the former rests on the judgment that some lives are not 'worth' living, which judgment can logically be made even if the patient is incapable of requesting euthanasia. Doctors are not automata who simply execute their patient's wishes, however autonomous. They are professionals who form their own judgment about the merits of any request for medical intervention. A responsible doctor would no more euthanatise a patient just because the patient autonomously asked for it any more than the doctor would prescribe anti-depressant drugs for a patient just because the patient autonomously requested them. The doctor, if acting professionally, would decide in each case whether the intervention was truly in the patient's best interests. A responsible doctor would no more kill a patient who had, in the doctor's opinion, a life 'worth' living any more than he would prescribe anti-depressants for a patient who, in the doctor's opinion, was not depressed. Consequently, the alleged justification of voluntary euthanasia rests fundamentally not on the patient's autonomous request *but on the doctor's judgment that the request is justified because the patient no longer has a life 'worth' living*. And, if a doctor can make this judgment in relation to an autonomous patient, he can, logically, make it in relation to an incompetent patient. Moreover, if death is a 'benefit' for competent patients suffering certain conditions, why should it be denied incompetent patients suffering from the same conditions?[1]

In its empirical form, the 'slippery slope' argument runs that even if a line can in principle be drawn between voluntary and non-voluntary euthanasia, a slide will occur in practice because the safeguards to prevent it cannot be made effective. A common illustration of the argument in this form is the story of decriminalised abortion in England, where the law allowing therapeutic abortion has conspicuously failed to prevent widespread abortion for social reasons.

The empirical argument is, of course, dependent on empirical evidence. Invaluable evidence about euthanasia in Holland has of late been provided by a large-scale survey carried out on behalf of a Commission appointed by the Dutch Government to investigate medical decision-making in Holland at the end of life. This chapter makes comprehensive use of this evidence.

The chapter comprises three parts. Part I outlines both the relevant law as laid down by the Dutch Supreme Court and the Guidelines for euthanasia prescribed by the KNMG and considers their alleged precision and

Part II summarises the evidence, including that contained in the above survey, which indicates widespread breach of those Guidelines, especially the practice of euthanasia without request. The final part examines the slide from voluntary to non-voluntary euthanasia in Dutch practice and the shift in Dutch opinion towards condonation of non-voluntary euthanasia. The chapter concludes that there is ample evidence from the Dutch experience to substantiate the relevance of the 'slippery slope' argument in both its forms. First, an important word about terminology.

A standard definition of 'euthanasia' is 'The intentional putting to death of a person with an incurable or painful disease'.[2] It is common to refer to euthanasia carried out by an act as 'active' euthanasia and euthanasia by omission as 'passive' euthanasia. A common further sub-division is between 'voluntary', 'non-voluntary' and 'involuntary' euthanasia, which refer respectively to euthanasia at the patient's request, where the patient is incompetent, and where the patient is competent but has made no request.

Dutch definitions of 'euthanasia' are, typically, markedly narrower, such as 'the purposeful acting to terminate life by someone other than the person concerned upon request of the latter'.[3] It will be apparent that this is narrower than the usual definition in two respects: it is limited to cases of *active*[4] killing where there is a *request by the patient*. In short, the Dutch definition corresponds to what is normally called 'active, voluntary euthanasia'.

I. STRICT SAFEGUARDS?

A. The legal and professional guidelines

Taking the life of another person at his request is an offence contrary to Article 293 of the Penal Code (as amended in 1891) and assisting suicide is prohibited by Article 294. In 1984, however, in the *Alkmaar* case, the Dutch Supreme Court allowed a doctor's appeal against conviction for intentionally killing one of his elderly patients at her request. The Court held that the lower courts had wrongly failed to consider whether he had been faced with a 'conflict of duties'[5] (his duty to obey Article 293 on the one hand and his duty to relieve his patient's suffering on the other), whether 'according to responsible medical opinion'[6] measured by the 'prevailing standards of medical ethics'[7] a situation of 'necessity'[8] existed, and whether he had, therefore, been entitled to the defence of necessity, contained in Article 40.[9]

This decision is remarkable for a number of reasons. First, the necessity defence has traditionally been understood as justifying an ostensible breach of the law in order to *save* life (as by pushing someone out of the path of an oncoming car), not to take it. Secondly, the judgment fails to explain *why* the doctor's duty to alleviate suffering overrides his duty not to kill. Finally, the Court appears to abdicate to medical opinion the power to determine the circumstances in which killing attracts the necessity defence.

In a series of decisions straddling this landmark case, lower courts have laid down a number of conditions which have hitherto been understood as being required for a doctor successfully to avail himself of the necessity defence, though there is increasing uncertainty as to which, if any, are required. Subject to this important *caveat*, they were listed in 1989 (by Mrs Borst-Eilers, then Chairman of the Dutch Health Council) as follows:

(1) The request for euthanasia must come only from the patient and must be entirely free and voluntary.
(2) The patient's request must be well-considered, durable and persistent.
(3) The patient must be experiencing intolerable (not necessarily physical) suffering, with no prospect of improvement.
(4) Euthanasia must be a last resort. Other alternatives to alleviate the patient's situation must have been considered and found wanting.
(5) Euthanasia must be performed by a physician.
(6) The physician must consult with an independent physician colleague who has experience in this field.[10]

Moreover, having performed euthanasia, the doctor should *not* certify death by 'natural causes', which would involve the offence of falsifying a death certificate, but should call in the local medical examiner to investigate. The medical examiner should carry out an external inspection of the corpse, interview the doctor and file a report with the local prosecutor, who should decide whether to investigate further or to allow the body to be handed over to the next-of-kin.

Three months before the landmark Supreme Court decision in 1984, the KNMG published a Report setting out its criteria for permissible euthanasia.[11] They are substantially similar to the conditions just listed and require a voluntary request by the patient which is well considered and persistent; unacceptable suffering by the patient, and consultation by the doctor with a colleague working in the same institution and then with an independent doctor.[12] The KNMG subsequently formulated, in collaboration with the National Association of Nurses, certain 'Guidelines for Euthanasia'[13] which embody the above criteria.

B. 'Precisely defined' and 'strict'?

Before considering the evidence which indicates the extent to which the practice of euthanasia conforms to the above requirements, some comment is called for on the nature of those requirements and particularly on the extent to which they are capable of closely regulating the practice of euthanasia.

A leading Dutch defender of euthanasia has claimed (a claim reproduced with uncritical, almost robotic repetition in many newspaper articles on this subject) that the Guidelines are 'strict' and 'precise'.[14] However, even a cursory examination indicates that this is not the case. For one thing, it is not even possible precisely to identify the legal criteria, let alone define them: the Supreme Court omitted to lay down a precise list and lower courts have issued sets of criteria which are far from congruent. For another, as Professor Leenen, a leading Dutch health lawyer (and supporter of legalised euthanasia) has observed, concepts such as 'unbearable pain' (*a fortiori*, one might add, 'suffering') are open to subjective interpretation and are incapable of precise definition.[15] As for the assertion that the Guidelines are 'strict', this too is difficult to sustain, not only because of their imprecision but also because of the absence of any effective independent check on the doctor's decision-making to ensure that they are satisfied.

A hypothetical case may help highlight their inherent vagueness. A leading Dutch practitioner of euthanasia, who is highly respected in Holland, has said that he would be put in a very difficult position if a patient told him that he wanted euthanasia because he felt a nuisance to his relatives who wanted him dead so they could enjoy his estate. Asked whether he would rule out euthanasia in such a case, the doctor replied:

> I . . . think in the end I wouldn't, because that kind of influence – these children wanting the money now – is the same kind of power from the past that . . . shaped us all. The same thing goes for religion . . . education . . . the kind of family he was raised in, all kinds of influences from the past that we can't put aside.[16]

If such a leading practitioner of euthanasia, who had delivered many lectures on the subject inside and outside Holland (including lectures to the Dutch police on how to handle euthanasia cases) can interpret the Guidelines requiring an 'entirely free and voluntary request' and 'unbearable suffering' as possibly extending to such a case, little more need be said about their inherent vagueness and elasticity. In short, the Guidelines are simply incapable, because of their vagueness and the fact that they entrust the decision-making to the individual practitioner, of ensuring that euthanasia is carried out only in accordance with the criteria they specify. The empirical evidence which confirms the inability of the Guidelines effectively to regulate euthanasia is set out in Part II.

II. EUTHANASIA IN PRACTICE: THE EMPIRICAL EVIDENCE

A. The origins of the Remmelink Commission and the van der Maas Survey

The Dutch coalition government which assumed office in 1989 decided to appoint a Commission to report on the 'extent and nature of medical euthanasia practice'.[17] A Commission under the chairmanship of the Attorney-General, Professor Remmelink, was appointed on 17 January 1990 by the Minister of Justice and the State Secretary for Welfare, Health and Culture and asked to report on the practice by physicians of 'performing an act or omission . . . to terminate [the] life of a patient, with or without an explicit and serious request of the patient to this end'.[18]

To assist the discharge of this responsibility, the Commission asked P.J. van der Maas, Professor of Public Health and Social Medicine at the Erasmus University, to carry out a survey which would produce qualitative and quantitative information on the practice of euthanasia. The Commission and van der Maas agreed that the survey should embrace all medical decisions affecting the end of life so that euthanasia could be seen within that broader context. The umbrella term 'Medical Decisions Concerning the End of Life' ('MDELs') includes 'all decisions by physicians concerning courses of action aimed at hastening the end of life of the patient or courses of action for which the physician takes into account the probability that the end of life of the patient is hastened'.[19] MDELs comprise the administration, supply or prescription of a drug; the withdrawal or withholding of a treatment (including resuscitation and tube-feeding), and the refusal of a request for euthanasia or assisted suicide.[20] The Commission's Report[21] and the Survey[22] were published in Dutch in September 1991. One year later, the Survey was published in English.[23]

A previous paper of mine[24] suggested that the Dutch experience lends support to the 'slippery slope' argument in both its 'logical' and 'empirical' forms.[25] Do the Report and Survey require that suggestion to be qualified? The answer, on an uncritical reading of the Report, would be 'Yes'. But a reading of the Report in the light of its Survey yields a contrary answer. Indeed, taken together, the Survey and Report tend forcefully to confirm the application of the argument in both its forms.

B. The findings of the Survey and the conclusions of the Commission

After an outline of the Survey's findings about the incidence of euthanasia, consideration will be given to the light the Survey and the Report throw on the extent to which the criteria laid down by the courts and the KNMG have been observed in practice. Attention will focus on the Survey rather than the Report: the Report contains the Commission's conclusions in the light of the Survey but the Survey is a comprehensive empirical study which stands independently of the Report, and the conclusions drawn in the Report are not infrequently difficult to square with the findings of the Survey.

1. Methodology

Before turning to the Survey's findings, a summary of its methodology is appropriate. The Survey comprised three studies.

(i) The retrospective study.[26] A sample of 406 doctors was drawn from general practitioners, specialists (concerned with MDELs) and nursing home doctors, of whom 91% agreed to participate. The doctors were interviewed on average for two and a half hours and almost always by another doctor.[27] The respondent was asked about relevant types of decision. If he had made a decision of a given type, the last occasion on which he had done so was discussed in greater detail. At most, ten cases were discussed with each.[28]

(ii) The death certificate study.[29] This study examined a stratified sample of 8500 deaths occurring in Holland from July to November 1990 inclusive. The treating doctor was identified from each death certificate and was sent a short questionnaire which could be returned anonymously. The response rate was 73%.[30]

(iii) The prospective study.[31] Each of the doctors interviewed in the retrospective study was asked at interview if he would complete a questionnaire about each of his patients who died in the following six months. This study had several advantages: there would be little memory distortion because the questionnaire would be completed soon after the death; it would provide additional information to strengthen the quantitative basis of the interview study; and the carefully planned selection of respondents meant that the responses were representative of 95% of all deaths. The study ran from mid-November 1990 to the end of May 1991. Eighty per cent of those involved in the first study participated, completing over 2250 questionnaires.[32] In all, each of some 322

doctors supplied information about, on average, seven deaths.[33] The method of collection of data in all three studies was such that anonymity of participants could be guaranteed.[34]

2. The incidence of euthanasia

In 1990, the year covered by the Survey, thee were almost 130 000 deaths in Holland from all causes, of which 49 000 involved a MDEL.[35] Both the Report and the Survey adopted the Dutch definition of euthanasia as 'the intentional action to terminate a person's life, performed by somebody else than the involved person upon the latter's request'.[36] How many cases of 'euthanasia' so defined were there in 1990?

The three studies differed as to the incidence of euthanasia, yielding respective figures of 1.9%, 1.7% and 2.6% of all deaths. The researchers felt that the difference between the second and third estimates was 'probably due to the existence of a boundary area between euthanasia and intensifying of the alleviation of pain and/or symptoms'[37] and to the probability of the third study counting cases of pain alleviation as cases of 'euthanasia', thereby exaggerating its incidence.[38]

Of the three studies it is, however, arguably the third which produces the most accurate estimate of 'euthanasia'. As the authors of the Survey point out, the respondents in the second study had no information other than the questionnaire and an accompanying letter, whereas those in the third had participated in the physician interviews, discussing one or more cases from their practice and the crucial concepts in the questionnaire for over two hours with a trained interviewer. The authors, noting that a 'great number'[39] of interviewees commented that the interview had clarified their thinking about MDELs, suggest the possibility of a learning effect: familiarity with the questionnaire, in which the question about euthanasia followed those relating to other MDELs, may have led the respondents to reply negatively to the earlier questions knowing that the question about euthanasia was to come. The authors conclude that the most important fact was that the respondents in the third study 'changed their approach with respect to their intention when administering morphine due to their recent intensive confrontation with thinking about this complex of problems'.[40] If the thinking of participants in the third study had been clarified by their participation in the first study, their responses are surely more likely to have been reliable than those in the second study, particularly as, the second study being retrospective, there was less risk of memory distortion.

The authors' conclusion, however, is that in the light of all three studies, 'euthanasia' occurred in about 1.8% of all deaths, or about 2300 cases,[41] and that there were almost 400 cases of assisted suicide, some 0.3% of all deaths.[42] More than half the physicians regularly involved with terminal patients indicated that they had performed 'euthanasia' or had assisted suicide and only 12% of doctors said they would never do so.[43]

So much for euthanasia in its narrowest sense: intentional, *active* termination of life *at the patient's request*. But the authors of the Survey themselves go on, rightly, to consider euthanasia in a somewhat wider but still precise and realistic sense. They estimated that in a further 1000 cases (or 0.8% of all deaths) physicians administered a drug 'with the explicit purpose of hastening the end of life without an explicit request of the patient'.[44]

And beyond this, there lies a range of evidence yielded by the Survey, but not adequately considered by the authors in their commentary. For many other MDELs also involved an intent to hasten death. Palliative drugs were administered in 'such high doses . . . that . . . almost certainly would shorten the life of the patient'[45] in 22 500 cases (17.5% of all deaths).[46] In 65% (or 14 625) of these cases the doctor administered the medication merely 'Taking into account the probability that life would be shortened',[47] but in 30% (or 6750 cases) it was administered 'Partly with the purpose of shortening life'[48] and in a further 6% (or 1350 cases) 'With the explicit purpose of shortening life'.[49]

Moreover, doctors withdrew or withheld treatment without request in another 25 000 cases and, by the time of the Survey, some 90% of these patients, or 22 500, had died.[50] In 65% (or 16 250 cases) the treatment was withdrawn or withheld 'Taking into account the probability that life would be shortened',[51] but in 19% (or 4750 cases) 'Partly with the purpose to shorten life'[52] and in a further 16% (or 4000 cases) 'With the explicit purpose to shorten life'.[53]

Further, physicians received some 5800 requests to withdraw or withhold treatment when the patient intended at least in part to hasten death.[54] In 74% of these cases the doctor withdrew or withheld treatment partly with the purpose of shortening life but in 26% 'With the explicit purpose of shortening life'.[55] By the time of the interview, some 82% (or 4756) had died.[56] The above figures are reproduced in Table 1.

Thus, it becomes clear that, while the Commission stated that the figure of 2700 cases of 'euthanasia' and assisted suicide 'does not warrant the assumption that euthanasia in the Netherlands occurs on an excessive scale',[57] the total number of euthanasiast acts and omissions in 1990 was in reality far higher than the Commission claims. To clarify and confirm this conclusion it is necessary to look more closely at the definitions used by the authors of the Survey in classifying their data to produce the figure of 2700.

Table 1. *Medical decisions concerning the end of life in 1990*

Acts or omissions with intent to shorten life[a]		
Total deaths (all causes)	129 000	
'Euthanasia'[b]		*2 300*
Assisted suicide		*400*
Intentional life-terminating acts without explicit request[c]		*1 000 (1 000)*
Alleviation of pain/symptoms[d]	22 500	
With the 'explicit purpose' of shortening life		*1 350 (450)*
'Partly with the purpose' of shortening life		6 750 (5 058)
Withdrawal/withholding of treatment without explicit request[c]	25 000	
With the 'explicit purpose' of shortening life		*4 000 (4 000)*
'Partly with the purpose' of shortening life		4 750 (4 750)
Withdrawal/withholding of treatment on explicit request[f]	5 800	
With the 'explicit purpose' of shortening life		*1 508*
'Partly with the purpose' of shortening life		4 292
Sub-total[g]		*10 558 (5 450)*
Total[h]		26 350 (15 258)

[a]Cases of 'explicit' intent to shorten life are in italics; cases without explicit request in parentheses.
[b]No shortening of life occurred in 1% of these cases. Survey, 49, table 5.13.
[c]No shortening of life occurred in 4% of these cases. Ibid., 66, table 6.10.
[d]No shortening of life occurred in 8% of these cases. Ibid., 73, table 7.3.
[e]Ninety per cent of these patients (22 500) had died by the time of the interview and there had been no shortening of life in 20% of these cases. Ibid., 90, table 8.14.
[f]Eighty-two per cent of these patients (4756) had died by the time of the interview and there had been no shortening of life in 19% of these cases. Ibid., 82, table 8.6.
[g]This sub-total refers to cases where doctors 'explicitly' intended to shorten life by act or omission.
[h]This total refers to cases where doctors intended ('explicitly' or 'partly') to hasten death by act or omission. Both it and the preceding sub-total therefore include (as does the Survey) cases where life may not in fact have been shortened and cases in the two withdrawal/withholding of treatment categories where patients had not died by the time of the Survey.

The definition of euthanasia adopted by the Commission was the '*intentional* action to terminate a person's life, performed by somebody else than the involved person upon the latter's request'.[58] Similarly, the definition adopted in the Survey was 'the *purposeful* acting to terminate life by someone other than the person concerned upon request of the latter'.[59] These definitions echo that embraced by the central committee of the KNMG in its 1984 report on euthanasia as all actions 'aimed at'[60] terminating a patient's life at his explicit request. This report added that a majority of the committee had rejected a sub-division into 'active' and 'passive' as 'morally superfluous'[61] and undesirable: 'All activities or non-activities *with the purpose to terminate a patient's life* are defined as euthanasia'.[62]

The authors of the Survey distinguish the following states of mind:

> [acting with] the explicit purpose of hastening the end of life;
> [acting] partly with the purpose of hastening the end of life;
> [acting while] taking into account the probability that the end of life will be hastened.[63]

They explain that the first category, unlike the third, applied where the patient's death was the intended outcome of the action. The second category was used because sometimes an act was performed with a particular aim (such as pain relief) but the side effect (such as death) was 'not unwelcome'.[64] The authors felt that such an effect should be categorised as intentional because to count as *un*intentional a death 'should not in fact have been desired'.[65] The category related to a situation in which the 'death of the patient was not foremost in the physician's mind but neither was death unwelcome'[66] and was regarded by the author as a 'type' of intention.[67]

As Table 1 reveals, doctors are stated by the Survey to have intended to accelerate death in far more than the 2700 cases classified by the Commission as 'euthanasia' and assisted suicide. This total ignores the 1000 cases of intentional killing without request and, in addition, three further categories where there is said to have been some intention to shorten life: first, the 8100 (1350 + 6750) cases of increasing the dosage of palliative drugs; secondly, the 8750 (4000 + 4750) cases of withholding or withdrawing treatment without request and, finally, the 5800 (1508 + 4292) cases of withholding or withdrawing treatment on request.[68] Adding these 23 650 cases to the 2700 produces a total of 26 350 cases in which the Survey states that doctors intended, by act or omission, to shorten life. This raises the incidence of euthanasia from around 2% to over 20% of all deaths in Holland.

It could be argued that the 23 650 cases are not 'euthanasia' because they are not cases of intentional killing at the patient's request. There are, however, two counter-arguments. First, some of them clearly *are*. In relation, for example, to the 1350 cases in which it was the explicit purpose of the doctor to shorten life by increasing the dosage of palliative drugs, the Survey discloses: 'In all these cases the patient had at some time indicated something about terminating life and an explicit request had been made in two thirds of the cases'.[69] Indeed, the authors comment: 'This situation is therefore rather similar to euthanasia'.[70] It is unclear, therefore, why the Commission does not regard these as cases of 'euthanasia'; they seem to fall squarely within its definition. Interestingly, a member of the Commission (who in fact wrote the

Report) has subsequently agreed with the proposition that those cases where doctors had, with the explicit purpose of shortening the patient's life and at the patient's explicit request, administered palliative drugs, could properly be categorised as euthanasia.[71]

The second counter-argument is that the true scale of euthanasia can only properly be gauged when the Commission's abnormally narrow definition of 'euthanasia' is replaced by a standard definition such as 'when the death of a human being is brought about on purpose as part of the medical care being given to him'.[72] If this more realistic definition is applied, then the Survey's own presentation of the data suggests that there were a further 23 650 deaths by euthanasia.

However, there remains a further question about the proper interpretation of the Survey's definitions, and thus of its figures. Is it appropriate to include the 15 792 cases in which hastening death was only 'partly' the doctor's intention? These cases were distinguished in the Survey from those where the doctor merely foresaw the acceleration of death (where he proceeded 'Taking into account the probability that life would be shortened'[73]). If the doctor's purpose in these cases was, albeit partly, to hasten death, then it seems quite appropriate to regard them as instances of euthanasia. By analogy, if racial discrimination is the intentional (purposeful) treating of one person less favourably than another on racial grounds and, say, an employer takes advantage of a need to make redundancies in order to get rid of his black workers, he may be said to have acted partly with a view to doing just that, even though his primary purpose is to save his company by reducing expenditure on wages.

On the other hand, it is arguable that these are not necessarily cases in which the doctor's purpose was to hasten death. Notwithstanding the researchers' treatment of these as cases of purposeful killing, their explanation of this category and in particular their apparent understanding of the concept of 'purpose' in fact leave the matter unclear. The implication in their explanation that death in these cases was 'desired' does indeed suggest that the doctor intended to shorten life, but the reference to death as a 'not unwelcome' consequence suggests that death, while not regretted, may not, in some of these cases, have been any part of the doctor's purpose or goal.

Although it may well be that the doctor's intention in most if not all of these cases was to shorten life (a conclusion which would be consistent with the finding that no fewer than 88% of Dutch doctors had performed euthanasia or would be willing to do so[74]), the possibility that it was not cannot be ruled out. These cases are, therefore, regarded in this chapter as cases of intentional shortening of life subject to this *caveat*. However, the force of the following critique of Dutch euthanasia in no way depends on their inclusion. For even if they are discounted, the total number of life-shortening acts and omissions where the doctor's *primary* intention (more graphically but less precisely called 'explicit purpose' by the Survey) was to kill, and which are therefore indubitably euthanasiast, is 10 558. That figure is almost 4 times higher than the number of cases categorised as 'euthanasia' and assisted suicide by the Commission and amounts to over 8% of all deaths in Holland. In other words, almost 1 in 12 of all deaths in Holland in 1990 was intentionally accelerated by a doctor.

3. 'Dances with data'?

The authors of the van der Maas Survey recently argued that I (and a number of other commentators on Dutch euthanasia) have misinterpreted their findings.[75] One of their main criticisms (to which I shall limit myself in the interests of conciseness) is that I have inaccurately inflated the number of cases of euthanasia and assisted suicide disclosed by their Survey. I respectfully demur.

It will be recalled that van der Maas *et al.* concluded that there were 2300 cases of euthanasia and 400 cases of assisted suicide[76] and that what largely accounts for the discrepancy between their total of 2700 and mine of 10 558 is their peculiarly narrow definition of 'euthanasia' as '*active, voluntary* euthanasia' as contrasted with my standard definition of euthanasia as the intentional shortening of a patient's life, by act or omission. Their arguments for rejecting my total are quite unpersuasive. Their main argument is that 'intentions cannot carry the full weight of a moral evaluation on their own'[77] because 'intentions are essentially private matters. Ultimately only the agent "decides" what his intentions are, and different agents may describe the same actions in the same situations as performed with different intentions'.[78] And, they add, the agent's purpose may change over time, so what is to count as the 'definitive description'?[79]

This line of argument is remarkable. They agree that euthanasia is to be distinguished from other MDELs in that it involves the intentional ('purposeful') shortening of life; indeed, one of the welcome features of their meticulous Survey is the care they took to ascertain the doctors' state of mind when hastening death. They specifically *asked* whether the doctors shortened life with the 'explicit purpose' of so doing; or 'partly with the purpose' of so doing; or merely 'taking into account the probability' of so doing and the doctors *replied* that in some 10 558 cases it had been their *explicit intention to shorten life*. Why are the doctors' own answers not taken as the 'definitive description' of their intention? If the authors thought it impossible to discern the doctors' intention, why did they bother asking them?

The authors add that no doctor who performs euthanasia does so with the sole intent to kill: 'His or her intention can always be described as trying to relieve the suffering of his or her patient. This is exactly what infuriates Dutch physicians when, after reporting the case they are treated as criminals and murderers'.[80] However, while the doctor's ultimate intention may be to relieve suffering, he intends to do so by shortening the patient's life which is precisely why, in most jurisdictions, the doctor who performs euthanasia is liable for murder. If an heir kills his rich father by slipping a lethal poison into his tea, would they deny that this was murder on the ground that the heir's intention was not to kill and 'can always be described as' trying to accelerate his inheritance?

They continue that it is wrong to rest the moral evaluation entirely on intention: 'For a moral evaluation, more is to be taken into account, such as the presence of a request of the patient, the futility of further medical treatment, the sequelae of the decision to stop treatment (e.g. will this cause heavy distress?), the interests of others involved such as family and so on'.[81] Yet more muddle. The question at issue here is not the *moral evaluation* of cases of euthanasia but their *incidence*, and this is a matter of definition, not evaluation. And standard definitions reckon as euthanasia cases where the doctor, by act or omission, intentionally shortens life.

A further argument they advance is that if the 'context' is taken into account, it can be questioned whether the intentions were euthanasiast. As an example they cite the 6% of cases of alleviation of pain and symptoms in which doctors stated that their explicit intention was to shorten life. The authors seek to distinguish these cases from euthanasia on the ground that they involve a failure of palliative care followed by the use of higher doses which may lead to a point at which 'the physician realises that he or she actually hopes that the patient dies'.[82] His or her intention is 'not necessarily'[83] the same as with euthanasia, where the physician would surely try another lethal drug if the first failed, which would 'never'[84] happen with the administration of opioids.

This argument, too, fails. First, in these 6% of cases doctors stated it was their *explicit*, not partial, intention to shorten life; the authors give no reason to doubt the accuracy of this response. Secondly, the argument appears to rest on the unsubstantiated speculation that, had the higher dose failed to shorten life, the doctor would not have resorted to another method. Even if this were so, the argument is specious, resting on a patent *non sequitur*. If A attempts to kill B by method M1, which fails, his decision not to resort to method M2 in no way establishes he did not intend to kill by method M1.

In sum, the arguments advanced by van der Maas *et al.* against my total of 10 558 backfire, succeeding only in highlighting the inaccurate basis on which they have calculated their own total of 2700.

C. Conformity with the Guidelines?

How many of the 10 558 (or, if partly intended life-shortening is included, 26 350) euthanasiast acts and omissions satisfied the Guidelines laid down by the courts and the KNMG? More specifically, in how many cases was there a 'free and voluntary' request which was 'well-considered, durable and persistent'? In how many was there 'intolerable' suffering for which euthanasia was a 'last resort'? And in how many cases did the doctor consult with a colleague and report the case to the legal authorities, whether prosecutor, police or local medical examiner?[85]

1. An 'entirely free and voluntary' request which was 'well-considered, durable and persistent'

Doctors stated that in the '2700' cases of euthanasia and assisted suicide there was an 'explicit request'[86] in 96%; which was 'wholly made by the patient'[87] in 99% of all cases and 'repeated'[88] in 94%; and that in 100% of cases the patient had a 'good insight'[89] into his disease and its prognosis. Oddly, no specific question was put about the voluntariness of the request and there is no evidence of any mechanism to ensure that the request was voluntary. Moreover, the request was purely oral in 60% of cases[90] and, when made to a general practitioner (GP) in cases where a nurse was caring for the patient, the GP more often than not failed to consult her.[91]

There is no way of gauging the accuracy of the doctors' statements, which are uncorroborated, about the patients' requests. Even if they are true, however, the Survey data show that in the 10 558 cases in which it was the doctor's primary purpose to hasten death, there was in the majority (52%) no explicit request from the patient. Similarly, in a majority (58%) of the 26 350 cases in which it was the doctor's primary or secondary intention to shorten life, the doctor shortened life without the patient's explicit request.

(i) 'Life-terminating acts without the patient's explicit request'. In the light of the three studies, the Survey concludes:

> On an annual basis there are, in the Netherlands, some thousand cases (0.8% of all deaths) for which physicians prescribe, supply or administer a drug with the explicit purpose of hastening the end of life without an explicit request of the patient.[92]

In over half these cases, the decision was discussed with the patient or the patient had previously indicated his wish for the hastening of death, but in 'several hundred cases there was no discussion with the patient and there also was no known wish from the patient for hastening the end of life'.[93] Virtually all cases, state the authors, involved seriously ill and terminal patients who obviously were suffering a great deal and were no longer able to express their wishes, though there was a 'small number'[94] of cases in which the decision could have been discussed with the patient.

The fact that doctors administered a lethal drug without an express request in 1000 cases – almost half as many as they did on request – is striking. So too is the Commission's reaction to this statistic. The Commission observes that the ('few dozen'[95]) cases in which the doctor killed a *competent* patient without request 'must be prevented in future',[96] and that one means would be 'strict compliance with the scrupulous care'[97] required for euthanasia 'including the requirement that all facts of the case are put down in writ[i]ng'.[98] However, the Commission *defends* the other cases of unrequested killing, stating that 'active intervention'[99] by the doctor was usually 'inevitable'[100] because of the patient's 'death agony'.[101] That is why, it explains, it regards these cases as 'care for the dying'.[102] It adds that the ultimate justification for killing in these cases was the patient's 'unbearable suffering'.[103]

The Commission's assertion that most of the 1000 patients were incompetent patients in their 'death agony' should not pass unchallenged. The physician interviews indicate that 14% of the patients were totally competent and a further 11% partly competent;[104] that 21% had a life expectancy of one to four weeks and 7% of one to six months (the Survey classed patients as 'dying' if their life had been shortened only by 'hours or days', not by 'weeks or months'[105]) and that doctors did not list 'agony' as a reason for killing these patients. The reasons given by doctors were the absence of any prospect of improvement (60%); the futility of all medical therapy (39%); avoidance of 'needless prolongation'[106] (33%); the relatives' inability to cope (32%); and 'low quality of life'[107] (31%). Pain or suffering was mentioned by only 30%.[108] And, even in relation to these 30%, if they were essentially cases of increasing pain or symptom treatment to shorten life, why did the doctors not classify them under that heading?[109]

In short, the Commission's defence of these 1000 cases would appear to be based on a shaky factual foundation and its attempted ethical justification amounts to little more than a bare assertion that killing without request, a practice in breach of cardinal criteria for permissible euthanasia, is morally acceptable. On the basis of this assertion, it proceeds to recommend that doctors should report such cases in the same way as they report cases of voluntary euthanasia.[110]

The Government has implemented the Commission's recommendation that euthanasia without request should be reported by incorporating the reporting procedure into the law regulating the disposal of the dead. The procedure makes it clear that it applies whether or not the patient requested euthanasia.[111]

(ii) Other cases of intentional life-shortening without explicit request. In addition to the 1000 cases of active life termination without explicit request there were many more in which the patient made no explicit request that his life be shortened.

In 59% (or 4779) of the 8100 cases in which doctors are said to have intended to hasten death by pain-killing drugs, the patient had 'never indicated anything about terminating life'.[112] and there had been no explicit request in a further 9% (or 729),[113] making 5508 cases in which there had been no explicit request.[114]

Additionally, in 8750 cases treatment is said to have been withheld or withdrawn without explicit request and intentionally to shorten life.[115] The Commission would have it that these were cases of omitting to provide futile treatment. It states:

> After all, a doctor has the right to refrain from (further) treatment, if that treatment would be pointless according to objective medical standards. The commission would define a treatment without any medical use as therapeutical interference that gives no hope whatsoever for any positive effect upon the patient. To the application of this kind of futile medicine, no one is entitled. It is undisputed that the medical decision whether a particular action is useful or not, belongs to normal medical practice.[116]

The Commission appears confused. First, the Survey did not use the concept of futile treatment in relation to withdrawal of treatment as the authors felt its meaning was open to 'variable' interpretation.[117] Secondly, the preamble to the relevant questions suggests that they were not asking about the withdrawal of futile treatment, that is, treatment which was unlikely or incapable of achieving its normal therapeutic purpose, but rather about the withdrawal of treatment which was preserving 'futile' lives, that is, lives which were not thought to be worth preserving:

> In most instances this [decision to withhold or withdraw treatment] concerns situations in which the treating physician does not expect or does not observe sufficient success. However, there are situations in which a considerable life-prolonging effect can be expected from a certain treatment while the decision can nevertheless be made to withhold such treatment or to withdraw it. This implies that under such circumstances considerable prolongation of

> life is considered undesirable or even futile. 'Considerable' is taken to mean more than one month.[118]

That the questions were concerned with 'futile' lives rather than ineffectual treatment is further suggested by the authors' explanation of this series of questions:

> Briefly, two types of situations are discussed here. On the one hand therapies are involved which will probably meet with little or no success. Such treatment can be withdrawn or withheld for this reason. On the other hand there are cases in which therapies which can have a considerable (more than one month) life-prolonging effect but in which prolongation of life is undesirable or pointless and treatment is withdrawn or withheld for this reason.[119]

They add that doctors were asked to discuss 'only the second type'[120] of situation.

Thirdly, it seems clear that the question was so understood by at least some of the respondents, 35% of whom replied that their (primary or secondary) intention was to hasten death, not to withdraw a futile treatment.[121]

That the lives of so many patients were shortened without explicit request is striking. Hardly less striking is the fact that by no means all of the patients killed without request were incompetent. It will be recalled that of the 1000 actively killed without request, 14% were (according to the physician interviews) totally competent and a further 11% partly competent. Van der Wal has aptly commented that in these cases the right to self-determination was 'seriously undermined'.[122] Moreover, of the 8100 patients whose deaths are said to have been intentionally accelerated by palliative drugs, 60% (or 2867) of those who had never indicated anything about life termination were competent.[123] Finally, the patient was totally competent in 22%, and partly competent in a further 21%, of all the cases where treatment was withheld or withdrawn without request.[124]

The Commission concludes that the Survey 'disproves the assertion often expressed, that non-voluntary active termination of life occurs more frequently in the Netherlands than voluntary termination'.[125] However, if intentional termination by omission is included, as it should be if an accurate overall picture is to be presented, the Survey indicates that non-voluntary euthanasia is in fact more common than voluntary euthanasia. As Table 1 illustrates, the Survey discloses that in 1990 doctors intentionally sought to shorten more lives without than with the patient's explicit request. It was their primary aim to kill 10 558 patients, 5450 (52%) of whom had not explicitly asked to have their lives shortened. If one includes cases in which the patient's death is referred to as part of what the doctor aimed to achieve, then the total number of intentional killings by doctors may not be far short of 26 350, in 15 258 (58%) of which the patient had not explicitly asked for death to be hastened.

2. 'Intolerable suffering with no prospect of improvement' when euthanasia was a 'last resort'

(i) 'Intolerable suffering'. The Survey throws considerable doubt on whether euthanasia was confined to patients who were 'suffering unbearably' and for whom it was a 'last resort'.[126] For example, doctors were asked in interview which reason(s) patients most often gave for requesting euthanasia. Their replies to this question (and to that about the most important reasons for killing without request[127]) show that in most cases, 57%, it was 'loss of dignity';[128] in 46% 'not dying in a dignified way';[129] in 33% 'dependence'[130] and in 23% 'tiredness of life'.[131] Only 46% mentioned 'pain'.[132]

One recent case concerned a 50-year-old woman who had lost two sons, one to suicide, the other to cancer, and who repeatedly asked her psychiatrist, a Dr Chabot, to help her die. Dr Chabot assisted her to commit suicide and was prosecuted but acquitted. The prosecution's appeal to the Court of Appeal was unsuccessful but an appeal to the Supreme Court resulted in the doctor's conviction on the ground that the doctor should have ensured that one of the doctors he had consulted had personally examined the patient. A novel and disturbing feature of the case is that the woman was not terminally or, indeed, even physically ill. The suffering which was considered sufficient to warrant assisted suicide was purely mental, resulting from a 'depression in a narrower sense without psychotic characteristics in the context of a complicated grieving process'.[133]

In relation to cases of withholding or withdrawal of treatment without explicit request and with intent to hasten death, the basis for the decision appears to have been simply a belief that, in the words of the preamble to the question put, 'considerable prolongation of life'[134] was considered 'undesirable or even futile'.[135]

That Dutch doctors regard 'unbearable suffering' as an essential criterion is, moreover, hardly confirmed by the agreement of two thirds of those interviewed with the proposition that 'Everyone is entitled to decide over their own life and death'.[136]

(ii) A 'last resort'. Nor does it appear that euthanasia was invariably a 'last resort'. Doctors said that treatment alternatives remained in 1 in 5 cases (21%) but that, in almost all of these cases, they were refused.[137] One in three GPs who decided that there were no alternatives had not sought advice from a colleague.[138] When asked to rank the Guidelines in order of importance, only

64% of respondents said absence of treatment alternatives was '(very) important'.[139]

Moreover, even in the 4 out of 5 cases in which the doctors said there were no treatment alternatives, this appears to mean 'alternatives to the current treatment' rather than 'alternatives to euthanasia', an interpretation supported both by the question asked ('Were alternatives available to the treatment given? Here I consider other therapeutic possibilities or possibilities to alleviate pain and/or symptoms'[140]) and by the doctors' response to another question about the aim of the treatment at the time when the decision to carry out euthanasia or assisted suicide was made. Seventy-seven percent replied it was palliative, 10% life prolonging, and 2% curative: only 14% said there was no treatment.[141] In other words, just because there might have been no treatment alternatives to the existing treatment does not mean that the existing treatment was not an alternative to euthanasia.

But even *if* palliative treatment given in 77% of cases was not preventing intolerable suffering and was so ineffectual that euthanasia was thought to be the only alternative, does this (and the fact that in 46% of cases pain was one of the reasons most frequently given by patients as a reason for wanting euthanasia) not raise questions about the quality of the palliative care that the patients were receiving? A report on palliative care published in 1987 by the Dutch Health Council concluded that a majority of cancer patients in pain suffered unnecessarily because of health professionals' lack of expertise.[142] Similarly, more recent research into pain management at the Netherlands Cancer Institute, Amsterdam, contains the 'critical and worrisome overall finding . . . that pain management was judged to be inadequate in slightly more than 50% of evaluated cases'.[143]

Interestingly, 40% of the Dutch doctors interviewed in the van der Maas Survey expressed agreement with the proposition that 'Adequate alleviation of pain and/or symptoms and personal care of the dying patient make euthanasia unnecessary'.[144] Yet the Commission concludes that its total of 2700 cases of 'euthanasia' and assisted suicide shows that 'euthanasia' is not being used as an alternative to good palliative medicine or terminal care.[145] This observation is quite unsupported by the data, which reveal not 2700 but over 10 500 unambiguously euthanasiast acts and omissions. It also sits uneasily with the Commission's later observation about the inadequacy of such care in Holland:

> The research report shows that the medical decision process with regard to the end of life demands more and more expertise in a number of different areas. First of all medical and technical know-how, especially in the field of the

treatment of pain, of prognosis and of alternative options for the treatment of disorders that cause insufferable pain.[146]

It adds:

> Especially doctors, but nurses as well, will have to be trained in terminal care . . . Optimal care for someone who is dying implies that the doctor has knowledge of adequate treatments for pain, of alternatives for the treatment of complaints about unbearable pain and that he is aware of the moment when he must allow the process of dying to run its natural course. Doctors still lack sufficient knowledge of this care . . . In a country that is rated among the best in the world when it comes to birth care, knowledge with regard to care for the dying should not be lacking.[147]

If there is such a lack of knowledge, does this not confirm and help to explain the Survey evidence which indicates that euthanasia is being used as an alternative to appropriate palliative care?[148]

3. Performed by a doctor who has consulted an independent colleague and reported the case to the legal authorities

(i) Consultation. A KMNG-proposed scheme of consultation with two colleagues, one of whom is independent, has never been put into effect. Doctors stated that they had consulted a colleague in 84% of cases of euthanasia and assisted suicide.[149] The Survey does not explain the form, substance or outcome of the consultations. Again, in respect of the 1000 acts of life termination without request – cases where it might be assumed that consultation assumed especial importance – only a minority (48%) of doctors consulted a colleague.[150] Moreover, 40% of GPs stated that they did not think that consultation was very important.[151]

(ii) Reporting. Only a minority of cases of 'euthanasia' were duly reported to the legal authorities. In almost 3 out of 4 cases (72%) doctors (3 out of 4 GPs and 2 out of 3 specialists) certified that death was due to 'natural causes'.[152] By so doing, they not only failed to comply with one of the Guidelines whose importance has been continually stressed by the KNMG, but they also committed the criminal offence of falsifying a death certificate.

Doctors gave as their three most important reasons for falsifying the certificate the 'fuss' of a legal investigation (55%); a desire to protect relatives from a judicial inquiry (52%); and a fear of prosecution (25%).[153]

Similarly, virtually all of the 1000 acts of life termination without request were certified as natural deaths. The most important reasons given by the doctors were the 'fuss' of a legal investigation (47%); the (remarkable) opinion that the death was in fact natural (43%); and the desire to safeguard the relatives from a judicial inquiry (28%).[154]

Interestingly, only 64% of doctors thought that each case of euthanasia should somehow be examined, and the most favoured form of review was by other doctors.[155]

III. THE SLIDE IN PRACTICE AND THE SHIFT IN OPINION

My earlier article suggested that the 'slippery slope' argument in both its logical and practical forms applies to the Dutch experience of euthanasia.[156] The Survey and the Report serve amply to reinforce that contention. The examination of the Guidelines in Part I of this paper concluded that they are vague, loose and incapable of preventing abuse. The Survey bears out this conclusion by indicating that cardinal safeguards – requiring a request which is free and voluntary; well-informed; and durable and persistent – have been widely disregarded. Doctors have killed with impunity. And on a scale previously only guessed at: the Survey discloses that it was the primary purpose of doctors to shorten the lives of over 10 000 patients in 1990, the majority without the patient's explicit request.

How the Remmelink Commission can so confidently conclude, in the light of the evidence unearthed by the Survey, that the 'medical actions and decision process concerning the end of life are of high quality'[157] is puzzling. The Commission's assessment is based solely on the doctors' uncorroborated replies, replies which disclose, surely far more reliably, wholesale breach of the Guidelines. In particular, the scale of intentional life-shortening without explicit request and of illegal certification of death by natural causes must cast grave doubt both on the Commission's conclusion that decision-making is of 'high quality' and on van der Maas's opinion that the Survey shows that doctors are 'prepared to account for their decisions'.[158] As the 1000 cases of unrequested killings vividly illustrate, the existing system cannot realistically hope to detect the doctor who ignores the Guidelines since it essentially relies on him to expose his own wrongdoing.

Moreover, the Remmelink Report's narrow categories of 'euthanasia' and 'intentional killing without request' may suggest to those who have not considered it before a neat way of side-stepping the reporting procedure. A doctor might kill not by a lethal drug, which he would be required to report, but by an overdose of morphine or by withdrawing treatment, which he could claim with at least some show of legitimacy (in the unlikely event of being challenged) to be 'normal medical practice'.

Even though recent statistics indicate a significant increase in the number of cases reported (1424 in 1994[159]) it seems clear that the reporting procedure will continue to provide a wholly inadequate mechanism for regulating euthanasia and that the reports filed will continue to provide no more accurate a picture of the reality of euthanasia than they have hitherto done. Reports of killing without request promise to be particularly unrepresentative: how many doctors are likely to report a practice which has not (yet) been declared lawful by the courts?[160] Further, even if all cases were reported, this would still provide no guarantee of propriety; indeed, were all to be reported, it is doubtful whether prosecutors would have the resources to subject them even to the limited check which reports currently receive.

The Report uses the finding that doctors refused some 4000 serious requests[161] to argue that 'euthanasia' is not used excessively and as an alternative to good palliative care.[162] Leaving aside the evident shortcomings in Dutch terminal care, this is simply illogical, particularly when viewed against the 10 500 occasions on which it was the doctor's primary purpose to shorten life.

That statistic suggests rather the pertinence of the 'slippery slope' argument. The argument's relevance is indeed quite strongly suggested by the fact that doctors had as their primary aim the shortening of the lives of some 5500 patients without their explicit request (and are represented in the Survey as having had as their subordinate aim the shortening of the lives of upwards of a further 10 000 without their explicit request). The relevance is sufficiently striking even if one focuses simply on the 1000 cases involving the administration of a lethal drug without explicit request. Nor were these patients killed by a minority of maverick doctors: a majority of doctors admitted that they either had killed without request or would be prepared to do so.[163]

In any event, it is now apparent that legal and medical authorities in Holland openly condone non-voluntary euthanasia in certain circumstances. The Remmelink Report defends, it will be recalled,[164] the vast majority of the 1000 killings without request as 'care for the dying'.[165] Stating that the absence of a request only serves to make the decision more difficult than when there is a request, it adds:

> The ultimate justification for the intervention is in both cases the patient's unbearable suffering. So medically speaking, there is little difference between these situations and euthanasia, because in both cases patients are involved who suffer terribly. The absence of a special request for the termination of life stems partly from the circumstance that the party in question is not (any longer) able to express his will because he is already in the terminal stage, and partly because the demand for an explicit request is not in order when the

> treatment of pain and symptoms is intensified. The degrading condition the patient is in, confronts the doctor with a case of force majeure. According to the commission, the intervention by the doctor can easily be regarded as an action that is justified by necessity, just like euthanasia.[166]

The classification of killing without request as 'care for the dying' could be criticised as tendentious euphemism and is inconsistent even with established Dutch terminology.[167] Moreover, in view of the importance which has long been attached by many Dutch proponents of euthanasia to the need for a request by the patient, it is remarkable that the Commission, rather than setting out a reasoned ethical case to substantiate its opinion that killing without request can be justified, should do scarcely more than simply assert that a request is no longer essential in all cases.

Nevertheless, the Dutch Parliament has implemented the Commission's recommendation that the reporting procedure for euthanasia should clearly allow for such cases. It has amended the Burial Act 1955 to set out the reporting procedure in statutory form, a form which makes it clear that the procedure is to be followed even in cases of euthanasia without request.[168] The amendment, which was passed in 1993 and came into force in June 1994, has not made euthanasia lawful but has enshrined the reporting procedure in statutory form.

Moreover, a committee of the KNMG set up to consider non-voluntary euthanasia has condoned the killing, in certain circumstances, of incompetent patients including babies and patients in persistent coma and has canvassed opinion on the killing of patients with severe dementia.[169] It is surely only a matter of time before such 'responsible' medical opinion receives judicial approval. Indeed, if the criterion for the availability of the defence of necessity is what accords with 'responsible' medical opinion, it is difficult to see how the courts could deny it. The authors of the van der Maas Survey, referring to the 1000 killings without explicit request, state that legally speaking there is no question that these cases should be seen as anything other than murder but that 'the possibility that a court will accept an appeal to force majeure cannot be ruled out'.[170] Similarly, Leenen has recently expressed the opinion (which seems to contradict his earlier opinion,[171] to which he does not refer) that in 'exceptional' cases non-voluntary euthanasia attracts the necessity defence.[172] The approval of the courts may not even be necessary: the Chief Prosecutors have already declined to prosecute in a number of cases of killing without request.

One such case involved a patient in a permanent coma after a heart attack. The local Chief Prosecutor, mindful of the Remmelink Commission's recommendation that such cases should be dealt with in the same way as killing on request, decided against prosecution; after questions had been raised in Parliament, his decision was affirmed at a meeting of all the Chief Prosecutors in February 1992.[173]

Another case concerned a dying, comatose 71-year-old man who had not asked for his life to be shortened. At a meeting in November 1992 the Chief Prosecutors decided against prosecution since 'the action taken . . . amounted to virtually the same as suspending ineffectual medical treatment',[174] even though they regarded the case as 'potentially extending the boundaries of current practice'.[175]

The current and growing condonation of non-voluntary euthanasia contrasts markedly with earlier pronouncements on euthanasia. There was little support for non-voluntary euthanasia in 1984. As has been seen, the very definition of 'euthanasia' adopted by the Dutch incorporated the need for a request. Moreover, the KNMG Report of that year was careful to confine itself to euthanasia on request and three of its five Guidelines were concerned with ensuring not only that there was a request but that it was free, well-considered and persistent. In 1985, a State Commission on Euthanasia concluded that third parties should not be permitted to request euthanasia on behalf of (incompetent) minors and 'other persons incapable of expressing their opinion, such as the mentally handicapped or senile elderly people'.[176] Its Vice-Chairman, Professor Leenen, has since written that the Commission proposed an amendment to the Penal Code to prohibit the intentional termination of an incompetent patient's life on account of serious physical or mental illness and did so in order to 'underline the importance of the request of the patient'.[177] In 1989, Leenen reaffirmed that a request was 'central' to the Dutch definition, adding:

> *Without it the termination of a life is murder*. This means that the family or other relatives, parents for their children, or the doctor cannot decide on behalf of the patient. *People who have become incompetent are no longer eligible for euthanasia*, unless they have made a living will prior to their becoming incompetent, in which they ask for the termination of life.[178]

He added that Article 2 of the European Convention for the Protection of Human Rights and Fundamental Freedoms, which provides that everyone's right to life shall be protected by law, does not (in his view) prohibit the killing of a patient who freely wishes to die but that it '*prohibits the State and others from taking another's life without his request*'.[179] Rejecting the argument that euthanasia would undermine the public's trust in doctors, he stated: 'People's trust in health care will not decrease if they are sure that euthanasia will not be administered *without their explicit request*'.[180] Leenen was echoed in the same year by Henk Rigter, who wrote in the *Hastings Center Report*: 'In the absence of a patient request the perpetrator renders him or herself guilty of manslaughter or murder'.[181] An array of leading Dutch advocates of voluntary euthanasia wrote endorsing the accuracy of Rigter's paper, adding that 'problems concerning the termination of life of incompetent patients, either comatose or newborn, are *not* part of the euthanasia problem'.[182] One, the Director of the National Hospital Association, wrote that 'euthanasia' meant killing on request, adding:

> Consequently, it is impossible for people who do not want euthanasia to be maneuvred or forced into it. The requirement of voluntariness means no one need fear that his or her life is in danger because of age or ill health, and that those who cannot express their will, such as psycho-geriatric patients or the mentally-handicapped, shall never be in danger as long as they live.[183]

But how much longer will they be allowed to live in view of the common practice of, and growing support for, non-voluntary euthanasia? The argument that euthanasia cannot be forced upon competent or incompetent people, and that such conduct is not part of the euthanasia problem, because it does not fall within the definition of 'euthanasia', is hardly convincing. If an advocate of abortion were to define abortion as 'therapeutic' abortion and dismiss arguments that its legalisation might lead to abortion for social reasons, or to women being pressured into abortion, on the ground that these would not be 'abortion' and are not, therefore, 'part of the abortion problem', he would rightly be given short shrift. The suggestion, by leading Dutch advocates of euthanasia, that the moral debate about euthanasia can be resolved by definitional *fiat* serves only to illustrate the intellectual poverty of the case for euthanasia which has come to prevail in their country.

The widespread readiness to kill without any request contrasts starkly with the refusal of many serious requests for euthanasia, and serves further to underline the dispensable role of patient autonomy in the reality, if not the rhetoric, of the Dutch experience. As ten Have and Welie shrewdly point out, acceptance of euthanasia is not resulting in greater patient autonomy but in doctors 'acquiring even more power over the life and death of their patients'.[184]

In 1990 Professor Leenen observed that there is an 'almost total lack of control on the administration of euthanasia' in Holland.[185] The Report and the Survey serve only to confirm the accuracy of that observation.[186] The Commission's Report paints a reassuring picture of the euthanasia landscape revealed by the Survey, but the scene it depicts is grossly misleading. As Dan Callahan has pointed out, the reality is quite different: 'The Dutch situation is a regulatory Potemkin village, a great façade hiding non-enforcement'.[187] The hard evidence of the Survey indicates that, within a remarkably short time, the Dutch have proceeded from voluntary to non-voluntary euthanasia. This is partly because of the inability of the vague and loose Guidelines to ensure that euthanasia is only performed in accordance with the criteria laid down by the courts and the KNMG. It is also because the underlying justification for euthanasia in Holland appears not to be patient self-determination, but rather acceptance of the principle that certain lives are not 'worth' living and that it is right to terminate them. Indeed, the authors of the van der Maas Survey recently lent support to this thesis when they wrote:

> [Is] it not true that once one accepts euthanasia and assisted suicide, the principle of universalizability forces one to accept termination of life without explicit request, at least in some circumstances, as well? In our view the answer to this question must be affirmative.[188]

An objection might be raised that the number of cases has remained static and that the evidence reveals not a slope but a plateau. This objection fails, however, to dent the slippery slope argument in its logical form. Indeed, even the empirical form of the argument is, arguably, not dependent on showing a statistical *in*crease in non-voluntary euthanasia over time. Even if the proportion of non-voluntary euthanasia cases remained stable from the time voluntary euthanasia gained approval, this would hardly disprove either the logical connection or the ineffectiveness of the safeguards; quite the contrary. There would appear, in any event, to be no empirical evidence to support the hypothesis of a plateau. Moreover, the hypothesis seems particularly implausible in the light of the available statistical evidence and the clear shift in opinion since 1984 in favour of the non-voluntary termination of life.

That the evidence from Holland lends support to the 'slippery slope' arguments should come as no surprise. Some twenty years ago a perspicacious warning about the dangers of venturing onto the slope was sounded by Dr John Habgood, now Archbishop of York and a member of the House of Lords Select Committee on Medical Ethics which reported early in 1994:[189]

> Legislation to permit euthanasia would in the long run bring about profound changes in social attitudes towards death, illness, old age and the role of the medical profession. The Abortion Act has shown what happens. Whatever the rights and wrongs concerning the present practice of abortion, there is no doubt about two consequences of the 1967 Act:
> (a) The safeguards and assurances given when the Bill was passed have to a considerable extent been ignored.
> (b) Abortion has now become a live option for *anybody* who is pregnant. This

does not imply that everyone who is facing an unwanted pregnancy automatically attempts to procure an abortion. But because abortion is now on the agenda, the climate of opinion in which such a pregnancy must be faced has radically altered.

One could expect similarly far-reaching and potentially more dangerous consequences from legalized euthanasia.[190]

However, the patent reality of the slide in Holland may not yet be fully appreciated outside (or, indeed, inside) that country. The slide was not *explicitly* identified and criticised by the House of Lords Select Committee on Medical Ethics, even though a delegation from the Committee visited Holland in October 1993. Perhaps the delegation was influenced by the statement made to them by a Ministry of Justice spokesman that 'the government held strongly to the position that euthanasia was not possible for incompetent patients'.[191] This statement was made eight months after the proposed change in the law to provide a mechanism for the reporting of non-voluntary euthanasia had been approved by the Second Chamber of the Dutch Parliament and one month before its approval by the First Chamber. If euthanasia was 'not possible' for incompetent patients, why was the government providing for its reporting?

A welcome recognition of the slide is, however, clearly implicit in the Committee's rejection of the legalisation of euthanasia, in the light of the Dutch experience, on the ground, *inter alia*, 'that it would not be possible to frame adequate safeguards against non-voluntary euthanasia'.[192] Moreover, in the debate on the motion to receive the Report in the Lords, the Committee's Chairman, Lord Walton, observed that those members of the Committee who had visited Holland returned from the visit 'feeling uncomfortable, especially in the light of evidence indicating that non-voluntary euthanasia . . . was commonly performed'.[193] He added that they were 'particularly uncomfortable'[194] about the case of the woman of 50 suffering from mental stress who had been assisted in suicide by her psychiatrist. His Lordship could, of course, have gone much further but took the view (without saying why) that it would not be proper for him to criticize the decisions of the 'medical and legal authorities in another sovereign state'.[195]

Another member of the Committee to comment unfavourably on the Dutch experience, Lord Meston, said:

> it did not seem possible to find any other place beyond the existing law for a firm foothold on an otherwise slippery slope. The evidence of the Dutch experience was not encouraging: in the Netherlands, which apparently lacks much in the way of a hospice movement, there seems to be a gap between the

> theory and practice of voluntary euthanasia. One cannot escape the fear that the same could happen here, with pressures on the vulnerable sick and elderly, who may perceive themselves to have become a burden on others, and pressures on the doctors and nurses from relatives and from those who are concerned with resources.[196]

Of course, the reality of the slippery slope may not have been lost on at least some Dutch advocates of voluntary euthanasia, who may have thought it tactically desirable to maintain a discreet silence about it. Professor Alexander Capron, reporting on a euthanasia conference in Holland at which this point was conceded, has written that the Dutch proponents of euthanasia began with a narrow definition of euthanasia 'as a strategy for winning acceptance of the general practice, which would then turn to . . . relief of suffering as its justification in cases in which patients are unable to request euthanasia'.[197] He adds: 'It was an instance, or so it seemed to me, when the candour of our hosts was a little chilling'.[198]

CONCLUSION

The evidence marshalled in this chapter indicates, consistently with that unearthed by others,[199] that the Dutch euthanasia experience lends weighty support to the slippery slope argument in both its forms. Within a decade, the so-called strict safeguards against the slide have proved signally ineffectual; non-voluntary euthanasia is now widely practised and increasingly condoned in the Netherlands.

As this book first went to press in 1995, it was reported that a Dutch court had, as predicted above, held that non-voluntary euthanasia could be lawful. The Alkmaar District Court held (in a case referred to in note 175) that a doctor charged with murder for killing a disabled newborn at its parents' request enjoyed the defence of necessity. In 1996, two Courts of Appeal affirmed the availability of the defence in such cases.[200] In the same year, a second survey by van der Maas was published, which served to confirm the lack of effective regulation as well as the extent of the Dutch descent down the slippery slope.[201] For inhabitants of such a flat country, the Dutch have indeed proved remarkably fast skiers.

NOTES

1 For an exposition of the argument in its logical form see Luke Gormally's chapter in this book. See also Yale Kamisar, 'Some Non-Religious Views against Proposed "Mercy-Killing" Legislation' (1958) 42 *Minnesota Law Review* 969.

2 *Stedman's Medical Dictionary* (25th ed., 1990) 544. See also n. 72.

3 P.J. van der Maas *et al.*, *Euthanasia and other Medical Decisions Concerning the End of Life* (Amsterdam: Elsevier, 1992) 5. Hereafter 'Survey'. Also published in (1992) 22(1)/(2) *Health Policy*. A summary of the Survey appears in (1991) 338 *Lancet* 669.

4 Though a Report of the KNMG on euthanasia states: 'All activities or non-activities with the purpose to terminate a patient's life are defined as euthanasia'. 'Vision on Euthanasia' (a translation by the KNMG in 1986 of its Report 'Standpunt inzake euthanasie' published in (1984) 39 *Medisch Contact* 990) 15.

5 *Nederlandse Jurisprudentie* ('*N.J.*') (1985) No. 106, 451 452. See also I. J. Keown, 'The Law and Practice of Euthanasia in The Netherlands' (1992) 108 *Law Quarterly Review* 51, 51–57.

6 *N.J.* (1985) No. 106, 453.

7 Ibid.

8 Ibid.

9 Ibid.

10 Keown, op. cit. n.5, 56.

11 Op. cit. n.4.

12 Ibid., 8–11.

13 'Guidelines for Euthanasia' (translated by W. Lagerwey) (1988) 2 *Issues in Law & Medicine* 429. Hereafter 'Guidelines'.

14 Henk Rigter, 'Euthanasia in The Netherlands: Distinguishing Facts from Fiction' (1989) 19(1) *Hastings Center Report* 31.

15 H. J. J. Leenen, 'The Definition of Euthanasia' (1984) 3 *Medicine and Law* 333, 334.

16 Interview by author with Dr Herbert Cohen, 26 July 1989.

17 Survey, 3.

18 Ibid., 4.

19 Ibid., 19–20.

20 Ibid., 20.

21 *Medische beslissingen rond het levenseinde. Rapport van de Commissie onderzoek medische praktijk inzake euthanasie* ('s-Gravenhage: Sdu Uitgeverij, 1991). Hereafter 'Report'.

22 *Medische beslissingen rond het levenseinde. Het onderzoek voor de Commissie Onderzoek Medische Praktijk inzake Euthanasie* ('s-Gravenhage: Sdu Uitgeverij, 1991).

23 Op. cit. n.3. Oddly, the Report has not been translated, though a brief English summary has been produced by the Ministry of Justice: *Outlines [sic] Report Commission Inquiry into Medical Practice with regard to Euthanasia* (nd). Hereafter 'Outline'. Dr Richard Fenigsen's unpublished 'First Reactions to the Report of the Committee on Euthanasia' (1991) contains a translation of key passages of the Report. I am grateful to Dr Fenigsen for permission to rely on his translation. His paper 'The Right of the Dutch Governmental Committee on Euthanasia' is published in (1991) 7 *Issues in Law & Medicine* 3.

24 Op. cit. n.5.

25 Ibid., 61–78.

26 See generally Survey, Part II (chapters 4–10).

27 Ibid., 14–17; 191. The authors considered whether those who refused to participate formed a select group which could lead to serious bias and concluded that, in the light of the total number of refusals (41) and the variety of reasons for refusing (mainly lack of time) this could hardly be so. The 15 who indicated that they disapproved of the Survey, did not wish to comment or opposed euthanasia could only have introduced a 'very modest' bias. Ibid., 228. This reasoning is unpersuasive: does the conclusion excluding bias not depend on answers which are unverified? Is it not possible that some of the 41 who declined to participate frequently performed euthanasia and equally possible that some of these cases fell outside the Guidelines?

28 Ibid., 33.

29 See generally ibid., Part III (chapters 11–13).

30 Ibid., 15; 121–125; 191.

31 See generally ibid., Part IV (chapters 14–15).

32 Ibid., 15; 149–151; 192.

33 Ibid., 160.

34 Ibid., 16.

35 Report, 14.

36 Ibid., 11 (see also Outline, 2); 'the purposeful acting to terminate life by someone other than the person concerned upon request of the latter'. Survey, 5; see also ibid., 23; 193.

37 Survey, 178.

38 Ibid.

39 Ibid., 162.

40 Ibid.
41 Ibid., 178.
42 Ibid., 179.
43 Ibid., 40, table 5.3.
44 Ibid., 182. The third study returned a figure of 1.6%. Ibid., 181.
45 Ibid., 71. The authors were not concerned with cases where palliative drugs were used which had no chance of shortening life. Ibid., 72. Life was shortened by up to one week in 70% of cases and by one to four weeks in 23%. Ibid., 73 table 7.3.
46 Ibid., 183.
47 Ibid., 72, table 7.2.
48 Ibid.
49 Ibid.
50 Ibid., 85; 90, table 8.14.
51 Ibid., 90, table 8.15.
52 Ibid.
53 Ibid.
54 Ibid., 81.
55 Ibid., 84, table 8.7.
56 Ibid., 82, table 8.6.
57 Report, 31; Outline, 2.
58 See n.36. (Emphasis added.)
59 Ibid. (Emphasis added.)
60 Op. cit. n.4, 15.
61 Ibid.
62 Ibid. (Emphasis added.)
63 Survey, 21. They state, confusingly, that death 'may not' have been intended in the third category.
64 Ibid.
65 Ibid.
66 Ibid.
67 Ibid.
68 By no means all of the patients from whom treatment was withdrawn on request were terminal. Life was shortened by one to four weeks in 16%, by one to six months in 43% and even longer in 13%. Ibid., 82, table 8.6. Moreover, three of the four reasons most frequently given by the patient for requesting withdrawal – 'loss of dignity' (31%), 'tiredness of life' (28%) and 'dependence' (24%): ibid., 82, table 8.4 – appear (unlike the remaining reason – 'burden of treatment' (43%)) quite consistent with a suicide intent. However, as the respondent doctors were not given the opportunity of stating that they withheld or withdrew treatment merely foreseeing that life would be shortened, the figures indicating that doctors intended to shorten life in *all* cases should be treated with some caution, and their categorisation here as cases of euthanasiast omissions is subject to this *caveat*.
69 Ibid., 72.
70 Ibid.
71 Interview by author with Mr A. Kors, Ministry of Justice, The Hague, 29 November 1991.
72 *Euthanasia and Clinical Practice: The Report of a Working Party* (The Linacre Centre, 1982) 2. See also *Dictionary of Medical Ethics* (A. S. Duncan, G. R. Dunstan, R. B. Welbourn eds; 1981) 164 ('. . . "mercy killing", the administration of a drug deliberately and specifically to accelerate death in order to terminate suffering'); and text at n.2.
73 Survey, 73, table 7.2; ibid., 90, table 8.15.
74 Ibid., 40, table 5.3.
75 P.J. van der Maas *et al.*, 'Dances with Data' (1993) 7 *Bioethics* 323.
76 See text at nn.41–42.
77 Op. cit. n.75, 325.
78 Ibid.
79 Ibid.
80 Ibid.
81 Ibid., 325–326.
82 Ibid., 326.
83 Ibid.
84 Ibid.
85 Ninety-eight per cent of doctors stated that they were aware of the 'rules of due care' formulated by the KNMG, the Health Council and the Government. When asked what they were, 89% mentioned consultation but only 66% the need for a seriously considered request; 42% a voluntary request; 37% 'unacceptable' suffering; and 18% a long-standing desire to die. Survey, 95–96, table 9.1. When shown 14 Guidelines, however, and asked to rank them in importance, 98% mentioned voluntariness and only 67% consultation. Ibid., table 9.2.
86 Ibid., 50, table 5.15.
87 Ibid.

88 Ibid.
89 Ibid.
90 Ibid., 43. A smaller, postal survey of euthanasia by nursing home physicians between 1986 and 1990 revealed that in over 1 in 5 cases euthanasia was administered less than a week after the first discussion with the patient (in 7% of cases in less than a day) and in 35% of cases less than a week after the first request. M. T. Muller *et al.*, 'Voluntary Active Euthanasia and Physician-Assisted Suicide in Dutch Nursing Homes: Are the Requirements for Prudent Practice Properly Met?' (1994) 42 *Journal of the American Geriatrics Society* 624, 626, table 2. Hereafter 'Muller'.
91 Survey, 108, table 10.3. (By contrast, 96% of specialists and nursing home doctors consulted nursing staff. Ibid.) Further, two thirds of GPs said they felt it was up to the doctors in certain circumstances to raise the topic of euthanasia. Ibid., 101.
92 Ibid., 182.
93 Ibid.
94 Ibid.
95 Outline, 3.
96 Ibid.
97 Ibid.
98 Ibid.
99 Ibid.
100 Ibid.
101 Ibid.
102 Ibid.
103 Ibid.
104 Seventy-five per cent of the patients were 'totally unable to assess the situation and take a decision adequately'. However, 14% were totally, and 11% partly ('not totally') able to do so. Survey, 61, table 6.4. The authors describe a person 'not totally able' as 'partially able to assess the situation and on this basis adequately take a decision'. Ibid., 23. According to the death certificate study, 36% were competent. Loes Pijnenborg *et al.*, 'Life-terminating Acts without Explicit Request of Patient' (1993) 341 *Lancet* 1196, 1197, table II.
105 Survey, 66, table 6.10. According to the Survey's (tentative) definition of 'dying' (ibid, 24), therefore, in only 29% of the 2700 cases of euthanasia and assisted suicide was the patient dying. Ibid., 49, table 5.13.
106 Ibid., 64, table 6.7.
107 Ibid.
108 Ibid. Surprisingly, no question was asked about the doctor's intention which, as the authors note, 'complicates the interpretation of the results'. Ibid., 57.
109 Henk Jochemsen, 'Euthanasia in Holland: An Ethical Critique of the New Law' (1994) 20 *Journal of Medical Ethics* 212 at 213.
110 Outline, 6. The Commission excepted from this recommendation cases where 'the vital functions have already and irreversibly begun to fail' on the ground that in such cases a natural death would have ensued anyway. Ibid. The Government has rejected this exception: see Gevers, op. cit. n.111, 140.
111 J. K. M. Gevers, 'Legislation on Euthanasia: recent Developments in the Netherlands' (1992) 18 *Journal of Medical Ethics* 138, 139–40. See text at n.168.
112 Survey, 76, table 7.9.
113 Ibid.
114 In 17% of cases, the patient had indicated something about life termination but the 'request was not strongly explicit'. Ibid. If these cases are included, the number of cases of life shortening without explicit request becomes 6885. In only 15% of cases, therefore, was there a 'strongly explicit' request. Ibid.
115 See text at nn.52–53. In 18% of cases the patient had 'indicated something at some time about terminating life' and in a further 13% there had been some discussion with the patient. Survey, 88, table 8.11.
116 Outline, 3–4.
117 Survey, 24.
118 Ibid., 84–85.
119 Ibid., 85.
120 Ibid.
121 See text at nn.52–53.
122 Gerrit van der Wal, 'Unrequested Termi-

nation of Life: Is It Permissible?' (1993) 7 *Bioethics* 330, 337.

123 Survey, 77.

124 Ibid., 88. The Survey does not appear to provide separate figures for those whose lives were intentionally shortened.

125 Outline, 3; Report, 33.

126 The Commission states that Dutch doctors regard the 'intolerable suffering of the patient and/or his natural desire for a quiet death' as the only grounds on which to perform euthanasia. Ibid., 32. The reference to these grounds in the alternative, without disapproval, is revealing: it confirms that neither all doctors nor the Commission regard both as essential for euthanasia to be permissible.

127 See text at nn.106–108.

128 Survey, 45, table 5.8.

129 Ibid.

130 Ibid.

131 Ibid.

132 Similarly, Muller found that the most common main reason for requesting euthanasia was not 'unbearable suffering' but 'fear of/avoidance of deterioration of condition'. Muller, 626, table 3. Nor is this clearly defined. Muller *et al.* observe that it means the 'gradual effacement and loss of personal identity that characterizes the end of stages [*sic*] of many terminal illnesses'. Ibid., 628. Further, earlier in the paper (at 624) they state that requests arising from fear of pain 'must be refused'. This makes it even more difficult to understand why fear of deterioration should be acceptable.

133 'een depressie in engere zin, zonder psychotische kenmerken, in het kader van een gecompliceerd rouwproces'. Hoge Raad, 21 June 1994, Strafkamer, nr. 96.972. para. 4.5. The Supreme Court rejected the prosecution's submissions that necessity required somatic pain and that a psychiatric patient could not make a genuine request for death. It held, however, that in cases where the suffering was not somatic, a proper factual basis for the necessity defence could be laid only where the patient had been examined by an independent doctor who had assessed the gravity of the suffering and possibilities for its alleviation. As the Appeal Court had not made such a finding in this case it had not been in a position to conclude that a situation of necessity existed. Although the doctor's conviction was restored, he was not punished. For commentaries on the case see T. Schalken, *N.J.* (1994) No. 656, 3256–59; J.H. Hubben, *Nederlands Juristenblad* (1994) No. 27, 912; H.J.J. Leenen, *Tijdschrift voor Gezondheidsrecht* (1994) No. 1, 48.

134 Survey, 85.

135 Ibid. For example, the evidence in relation to the 8750 cases in which doctors stated that they withheld or withdrew treatment without request with intent to shorten life does not indicate that all the patients were suffering unbearably and that euthanasia was a last resort. For one thing, 58% were incompetent, so how was the doctor able to assess the extent of the patients' suffering (if any), particularly as the patients' conditions varied? Survey, 88, table 8.12.

136 Ibid., 102, table 9.7.

137 Ibid., 45, table 5.7.

138 Ibid., 43. Even in those cases where the doctors (two thirds of GPs and 80% of specialists) did consult, there is nothing to suggest that the colleague consulted was a specialist in palliative medicine.

139 Ibid., 96, table 9.2.

140 Ibid., 43.

141 Ibid., 45, table 5.6. Why 14% were receiving no treatment is unexplained.

142 Op. cit. n.5, 65. The British Medical Association Working Party on Euthanasia commented that palliative care in Holland is not as advanced as in Britain. *Euthanasia* (London: BMA, 1988) 49.

143 Karin L. Dorrepaal *et al.*, 'Pain Experience and Pain Management among Hospitalized Cancer Patients' (1989) 63 *Cancer* 593, 598. Referring to this study, Zbigniew Zylic, Medical Director at Holland's newest hospice, comments that it does not warrant a general judgment about terminal care in Holland but should be

taken as a warning and a stimulus for further studies. He notes that 'cancer pain treatment and symptom control does not receive enough attention and in many places, it is practised at a very poor level. As yet, there is no specific training available in palliative care'. 'The Story Behind the Blank Spot', (July/August 1993) 10 *American Journal of Hospice & Palliative Care* 30, 32. He adds that there are no comprehensive hospices in Holland because the high standard of care in hospitals and nursing-homes and the Government's policy to reduce institutional beds have combined to discourage the hospice system. While hospitals are officially encouraged to provide hospice care, the necessary resources are not provided. Zylic urges the establishment of more hospices. Ibid., 33–34.

144 Survey, 102, table 9.7.

145 Outline, 2; Report, 31.

146 Outline, 7.

147 Ibid.

148 An expert committee of the World Health Organization has concluded: 'now that a practicable alternative to death in pain exists, there should be concentrated efforts to implement programmes of palliative care, rather than a yielding to pressure for legal euthanasia'. *Cancer Pain Relief and Palliative Care* (Geneva: WHO, Technical Report Series No. 804, 1990). Dr Pieter Admiraal, one of Holland's leading practitioners of euthanasia, has written that 'in most cases, pain can be adequately controlled without the normal psychological functions of the patient being adversely affected'. 'Justifiable Euthanasia' (1988) 3 *Issues in Law & Medicine* 361, 362.

149 Survey, 47, table 5.9.

150 Ibid., 64, table 6.8. The reason given for not doing so in 68% of cases was that the doctor felt no need for consultation because the situation was clear. Ibid., 65. Before withholding or withdrawing a treatment without request, doctors consulted a colleague in 54% of cases. Ibid., 89, table 8.13. (When there was a request the figure was 43%. Ibid., 82, table 8.5.) Before administering palliative drugs in such doses as might shorten life, doctors consulted in 47% of cases. Ibid., 73, table 7.4.

151 Ibid., 96, table 9.2. Muller's survey revealed that, of the doctors consulted, only two thirds talked with the patient, only half studied the medical records and only 17% physically examined the patient. Muller, 627.

152 Survey, 49, table 5.14. Muller found that in 57% of cases doctors certified a natural death. Muller, 628, table 7.

153 Survey, 48. The authors add that 23 doctors actually stated that they had regarded the death as natural.

154 Ibid., 65. Deaths hastened by withholding or withdrawing a treatment without request were almost all certified as natural deaths. Ibid., 89. So too were all deaths hastened by the administration of palliative drugs, in over 90% of cases because the doctor felt the death was natural, but in 9% because he felt that reporting an unnatural death would be 'troublesome'. Ibid., 74.

155 Ibid., 97, table 9.3. See also ibid., 98. It merits mention that in a small number of cases the lethal drug was administered by someone other than the doctor, nurse or patient. See ibid., 140, table 13.10; 143; 193.

156 Op. cit. n.5.

157 Outline, 6. Remarkably, van der Maas also regards them of 'good quality'. Survey, 199. According to the replies to Muller's survey, all the requirements were met in only 41% of cases. Muller, 628. Even this figure, based as it is on self-serving replies, may well be too high.

158 Survey, 205.

159 *See Table at end of these notes.*

160 Op. cit. n.111, 140.

161 Survey, 52.

162 Outline, 2.

163 Survey, 58, table 6.1.

164 See text at nn.99–103.

165 A member of the Commission informed me that these killings came as a 'terrible shock' to its members, who had hoped that they did not exist. Interview by author with Mr A. Kors, 29 November

1991. This makes the Commission's defence of the bulk of these killings all the more puzzling.

166 Outline, 3.

167 See text at nn.178; 181.

168 See *Report of the Select Committee on Medical Ethics* (HL 21-I of 1993–94) appendix 3, 65.

169 Henk Jochemsen, 'Life-prolonging and Life-terminating Treatment of Severely Handicapped Newborn Babies . . .'(1992) 8 *Issues in Law & Medicine* 167; *Doen of laten*? (Utrecht: Nederlandse Vereniging voor Kindergeneeskunde, 1992) 13; 'Dutch Doctors Support Life Termination in Dementia' (1993) 306 BMJ 1364.

170 Johannes J. M. van Delden *et al.*, 'The Remmelink Study: Two Years Later' (1993) 23(6) *Hastings Center Report* 24, 25; cf. Loes Pijnenborg *et al.*, 'Life-terminating Acts without Explicit Request of Patient' (1993) 341 *Lancet* 1196, 1199, where they write that, when all the 'safeguards' are respected and 'only the best interests of the patient are taken into account' such killings are 'certainly not murder'.

171 See text at nn.177–180.

172 H. J. J. Leenen and Chris Ciesielski-Carlucci, '*Force Majeure* (Legal Necessity): Justification for Active Termination of Life in the Case of Severely Handicapped Newborns after Forgoing Treatment' (1993) 2(3) *Cambridge Quarterly of Healthcare Ethics* 271, 274.

173 Personal communication, Staff Office of the Public Prosecutor, The Hague, 12 February 1993.

174 Ibid.

175 Ibid. A third case involved the killing of a 4-year-old handicapped child who was dying. Charges were dropped 'in view of the specific and unusual circumstances of the case, despite the fact that the patient had not expressly requested intervention'. Ibid. It has since been reported that two doctors who allegedly killed gravely ill newborns are to be prosecuted by order of the Minister of Justice in order to ascertain the law relating to non-voluntary euthanasia. *The Times*, 23 December 1994.

176 H. J. J. Leenen, 'Euthanasia, Assistance to Suicide and the Law: Developments in the Netherlands' (1987) 8 *Health Policy* 197, 204.

177 Ibid.

178 H. J. J. Leenen, 'Dying with Dignity: Developments in the Field of Euthanasia in the Netherlands' (1989) 8 *Medicine and Law* 517, 520. (Emphasis added.)

179 Ibid., 519. (Emphasis added.)

180 Ibid. (Emphasis added.)

181 Op. cit. n.14, 31.

182 Letters (1989) 19(6) *Hastings Center Report* 47–48. (Original emphasis.)

183 Ibid., 48.

184 Henk A. M. J. ten Have and Jos V. M. Welie, 'Euthanasia: Normal Medical Practice?' (1992) 22(2) *Hastings Center Report* 34, 38. See also Jos V. M. Welie, 'The Medical Exception: Physicians, Euthanasia and the Dutch Criminal Law' (1992) 17 *Journal of Medicine and Philosophy* 419, 435.

185 'Legal Aspects of Euthanasia, Assistance to Suicide and Terminating the Medical Treatment of Incompetent Patients' (Unpublished paper delivered at a conference on Euthanasia held at the Institute for Bioethics, Maastricht, 2–4 December 1990) 6.

186 The author of the Remmelink Report agreed that there was no control over cases which had not been reported and that, even in relation to the reported cases, the prosecutor did not know whether the doctor was telling the truth. He maintained that euthanasia occurred even if the law prohibited it, as was the case outside Holland, and that it was preferable to try to control it. Interview by author with Mr A. Kors, 29 November 1991.

187 *The Troubled Dream of Life* (New York: Simon & Schuster, 1993) 115.

188 Op. cit. n.170, 26. (Footnote omitted.)

189 *Report of the Select Committee on Medical Ethics* HL Paper 21-I of 1993–94.

190 Rt Rev. J. S. Habgood, 'Euthanasia – A Christian View' [1974] 3 *Journal of the Royal Society of Health* 124, 126. The

Abortion Act 1967 decriminalised abortion where, in the opinion of two registered medical practitioners, the continuance of the pregnancy involved risk to the life, or to the physical or mental health of the mother, greater than if the pregnancy were terminated, or where there was a substantial risk that if the child were born it would be seriously handicapped.

191 Op. cit. n.189, appendix 3, 68.

192 Ibid., 49.

193 (1993]94) 554 Parl. Deb. H.L. col. 1345, 1346.

194 Ibid. See text at n.133.

195 (1993]94) Parl. Deb. H.L. col. 1346.

196 Ibid., col. 1398. In a recent decision of the Canadian Supreme Court rejecting an alleged right to assisted suicide in Canadian law, Mr Justice Sopinka, delivering the majority judgment, noted the 'worrisome trend' in Holland toward euthanasia without request, which supported the view that 'a relaxation of the absolute prohibition takes us down the "slippery slope"'. *Rodriguez* v. *Attorney-General* (1994) 107 D.L.R. (4th) 342 at 403.

197 Alexander Morgan Capron, 'Euthanasia and Assisted Suicide' (1992) 22(2) *Hastings Center Report* 30, 31.

198 Ibid.

199 See e.g., Carlos F. Gomez, *Regulating Death: Euthanasia and the Case of the Netherlands* (New York: Free Press, 1991); Herbert Hendin, *Seduced by Death* (New York, W. W. Norton, 1997); the colloquy in (1992) 22(2) *Hastings Center Report*; cf. Margaret Battin 'Voluntary Euthanasia and the Risks of Abuse: Can We Learn Anything from the Netherlands?' (1992) 20 *Law, Medicine & Health Care* 133.

200 Henk Jochemsen 'Euthanasia in the Netherlands' *Issues in Law and Medicine* (forthcoming).

201 Herbert Hendin *et al.* 'Physician-assisted Suicide and Euthanasia in the Netherlands (1997) *JAMA* 1720.

Note 159. *The following table of disposals in euthanasia cases has been translated from the annual report of the public prosecutor for 1994 (Jaaverslaag Openbaar Ministerie 1994,* Ministerie van Justitie, Den Haag, 1995).

Year	Non-prosecution	Prosecution	Non-prosecution after judicial investigation	Prosecution taken further
1984	16	1	0	0
1985	26	4	1	0
1986	81	0	1	2
1987	122	2	1	1
1988	181	2	1	0
1989	336	1	1	0
1990	454	0	0	0
1991	590	1	0	0
1992	1318	4	1	0
1993	1303	15[a]	1	0
1994	1417	7	12	2

[a]The relatively high number of decisions not to prosecute following judicial investigation concerns cases which were reconsidered taking account of the *Chabot* decision (see text at n. 133).

17

Advance directives: a legal and ethical analysis

STUART HORNETT

ADVANCE DIRECTIVES occupy an important place in the debate about the limits of patient autonomy, the right to refuse life-saving medical treatment and euthanasia. In February 1994, the House of Lords Select Committee on Medical Ethics[1] strongly endorsed the use of advance directives as a way of enabling patients to express in advance their individual preferences and priorities for medical treatment in the event that they should subsequently become incompetent. The Committee felt that the preparation of advance directives could often stimulate healthy dialogue between doctor[2] and patient about health care choices, assist health carers in decisions about appropriate treatment and provide secure knowledge for patients that their wishes have been properly documented.

With advance directives entering the public domain in increasing numbers[3] and the recommendation by, amongst others, the Law Commission for legislation to define and regulate their use[4] the legal and ethical debate over the effect, use, limitations and general desirability of advance directives continues to intensify. This chapter attempts to examine the present status of advance directives in English law and explore a number of the important legal and ethical questions to which they give rise.

THE NATURE AND FORM OF ADVANCE DIRECTIVES

An advance directive is essentially a stipulation made by a competent person about the medical treatment he should or should not receive in the event of his becoming incompetent to make or communicate treatment choices. Advance directives can take the form of a document (often known as a 'living will') which sets out an individual's wishes regarding what measures should or should not be taken after the onset of incompetence and the occurrence of certain medical conditions or 'triggering events'. Alternatively, an individual may confer an enduring power of attorney by which he appoints an agent to make decisions on his behalf during any future period of incompetence.

Although the precise form and effect of advance directives vary, the two key concepts which underpin them are that (*a*) a patient has the right to refuse medical treatment, including life-saving and life-sustaining treatment, which refusal should be respected and complied with by the patient's doctor and (*b*) a person can make valid and enforceable treatment decisions in anticipation of incompetence (either by making them himself or delegating that power to a proxy).

These two propositions form the conceptual basis of advance directives. As regards the first, advance directives are almost invariably directed at the non-provision during terminal illness of life-sustaining measures, including specific treatments and operations, artificial life support and sometimes artificial nutrition, hydration and palliative care. Although an advance directive could purport to request treatment, it could not thereby place the doctor under a duty to provide it.

As regards the second proposition, the execution of an advance directive entails making a decision in the present about treatment to be received or refused in the future (an anticipatory decision). However, the concept of an anticipatory decision is not *per se* remarkable for, in a temporal world, all decisions about treatment will, to a greater or lesser extent, precede its delivery. What truly distinguishes decisions contained in an advance directive from other treatment decisions is that an advance directive entails an individual making a decision while in a competent state about treatment to be received or rejected if that individual falls into an incompetent state. The very *raison d'être* of an advance directive is that an individual's pre-incompetent wishes are to take effect if and insofar as that individual is at a later date legally incompetent to make treatment decisions.

THE LEGAL STATUS OF ADVANCE DIRECTIVES

Unlike the United States[5] and parts of Canada[6] and Australia,[7] the United Kingdom has no legislative framework giving effect to advance directives or defining their legal scope. The House of Lords Committee considered that legislation for advance directives in England was unnecessary, particularly as doctors were increasingly recognising their ethical obligations to comply with advance directives and because of the development of case law affording them legal recognition.[8] Although there has yet to be a definitive court decision on the validity and scope of standard advance directives, a considerable amount can be gleaned from both basic common law principles and a number of recent court decisions germane to the issue, both of which suggest that English law does to a considerable extent accept the two underlying propositions on which the enforceability of advance directives depends.

The right to refuse treatment

The common law has always recognised the basic liberty of a person to refuse a touching, be it in the medical context or otherwise. In *Sidaway* v. *Board of Governors of the Bethlem Royal Hospital*,[9] Lord Scarman described the existence of a patient's right to make his own decisions about treatment as 'a basic human right protected by the common law'.[10] In another House of Lords decision, Lord Goff summarised the law in these terms:

> every person's body is inviolate . . . everybody is protected not only against physical injury but against any form of physical molestation . . . 'every human being of adult years and sound mind has the right to determine what shall be done with his own body; and a surgeon who performs an operation without his patient's consent commits an assault'.[11]

It is quite clear that the common law prohibits intentional, non-consensual touching[12] and a doctor who treats a competent patient without consent commits a civil and criminal battery. A doctor will act within the law if he treats a patient who, having been informed in broad terms of the nature and consequences of the procedure,[13] consents to it. Treatment without consent is unlawful unless a doctor can establish the lawfulness of his action in some other way, for example through statutory justification or by the defence of necessity which will apply, for example, where an unconscious patient needs treatment although not where the treatment is contrary to the known wishes of the patient.[14]

These basic principles hold good even if the treatment might prolong or save the patient's life. So much was made clear by the Court of Appeal in *Re T (Adult: Refusal of Treatment)*.[15] T was a woman admitted to hospital after a traffic accident who, after being visited by her mother, a devout Jehovah's Witness, stated that she did not wish to have a blood transfusion. She later lapsed into unconsciousness and a blood transfusion became necessary to save her life. On an application for a declaration that the transfusion would be lawful notwithstanding T's refusal, the High Court and Court of Appeal ruled that an adult patient could refuse life-saving treatment irrespective of the wisdom of such a choice but that, in the instant case, T's refusal was not effective because her physical and mental state combined with pressure exerted by her mother to vitiate her refusal. In the Court of Appeal, Lord Donaldson, Master of the Rolls, set out a number of propositions which form the basis of the present law:

1 *Prima facie*, every adult has the right and capacity to decide whether or not he will accept medical treatment, even if a refusal may risk permanent injury to his health or even lead to premature death. Furthermore, it matters not whether the reasons for the refusal are rational or irrational, unknown or even non-existent. This is so notwithstanding the very strong public interest in preserving the life and health of all citizens. However, the presumption of capacity to decide – which stems from the fact that the patient is an adult – is rebuttable.
2 An adult patient may be deprived of his capacity to decide by long-term mental incapacity or by temporary factors such as unconsciousness, confusion, the effects of fatigue or shock, pain or drugs.
3 If an adult patient does not have the capacity to decide whether to accept treatment at the time of the purported refusal and still does not have that capacity, it is the duty of the doctors to treat him in whatever way they consider in the exercise of clinical judgment to be in his best interests.
4 Doctors faced with a refusal of consent have to give very careful and detailed consideration to the patient's capacity to decide at the time when the decision was made. It may not be a case of capacity or no capacity; it may be a case of reduced capacity. What matters is whether at the time the patient's capacity is reduced below the level needed in the case of a refusal of that importance, for refusals can vary in importance. Some may involve a risk to life or of irreparable damage to health; others may not.

These propositions recently received support in the land-mark decision of the House of Lords in *Airedale NHS Trust* v. *Bland*[16] in which Lord Keith declared that 'a person is completely at liberty to decline to undergo treatment, even if the result of his so doing will be that he will die'.[17] It can be confidently stated, therefore, in the light of the foregoing authorities, that the law recognises the basic right of a competent adult to refuse medical treatment even if that refusal will lead to death. A doctor who treats a patient in this situation acts unlawfully even if, judged objectively, he is acting in his patient's best interests.

The first conceptual requirement for the legal recognition of advance directives would therefore seem to be satisfied. What of the second: does the law recognise the validity of an anticipatory refusal of treatment?

Anticipatory refusals

Dicta in a number of cases would suggest that this is so. Moreover, a recent case in the High Court has expressly so held. In *Re T*, Lord Donaldson stated that a refusal can take the form of a declaration of intention never to consent in some future circumstances.[18] In the Court of Appeal in *Bland*, Lord Justice Butler-Sloss agreed *sub silentio* with the proposition of all counsel in the case that:

> [T]he right to reject treatment extends to deciding not to accept treatment in the future by way of advance directive or 'living will'. A well known example of advance directive is provided by those subscribing to the tenets of the Jehovah's Witnesses who make it clear that they will not accept blood transfusions: see, for example, *Malette* v. *Shulman* (1990) 67 D.L.R. (4th) 321.[19]

In the House of Lords in *Bland*, Lord Keith stated that the right of a person to refuse treatment:

> extends to the situation where the person, in anticipation of his, through one cause or another, entering into a condition such as PVS [persistent vegetative state], gives clear instructions that in such event he is not to be given medical care, including artificial feeding, designed to keep him alive.[20]

Lord Goff maintained in relation to a patient's right to refuse treatment:

> Moreover the same principle applies where the patient's refusal to give his consent has been expressed at an earlier date, before he became unconscious or otherwise incapable of communicating it; though in such circumstances especial care may be necessary to ensure that the prior refusal of consent is still properly to be regarded as applicable in the circumstances which have subsequently occurred.[21]

Neither *Re T* nor *Bland* was concerned directly with the validity of an advance directive. The nearest the English courts have come to specifically adjudicating on the effect of an advance directive is in the recent High Court case of *Re C (Refusal of Medical Treatment)*.[22]

This case concerned C, a 68-year-old patient in a secure hospital, who was diagnosed as suffering from chronic paranoid schizophrenia. He developed gangrene in his leg and the prognosis was that he would die if his leg were not amputated below the knee. C refused and made it clear that he did not want the operation to be performed at any time in the future, i.e. he made an oral advance directive. Although the hospital agreed to abide by his refusal for the time being, it refused to undertake that it would not amputate his leg at some time in the future. C applied to the court for an injunction to restrain the hospital from amputating his leg then or at any time in the future without his express consent.

Applying the presumption adumbrated by Lord Donaldson in *Re T*, Mr Justice Thorpe found that although C's capacity was impaired by his schizophrenia, it had not been established that C did not understand the nature, purpose and effect of the treatment he was refusing. Relying on *Re T* and *Bland*, Thorpe J. held that the court could grant injunctive or declaratory relief to enforce C's oral direction and prevent the hospital amputating his leg in the future without his express written consent and granted a declaration in those terms.

The decisions in *Re T, Bland* and *Re C*, together with those in other common law jurisdictions,[23] show that the common law does, in principle, recognise the two basic concepts which underpin advance directives, namely, that a patient may refuse life-saving treatment even if it results in death and that such a decision may take an anticipatory form and will bind a patient's doctors in the same way as any other competent decision.

THE LEGAL FRAMEWORK FOR ADVANCE DIRECTIVES

If, as has been suggested, advance directives are valid in English law, there remains a great deal to be resolved as to the precise scope of their validity and legal effect. In the absence of legislation, advance directives remain a creature of the common law and, in contrast to the United States where the impetus for the recognition of advance directives has often been found in Constitutional rights and the doctrine of informed consent,[24] the scope for going beyond basic common law principles in England is rather limited.

Nonetheless, if advance directives are to be regulated by the common law (perhaps in conjunction with medical codes of practice as was recommended by the House of Lords Select Committee[25]) judicial thought will need to be given to developing a coherent and satisfactory legal framework for their use. Thus far, the English decisions have imposed but few pre-conditions to the validity of advance directives, namely, that the decision to refuse treatment is (*a*) made while competent (and free from undue influence); (*b*) 'clearly established' and (*c*) 'applicable in the circumstances which have subsequently occurred'.[26]

The remainder of this chapter explores what other conditions, if any, the common law might impose and whether the courts have thus far given sufficient consideration to the legal and ethical difficulties advance directives pose.

Legal limits on form

It has been noted that one form some advance directives take is that of an enduring power of attorney, that is, a power purportedly vested in another person to make healthcare choices for an individual once he has lapsed into incompetence. While many advance directives contain such a power, it is most unlikely that they carry any legal force. While no English authority has considered the position as yet, there is nothing at common law to suggest that such enduring powers of attorney are lawful and the better view is that even if a patient could nominate an individual to take healthcare decisions for him while competent, that authority would lapse upon the onset of incompetence.[27] Further, it would also appear quite clear that section 3(1) of the *Enduring Powers of Attorney Act 1985* does not contemplate, and could not legitimately be construed as applying to, healthcare decisions.[28] As the law now stands, it is most unlikely that a doctor would have to abide by a refusal of treatment purportedly expressed for an incompetent patient by a proxy nominated in an advance directive.

Legal limits on substance

Insofar as advance directives are enforceable in English law, their validity derives from the common law's recognition that a person should be protected from non-consensual touching. It does not derive from any so-called right to die and none of the English authorities purport to recognise or establish such a right. Maintaining this distinction is essential if the law is not to fall into the trap of equating the liberty to refuse treatment with a 'right to die'.[29] Such a concept, if imported into English common law, would have profound ramifications not only for the legality of advance directives but for the lawfulness of euthanasia – the intentional shortening of patient's life by act or omission.

Active euthanasia

Even in *Bland*, a case which effectively sanctioned passive euthanasia in all but name,[30] the House of Lords made clear that active euthanasia remained unlawful.[31] In the absence of statutory intervention, therefore, any request in an advance directive for positive steps to be taken to hasten death would be completely unenforceable. Indeed, it would amount to an incitement to murder.

Positive treatment requests

Furthermore, as the law stands, even an advance directive that positively requests treatment is most probably unenforceable. In its 1992 statement on advance directives[32] the British Medical Association (BMA) justifiably expressed its concern that patients should not be able to insist in an advance directive on the provision of certain treatments which might be clinically inappropriate. If patients were able to do so, not only would that place them in a better position than a competent patient (who cannot, merely by asking for treatment, require it to be provided)[33] but it might require a doctor to provide inappropriate, futile or even dangerous treatment. So long as advance directives remain a creature of the common law, however, the BMA's fears are likely to be assuaged. The common law's acknowledgment of the need for consent does not allow a person to demand that certain treatments be administered and its recognition that individuals must be protected from unwanted touching does not imply any corresponding right to be treated in a certain manner, other than in accordance with good medical practice.[34] Consequently, if an advance directive requested, as opposed to refused, a specific treatment, it would impose no legal obligation on a doctor to provide it. The doctor's common law duty of care requires him to act in what he reasonably believes to be his patient's best interests in the light of available resources, not at the patient's *diktat*.

Suicidal requests

What if a patient's refusal of treatment expressed in an advance directive is made with a suicidal intent?

The recent English authorities have asserted the existence of a wide-ranging and apparently absolute right to refuse treatment and tube-feeding. In *Bland*, Lord Keith claimed that a patient of sound mind is *completely* at liberty to decline to undergo medical treatment even if a refusal will result in death[35] and these sentiments were echoed in other speeches in the House of Lords and the judgments in the Court of Appeal. In *Re T*, Lord Donaldson stated that a refusal could be based on irrational or non-existent reasons and the courts seem to have accepted that, in principle, a refusal should be respected irrespective of the intentions and motives of the decision maker or the objective ethical propriety of the decision. While prepared to recognise the public interest in preserving the life of its citizens, the recent authorities seem, as a matter of policy, to have come down firmly on the side of the individual's right to refuse treatment: 'the principle of the sanctity of human life must yield to the principle of self-determination'.[36]

Although one possibility has been specifically canvassed as an exception to that general principle, namely, a refusal which endangers the life of a viable fetus,[37] the English courts seem otherwise to have glossed over the possibility that individuals might refuse treatment with a suicidal intent or for other patently unethical reasons (for example, to abdicate responsibility for dependent third parties). The courts seem to have accepted that a decision made by a competent patient is sacrosanct and may not be impugned for being unethical. The courts do not appear to have appreciated that *if* such a choice is motivated by, for example, a suicidal intent, the traditional policy of the law as informed by the principle of the sanctity of human life would deny it legal force.

It might be said that a patient who refuses treatment can never do so in an unethical or suicidal way or, alternatively, that even if that were possible, the law should respect such decisions nonetheless. Yet, while it will often, indeed normally, be perfectly proper for a person to refuse medical treatment because it is futile or too burdensome (which is largely a matter for the subjective determination of the patient),[38] it does not follow that *every* refusal can be justified and should be given legal effect without having regard to the intention of the individual making the decision.

But can a patient commit suicide by refusing treatment or nutrition? In its report on living wills, the King's College Working Party took the view that even if a patient is not suffering from a terminal illness from which he would otherwise die, starvation is not suicide because 'the patient must *positively* do something to himself before his conduct would be so regarded'.[39] This, with respect, must be wrong. Is it really to be supposed that a diabetic who says to his doctor 'please don't give me my insulin: I want to die so my wife can claim my life insurance' makes anything other than a suicidal request? In *Bland*, both Sir Thomas Bingham, M. R., [40] and Lord Goff[41] doubted whether a refusal of treatment could amount to suicide. If their Lordships' statements were meant to include cases where the refusal is motivated by an intent to shorten life, they are also, with respect, wrong. So too is the US judge who asserted that declining life-sustaining treatment is not properly classified as an attempt to commit suicide because the refusal of medical intervention merely allows the underlying disease to take its natural course and death results not from the refusal but from the underlying condition.[42] The crucial determining factor is neither the method by which death occurs nor the nature of the treatment being rejected but the *intention* behind the choice. It is the *intention* that in ethics is crucial in defining the morality of the choice,[43] and in law, determines the nature of the act,[44] including, significantly, suicide.[45] Certainly as a matter of law, it seems irrelevant whether suicide be carried out through an act or omission: '[to] "commit suicide" is for a person voluntarily to do an act (or, as it is submitted, *to refrain from taking bodily sustenance*), for the purpose of destroying his own life'.[46] Since suicide used to be a felonious homicide at common law[47] until abolished by section 1 of the *Suicide Act 1961*, it can be assumed that it, like other types of homicide, could then, and can now, be committed by omission.[48]

As to the second possible objection – that even if individuals might make suicidal or unethical choices the law should nonetheless respect them – this ignores the law's interest in upholding and preserving human life. The law has never given free reign to an individual's autonomy, but has held it in tension with the claims and wider interests of society.[49] In *Re T* Lord Donaldson readily conceded that there was 'a very strong public interest in preserving the life and health of all citizens'[50] and in another case he spoke of the 'vast importance of the sanctity of human life'.[51] These sentiments have been echoed and endorsed by the courts on numerous occasions in various contexts. A judge in a leading American decision has explained the point in these terms:

> Whether based on common-law doctrines or on constitutional theory, the right to decline life sustaining treatment is not absolute. In some cases, it may yield to countervailing societal interests in sustaining the person's life. Courts and commentators have commonly identified four state interests that may limit a person's right to refuse medical treatment: preserving life, preventing suicide, safeguarding the integrity of the medical profession and protecting innocent third parties.[52]

Further examples of courts' recognition that personal autonomy is not absolute but must yield to the sanctity of human life include *Rex* v. *Rice*[53] where a dueller was found liable for murder notwithstanding his victim's consent; *McKay* v. *Essex A.H.A*[54] in which it was held that damages for 'wrongful life' were contrary to public policy and an abrogation of the 'sanctity of human life', and *Howe*[55] in which the House of Lords, emphasising the 'special regard that the law has for human life',[56] held that duress is no defence to murder. Moreover, notwithstanding the tenor of the speeches in *Bland*, English law does not recognise an absolute right to self-determination. In 1985 the Law Lords baldly refused to import the doctrine of 'informed consent', which is based on the right to self-determination, into English law.[57] Further, the law denies that there is any right to consent to be killed[58] or even to the infliction of bodily harm.[59] In *R* v. *Brown et al.*,[59] the

House of Lords held that consent was no defence to the infliction of bodily harm in the course of sadomasochistic sex, even though no permanent harm was occasioned. Lord Mustill (who sat in *Bland*) observed 'Believer or atheist, the observer grants to the maintenance of human life an overriding imperative, so strong as to outweigh any consent to its termination'.[60]

Furthermore, while suicide is no longer a criminal offence in England, it remains an offence under Section 2 of the *Suicide Act 1961* to aid and abet suicide, and in this respect the law retains its policy against intentionally taking one's life and encouraging others to do so. Moreover, notwithstanding the enactment of the *Suicide Act*, doctors will often be free, and sometimes obliged, to prevent patients from committing suicide.[61] Even those of a consequentialist viewpoint recognise the strong case for the legal discouragement of suicide in a variety of contexts[62] and the justification for such a policy need not even stem from the recognition of the sanctity of human life *per se* but, for example, from the adverse effect that a refusal of basic nursing care and nutrition by a patient might have on those caring for him.[63]

Of course, the courts' ability to exercise control over an individual will be much reduced outside the context of the hospital where neither the courts nor the doctors will be seised of the matter (as, for example, where an individual discharges himself from hospital to starve himself to death at home). The position is quite different, however, where an individual submits himself to the care of doctors and others whose primary professional duty is to act in his best interests and who then decides to starve himself to death while expecting his doctors to keep him comfortable in the process.

While it is doubtless the case that the emphasis of the law is, and should be, to allow individuals to make free choices about their healthcare, the law nevertheless has a legitimate and justifiable interest in scrutinising and, if necessary, curtailing such freedom. One criticism that might be levelled at the recent English authorities is that the courts have failed to accord sufficient weight to this wider interest, at least insofar as it impinges upon suicidal refusals and refusals which may otherwise be unlawful or contrary to public policy.

Inadequately informed refusals

The prerequisite that refusals have to be both clearly established and 'applicable' to present circumstances raises important questions as to how well informed an individual need be before the courts will give effect to his advance directive. One powerful objection to advance directives is that they require individuals to make decisions in the present about conditions which may or may not arise in the future and which that individual may never have before experienced. This is particularly so in the realm of terminal healthcare where people are likely to have an unduly pessimistic view of the quality of life attainable during the dying process and the latent qualities which that process can bring to the surface.[64]

While the BMA[65] has recommended that patients wishing to draft advance directives should receive proper medical advice and be told of the attendant medical benefits and risks,[66] it is nonetheless likely that many people who make advance directives will do so in either total or partial ignorance of the nature and effect of the medical conditions in respect of which they make refusals. Yet whether such ignorance will vitiate a refusal stated in an advance directive remains unclear. In *Re T*, Lord Donaldson rejected any concept of 'informed refusal' by which a refusal would amount to 'no refusal' if a patient were not properly informed in broad terms of the nature and effect of the procedure to which the refusal related.[67] Instead, he maintained that the failure to inform sounded in negligence only, albeit that the refusal might be rendered ineffective if information were deliberately withheld or the assumption upon which a refusal was based was falsified.[68]

While it is true that English law does not recognise the doctrine of informed consent,[69] there are nonetheless powerful arguments for incorporating some form of doctrine of informed refusal into the law[70] whereby a doctor would be entitled to treat a patient if there was evidence which cast doubt on whether an advance directive truly reflected that patient's informed wishes. Informed consent and informed refusal are not symmetrical concepts and the reasons for rejecting a doctrine of informed consent do not necessarily apply to informed refusal. The consequences of refusing life-saving treatment are patently more severe than the consequences of consenting to (most) treatments and while it may be logical for Lord Donaldson to hold that a failure to perform a duty (to inform) sounds in negligence and does not vitiate a refusal, that gives no redress to a patient who, as a result of ignorance, refuses a life-saving treatment and dies. Redress is of course open to the patient who is treated without being adequately informed of the nature of the treatment. Furthermore, one good reason why the English courts have rejected the doctrine of informed consent is that a failure to inform might give rise to an action in battery against a doctor who treats an inadequately informed patient whereas the more appropriate remedy lies in negligence since this allows the application of the *Bolam* test[71] to the doctor's decision to treat. However, rather than expose doctors to battery actions, the doctrine of informed refusal might help to *protect* from such an action a doctor who treats a patient in the honest belief that that patient has been inadequately informed about the nature and effect of the condition he is suffering from and the consequences of refusing treatment.

Given that most individuals will execute advance directives away from hospital and in all likelihood without medical advice, there are good reasons why the courts should be particularly vigilant to safeguard against ill thought out, misconceived and medically inappropriate refusals, subject them to strict scrutiny and, where appropriate, deny them validity.[72]

ANTICIPATORY DECISIONS: THE FALLACY OF ABSOLUTE AUTONOMY

A further issue to which the English courts have hitherto given little attention is the inherent difficulty of respecting an individual's so-called right to self-determination through a binding anticipatory decision. It has been suggested by one commentator that since an incompetent person does not possess a presently exercisable capacity for self-determination, it is fallacious to speak of such a person possessing the right to self-determination or of respecting his autonomy through the agency of an advance directive.[73]

However, one need not go that far to expose what is perhaps the most subtle theoretical flaw with advance directives, namely, that in purporting to recognise a patient's autonomy in the here and now, upholding an anticipatory decision can in fact deny an individual that autonomy in the future. This can be well illustrated by considering in what circumstances an advance directive can be revoked. No difficulty will arise if a patient revokes an advance directive while in a competent state: the revocation will be effective. What, though, if a patient purports to revoke an advance directive *after* having lapsed into an incompetent state? On the face of it, the issue comprises a simple choice: either an incompetent refusal will be sufficient to revoke an advance directive or it will not. In the United States a number of states have decided that as a matter of policy, revocation procedures should not be too burdensome and their statutes allow incompetent revocations.[74] But is this consistent with the very rationale of advance directives, namely that a pre-incompetence refusal should bind and override a subsequent incompetent request? In short, no. If a decision can be revoked by an incompetent request, how can it be said that a previous, competent refusal (perhaps made in contemplation of a later incompetent request) has been accorded any meaningful legal recognition?

In this respect, the American statutes that allow revocation by a mentally incapacitated person fail to carry through what they purport to do. Yet, at the same time, the conundrum that faced the various legislatures highlights the very troubling consequences of giving full legal effect to binding anticipatory decisions contained in advance directives. *Re C*, discussed earlier, is a case in point. C's condition was such that he fluctuated between competence and incompetence. What if C were to lapse into incapacity, his gangrene were to return and C *then* were to change his mind and consent to the amputation? Quite simply, the operation could not be performed. C's doctors might all agree that the operation should proceed – for it would save C's life and C, now being perfectly happy with life, could plead for the operation to proceed. Nonetheless, so long as C remained incompetent, the operation could not be performed even if, contrary to everybody's then *present* wishes, C's death would result. No liberty to apply to vary the order was given on the basis that that might deny C his right to self-determination. Therefore, in purporting to respect C's autonomy, Mr Justice Thorpe locked him into his competent refusal and bound him to it for the future, possibly until his death.

If the consequence of recognising advance directives leads to a situation such as this, where even ardent proponents of autonomy-based jurisprudence seem to cavil at the prospect of denying treatment to someone who enjoys life and requests treatment to sustain or save that life but nonetheless must forgo it in view of a previous competent refusal,[75] there is much force in the criticism that far from providing a framework for patient autonomy, advance directives (taken to their logical conclusion) may well prove not so much a good servant as a bad master. Professor Dworkin nonetheless maintains that to provide treatment to an incompetent patient who presently requests treatment contrary to a previous competent refusal violates, rather than respects, that individual's autonomy. But this position must be predicated on the assumption that a person only has autonomy while competent, otherwise, a subsequent incompetent request could override a previous competent refusal. Dworkin's argument therefore proves too much: how can it be right to speak of respecting the autonomy of an incompetent individual when that individual in fact has no autonomy? And if that is correct, wherein lies the justification for treating such an individual otherwise than in accordance with good medical practice?

CONCLUSION

Should advance directives be given full legal recognition? In the light of the potential clinical problems that they create for doctors;[76] the questionable premise upon which anticipatory decisions are given effect and the danger of ill-informed refusals being made by individuals, there is much to commend the argument that advance directives should inform but not bind the doctor.[77] Some of the problems at which advance directives are aimed would no doubt be better solved by a greater understanding by doctors of the fears patients have of being overtreated and kept alive 'at all costs' and a better appreciation of patients' desires to avoid burdensome and unnecessary treatments. It may be that the development of a suitable Code of Practice commended by the House of Lords Select Committee[78] will assist in this respect.

Assuming the current trends in the law continue, however, it remains to be seen whether the English courts will be able to adopt advance directives and fashion them into useful tools for promoting an individual's treatment choice while at the same time respecting the need to safeguard those individuals from uninformed and suicidal decisions, the needs and concerns of doctors and healthcarers and the wider interests of society and public and legal policy. What the courts must not do is blithely to enforce advance directives without a full consideration of the medical, social, ethical and policy implications of so doing and, moreover, without exploring what limits should be placed upon their operation. It is regrettable that neither the courts, nor the House of Lords Select Committee, nor the Law Commission, nor the BMA appear adequately to have addressed the problems with advance directives, some of them quite fundamental, which have been outlined in this chapter. There is, therefore, cause for concern that advance directives, hailed by many as a panacea, may well prove something of a Pandora's Box.

NOTES

1 *Report of the Select Committee on Medical Ethics* HL Paper 21-I of 1993–94 at paras. 263–267.

2 In this paper 'doctor' should be read to include any healthcare provider. Also, 'he' includes 'she'.

3 Examples include the Voluntary Euthanasia Society Advance Directive and the Terrence Higgins Trust Living Will. For a further precedent see Vol. 31 *Butterworth's Encyclopedia of Forms and Precedents* at para. 2269.

4 Law Commission, *Mentally Incapacitated Adults and Decision-Making; Medical Treatment and Research* (Consultation Paper No. 129, (1993)) at 31. The Commission's *Report on Mental Incapacity* (Report No. 231, 1995) was published after this chapter was completed. It is not addressed in this chapter, whose focus is the existing law.

5 See C. Condie, 'Comparison of the Living Will Statutes of the Fifty States' (1988) 14 *J.C.L.* 105; G. Gefland, 'Living Will Statutes: The First Decade' (1987) 5 *Wisconsin L.R.* 738; S. Vile, 'Living Wills in New York: Are they Valid?' (1987) 38 *Syracuse L.R.* 1369.

6 See, e.g., *Ontario Consent to Treatment Act 1992; Manitoba Health Care Directives Act 1992.*

7 See, e.g., *South Australia Natural Death*

Act 1983; Northern Territory Natural Death Act 1988.

8 *Op. cit.* n. 1 at para. 264.

9 [1985] A.C. 871.

10 *Op. cit.* at 882.

11 *F* v. *West Berkshire Health Authority* [1990] 2 A.C. 1 at 72–73 citing Mr Justice Cardozo in *Schloendorff* v. *Society of New York Hospital* (1914) 211 NY 125 at 126.

12 *Collins* v. *Wilcock* [1984] 1 W.L.R. 1172 (criminal liability); *Wilson* v. *Pringle* [1986] 2 All E.R. 440 (civil liability).

13 *Chatterton* v. *Gerson* [1981] 1 All E.R. 257 at 265.

14 *F* v. *West Berkshire Health Authority* [1990] 2 A.C. 1 at 76.

15 [1992] 3 W.L.R. 782.

16 [1993] A.C. 789 and see now *Frenchay Healthcare National Health Service Trust* v. *S* [1994] 1 W.L.R. 601 (C.A.).

17 *Op. cit.* at 857. See also Lord Goff at 864 and Lord Mustill at 891.

18 [1992] 3 W.L.R. 782 at 796.

19 [1993] A.C. 789 at 816.

20 *Op. cit.* at 857.

21 *Op. cit.* at 864.

22 [1994] 1 F.L.R. 31.

23 *Fleming* v. *Reid* (1991) 82 D.L.R. (4th) 298; *Malette* v. *Shulman* (1990) 67 D.L.R. (4th) 321; *Re Conroy* 486 A 2d 1209 (1985).

24 *Re Quinlan* 355 A 2d 647 (1976); *Re Conroy* 486 A 2d 1209 (1985); *Bouvia* v. *Superior Court* 225 Cal. Rptr. 297 (1986); Note, 'The Living Will: The Right to Death With Dignity?' (1976) 26 *Case Western L. Rev.* 485.

25 *Op. cit.* n. 1 at para. 265.

26 *Op. cit.* n. 4 at 28; *Airedale NHS Trust* v. *Bland* [1993] A.C. 789 at 864, *per* Lord Goff.

27 *The Living Will – Consent to Treatment at the End of Life* (Report under the auspices of Age Concern and Centre of Medical Law and Ethics, King's College, London) (1988) at 49; see also *op. cit.* n. 4 at 85–96.

28 See *Re W (EEM)* [1971] Ch. 123; *F* v. *West Berkshire Health Authority* [1990] 2 A.C. 1 at 58–60, construing a similarly phrased provision in Part VII of the *Mental Health Act 1983*.

29 Germain G. Grisez and Joseph M. Boyle, *Life and Death with Liberty and Justice* (London, 1979) at 97.

30 See John Keown, 'Doctors and Patients: Hard Case, Bad Law, "New Ethics"' (1994) 52 *C.L.J.* 209; John Finnis, '*Bland*: Crossing the Rubicon?' (1993) 109 *L.Q.R.* 329.

31 See, for example, [1993] A.C. 789 at 865, *per* Lord Goff. See also *R* v. *Cox* (1992) 12 B.M.L.R. 38.

32 British Medical Association, *Statement on Advance Directives* (1992) at 4–10. Hereafter '*Statement* (1992)'. See also its *Statement on Advance Directives* (1994) at 2. Hereafter '*Statement* (1994)'.

33 See n. 34, *infra*.

34 *Re J (A Minor)* [1992] 3 W.L.R. 507 and see Lord Donaldson's comment in *Re R (A Minor)* [1991] 3 W.L.R. 592 at 599 that 'consent by itself creates no obligation to treat. It is merely a key which unlocks a door'.

35 [1993] A.C. 789 at 857.

36 *Op. cit.* at 864, *per* Lord Goff.

37 *Re T* [1992] 3 W.L.R. 782 at 786; see also *Re S (Adult: Refusal of Treatment)* [1992] 3 W.L.R. 806.

38 A good recent example of this was the case of Benny Agrelo, the 15-year-old American liver transplant patient who, without any wish to die and with no suicidal intent, refused to take painful and debilitating drugs on the basis that they caused him too much pain and distress with no guarantee of success (*The Times*, 17 June 1994).

39 *Op. cit.* n. 27 at 29, original emphasis.

40 [1993] A.C. 789 at 814.

41 *Op. cit.* 864. In a recent High Court decision concerning a prisoner on hunger-strike, Mr Justice Thorpe granted the Home Secretary a declaration that the Home Office, prison officials and doctors and nurses caring for the prisoner might lawfully abide by the prisoner's refusal to eat for so long as he retained the capacity to refuse. *Secretary of State for the Home Department* v. *Robb* [1995] 1 All E.R. 677. His Lordship held that there were no countervailing state interests in this case to set in the balance against the right to self-determination of an adult of sound

mind. The judge noted (at 682) that the interest of the state in preventing suicide 'is recognisable'. However, having stated (at 681) that *Bland* is authority for the proposition that a patient who dies by reason of refusing treatment does not commit suicide and that a doctor who complies with the refusal does not aid or abet suicide, the judge concluded (at 682) that the state interest in preventing suicide seemed to have no application to cases such as the instant case where the refusal 'does not constitute an act of suicide'. With respect, whether refusal of treatment can amount to suicide was not an issue in *Bland*.

42 *Re Conroy* 486 A 2d 1209 (1985) *per* Mr Justice Schrieber.

43 John Finnis, ' "Living Will" Legislation' in Luke Gormally (ed.) *Euthanasia: Clinical Practice and the Law* (London, 1994).

44 R v. *Adams* [1957] Crim. L.R. 365; R v. *Moloney* [1985] A.C. 905; *R* v. *Hancock* [1986] A.C. 455; *R* v. *Nedrick* [1986] 1 W.L.R. 1025. See also Lord Goff 'The Mental Element in the Crime of Murder' (1988) 104 *L.Q.R.* 30.

45 See *In re Davis, decd* [1968] 1 Q.B. 72 in which it was held '[s]uicide is not to be presumed. It must be affirmatively proved to justify the finding. Suicide requires an intention. Every act of self-determination is, in common language, "described by the word 'suicide', provided it be the intentional act of a party knowing the probable consequences of what he is about"' at 82 *per* Lord Justice Sellers citing Baron Rolfe in *Clift* v. *Schwabe* (1846) 3 C.B. 437 at 464.

46 *Strouds Judicial Dictionary* at 2674 citing *Clift* v. *Schwabe* (1846) 3 C.B. 437 (approved in *In re Davis, decd.* [1968] 1 Q.B. 72), emphasis added.

47 Stephen, *A History of the Criminal Law of England* (1883, 3 vols.) Vol. III, at 104; Hawkins, *Pleas of the Crown* (1716–1721, 2 vols.) Vol. I, ch. 27; *Russell on Crime*, 12th ed. (London, 1964) Vol. 1, 558.

48 *Archbold* (1994) at 19–101 to 102. East defined suicide as 'where any one wilfully *or* by any malicious act causes his own death', East, *Pleas of the Crown* (1803, 2 vols.) Vol. 1, 219 (emphasis added). *Quaere*, whether the 'wilfully or' would be otiose if suicide were only possible by a positive act. Cf. P. D. G. Skegg, *Law, Ethics and Medicine* (Oxford, 1984) 112 n. 59.

49 [1993] 3 W.L.R. 316 at 367, *per* Lord Goff.

50 [1992] 3 W.L.R. 782 at 799.

51 *Re J (A Minor)* [1990] 3 All E.R. 930 at 936.

52 *Re Conroy* 486 A 2d 1209 (1985) at 1223, *per* Mr Justice Schrieber.

53 (1803) 3 East 581.

54 [1982] Q.B. 1166.

55 [1987] 1 A.C. 417.

56 *Op. cit.* at 445.

57 *Sidaway* v. *Board of Governors of the Bethlem Royal Hospital* [1985] A.C. 871.

58 Glanville Williams, *Textbook of Criminal Law* (London, 1983) 2nd ed. at 579.

59 [1994] 1 A.C. 212.

60 *Op. cit.* at 261.

61 *Selfe* v. *Ilford and District Hospital Management Committee* (1970) 114 *Sol. Jo.* 935 and see Skegg, *op. cit.* n. 48, *supra*, at 110–113. See also the comment of Lord Denning in *Hyde* v. *Thameside A.H.A.*, *The Times* 16 April 1981 that, while no longer a crime, suicide is still 'unlawful'. This comment must, however, be treated with caution in the light of *Kirkham* v. *Chief Constable of the Greater Manchester Police* [1990] 2 Q.B. 283, which decided that it is contrary to public policy to award damages to the estate of a mentally unstable prisoner for a negligent failure to prevent his suicide, although Lord Justice Farquharson did observe (at 291) that the position 'may well be different where the victim is wholly sane' and Lord Justice Lloyd noted (at 292) that 'The court does not condone suicide'.

62 Jonathan Glover, *Causing Death and Saving Lives* (London, 1977) at 183.

63 See the comments of Andrew Grubb (1993) 1 *Med. L. Rev.* 84 at 85.

64 See the chapter by Robert Twycross elsewhere in this book. See also Julian Savulescu, 'Rational Desires and the Limitation of Life-Sustaining Treatment' in (1994) 8 *Bioethics* 191; Jim Stone, 'Advance Directives, Autonomy and Unintended

Death' in *op. cit.*, 223.

65 *Statement* (1992) at 3. See also *Statement* (1994) at 2–3.

66 The Terrence Higgins Trust Living Will recommends such a course.

67 [1992] 3 W.L.R. 782 at 798. In *Malette* v. *Shulman*, Mr Justice Donnelly at first instance rejected the concept of informed refusal, 47 D.L.R. 18 at 47. The Ontario Court of Appeal found it unnecessary to decide the point, 67 D.L.R. 321 at 336.

68 [1992] 3 W.L.R. 782 at 798.

69 *Sidaway* v. *Board of Governors of the Bethlem Royal Hospital* [1985] A.C. 871.

70 See Alan Newman Q.C., *Re: A Proposed Form of Declaration (an Opinion)* prepared for and published by the Voluntary Euthanasia Society (London, 1990).

71 *Bolam* v. *Friern Hospital Management Committee* [1957] 1 W.L.R. 582. See *Sidaway* v. *Board of Governors of the Bethlem Royal Hospital* [1985] 1 A.C. 871 at 891–895, *per* Lord Diplock.

72 See *Cruzan* v. *Director of the Missouri Department of Health* (1990) 110 S. Ct. 2841 for the strict approach adopted in Missouri.

73 Luke Gormally, 'The Living Will: The Ethical Framework of a Recent Report' in Luke Gormally (ed.) *The Dependent Elderly* (Cambridge, 1988).

74 See, e.g., *California Natural Death Act 1976 s. 7189*; Condie, *op. cit.* n. 5, *supra*, at 117.

75 See Ronald Dworkin, *Life's Dominion* (London, 1993) at 228–232.

76 Such as where a new and better treatment is developed after the execution of an advance directive which a patient had no opportunity of considering.

77 See *op. cit.* n. 1, *supra*, at para. 212.

78 *Op. cit.* n. 1, *supra*, at paras. 265–267.

18

Theological aspects of euthanasia

ANTHONY FISHER

CATHOLIC WRITERS on euthanasia usually offer a largely philosophical position, drawing upon that 'common morality' which is shared by all civilized societies, and eschewing the specifically religious or confessional. This allows them the better to engage in debate in a pluralist society and reflects the fact that morality can, in principle, be recognized by any reasonable person of good will, undeflected by distracting emotion, prejudice or convention. But because of our capacity for misdirection, and because we believe that the human situation is only adequately and reliably illuminated by the life and teachings of Jesus Christ, Catholics naturally look to the Church's scriptures and tradition for guidance. Morality is thus a matter not only for philosophy but for doctrine and theology. It is a guide to a life which both befits our human nature and reason, and responds to our divine calling (Finnis and Fisher, 1993). This chapter seeks to complement the more philosophical ones in the present volume, by showing the specific contribution which Catholic theology has to offer.

THE EUTHANASIA OF KING SAUL

The story of the death of Saul, the first king of Israel, is related in the books of Samuel. Saul was badly wounded in battle by a Philistine arrow. Afraid of being tortured and humiliated by his captors, he pleaded with his armour-bearer to kill him (1 Sam 31:1–4; 1 Chron 10:1–4). There are two versions of what happened next. According to the first, the man refused, so Saul committed suicide by falling on his own sword (1 Sam 31:5–6; 1 Chron 10:4).[1] In the other account a young Amelikite came upon the wounded Saul leaning on his spear, perhaps attempting suicide. Saul begged him, 'Stand beside me and slay me, for anguish has seized me and yet my life still lingers.' So the youth obliged (2 Sam 1:6–10) in what today we would call an act of voluntary euthanasia, assisted suicide or mercy-killing.

We might note a few points about this incident. First, to use our contemporary slogan, Saul was thought to be 'better off dead', or in current medico-legal parlance, death was 'in his best interest': in so far as these phrases can be given any coherent meaning at all, they mean that he might reasonably have hoped to die, to 'go to his fathers'. Secondly, everyone else was, more or less, better off with Saul being dead: David certainly was. Thirdly, the Amelikite who slew Saul seems to have done so with the best of motives: he was trusted by Saul and did nothing furtively; he formally mourned Saul's death and brought the crown and a full account to David. And fourthly, as the lad reported, 'I stood beside Saul and slew him, because I was sure that he could not live after he had fallen' or, to put it in a modern idiom, 'I stood by him and actively helped him have a peaceful death because I was sure he was terminally ill'. So Saul died at the hand of a merciful man, having asked for euthanasia, being terminally ill and in great suffering at the time.

Yet the undoubted conclusion of this story is that despite being done with the best will in the world, this was none the less a wicked act, deserving the severest of punishments.[2] When the lad arrived to tell David the news, no doubt expecting jubilation and personal reward, David did not rejoice even though Saul had been a great 'burden', indeed an enemy; instead he immediately rent his clothes, wept and fasted in a ritual demonstration of non-complicity and mourning, and had the youth punished for having killed his friend and the Lord's anointed (2 Sam 1:11–27).

CHOOSE LIFE

The so-called sanctity of life principle,[3] like the rest of Catholic morality, rests upon two complementary sources: revelation (or faith, theology) and reason (or natural law, philosophy). The God of the Bible is a living God who communicates his life to all living creatures, above all to the pinnacle of his creation, human beings (Gen 2:7; Ps 104:29–30; Isa 45:9–13; Zech 12:1).[4] Human beings are accorded great dignity, created uniquely as God's image and likeness, little less than gods themselves, intimately known by God, joined to him as in a marriage covenant, destined and oriented to him as their ultimate goal (Gen 1:26–31, 9:6; Job 12:10; Ps 8; Wis 2:23; Isa 57:16; Hos 2; Zech 12:1; 1 Cor 11:7; Eph 5; Rev 1:16; cf. Aquinas, *S Th* IIa IIæ 1–5). The Incarnation and Redemption further dignify human beings: the Son of God himself became human, and died to redeem all people and make them 'children of God'. I will return later to the significance of Christ's passion for our present issue. For now it is enough to note that in the Christian view of things, life is a trust given into our stewardship by God (CDF, 1980; *Catechism*, 1994: §2280); we are called to choose life not death, and the ways of life not of death; any killing demands justification and the taking of innocent human life is always contrary to God's law and to that trust (Gen 4:8–11; 9:1–6; Ex 20:13; 21:22–25; 23:7; Deut 5:17; 30:19; 2 Kings 8:12; 15:16; Jer 7:30–32; 19:4; 26:141–15; Mt 19:18 etc.).[5] As the Catholic Church has recently put it:

> Scripture specifies the prohibition in the fifth commandment: 'Do not slay the innocent and the righteous' (Ex 23:7). The deliberate murder of an innocent person is gravely contrary to the dignity of the human being, to the golden rule and to the holiness of the Creator. The law forbidding it is universally valid: it obliges each and everyone, always and everywhere. (*Catechism*, 1994: §2261)[6]

Even if motivated by 'mercy' or a concern for the 'best interests' of someone who is thought to be 'better off dead', no one should assume the rôle of the Author of Life and Death.[7]

In common with people of other religions and none, the Christian 'natural law' tradition teaches that human beings are of great and equal worth and ought to be respected by others and protected by society; life is a basic good of human beings, a reason for action, an aspect of their fulfilment, a good they share in common and part of their common good; human lives are of such intrinsic importance that no choice intentionally to bring about the death of an innocent[8] person can be right.[9] This sanctity of life principle has been much referred to in legal cases and most recently in the House of Lords Select Committee report on euthanasia. It is said to be deeply embedded in our law and ethics throughout the world, recognized in international human rights documents, and basic to our common morality. It has also informed medical ethics since at least as far back as Hippocrates: killing is amongst the ways in which healthcare workers may not deal with their patients. Thus classical medical ethics has held that physicians might not be called upon to act as public executioners (Emanuel, 1991, pp. 19–20). Likewise it has traditionally excluded both active and passive euthanasia. For these reasons the court and the General Medical Council held that Dr Nigel Cox had acted 'wholly outside' and 'contrary to' his duty as a doctor when he killed a patient even though (like King Saul) she was in severe pain and had asked to be killed.[10]

Most people regard killing someone arbitrarily, or simply for advantage or the convenience of others, as inconsistent with a recognition of that person's dignity and as obviously immoral. More difficult cases arise when a person asks to be killed, especially where that person is 'weary of life', or in great pain, or very dependent, or a strain on the financial and personal resources of others. Similarly when the person is living in a state of permanent unconsciousness: most people would sympathize with a family and doctors who hoped that such a patient would die sooner rather than later. The question is: should we hasten the death?

The theological answer to this seems to be a resounding no: 'you shall not kill'. But this is no mere superstitious taboo or perverse decree from on high. Rationally we must recognize that were we to say yes to medical killing we would have to abandon the sanctity of life principle: and that is exactly what the proponents of euthanasia always ultimately do.[11] Thus some deny that there is anything about human beings *per se* which is especially or equally valuable or deserving of respect: rather, they require certain qualifications, such as colour, creed, age, lack of handicap, or (as is presently fashionable) consciousness.[12] Others, aware of the dangers of this elitist and discriminatory move, argue instead that every person's right to life should be respected *in principle*, but that in some situations it might legitimately be compromised to serve other important 'values' such as the supposed 'best interests' or 'well-being' of the patient or (more often) the interests of the bystanders. This in turn highlights the fact that essential to respect for the precept against killing and to the killing–letting die distinction of classical and Christian medical ethics is a high view of human dignity and equality, and of our moral responsibilities in acting and forbearing to act with respect to it.

THE AGONY IN THE GARDEN: LIBERAL AUTONOMY V. THY WILL BE DONE

Having reviewed some implications of the death of the first king of Israel, we might turn now to the story of the death of the last: the Passion of Jesus Christ. Here God like David will rend his clothes asunder at the news of the killing of the king, tearing the veil of the Temple from top to bottom. But there is more to be gleaned for the purpose of the present debate than the principle of the sanctity of life.

The story begins with the agony in the garden (Mt 26:36–46 *et par*; Lk 22: 39–46). Jesus, contemplating the full horror of his suffering and death, is 'scared to death', falls to the ground shaking, and sweats blood. There is no Stoicism here, no romanticizing of sickness and death. Jesus enters into the full horror of human suffering: the pain and torment, the loneliness and abandonment. And like any of us would, he prays that this cup be taken from him. Yet he finishes his prayer, not like Saul asking to be speared (indeed, Jesus will be dead before the centurion arrives with that relief), but with the daily prayer of the Christian: 'Thy will be done' (Mt 26:39, 42 *et par*; cf. Mt 6:10 *et par*). Even the prospect of humiliation, pain and death does not dispense him from his obedience to the Father, the will of God, the law of the Lord.

This brings us to a second issue in the euthanasia debate and the one which receives the most attention in the press and the liberal philosophical academy: personal freedom or autonomy. Christian faith as well as secular bioethics have always required respect not only for the life of persons but for their free will. But 'autonomy' is now often equated with absolute freedom of self-determination, as when the House of Lords Committee (Lords 1994: §234), in keeping with recent legal trends, declared: 'We strongly endorse the right of the competent patient to refuse consent to *any* medical treatment, *for whatever reason*'. This sounds very reasonable in our individualistic, consumer culture; but, from a Catholic perspective, it is a distorted view of human dignity and freedom. First, because few sick people fit the somewhat idealized picture of the freely choosing agent: as the British Medical Association itself recognized, 'even apparently clear patient requests for cessation of treatment sometimes stem from ambivalence or may be affected by an undiagnosed depressive illness which, if successfully treated, might affect the patient's attitude' (Lords, 1994: §45). The Lords themselves expressed concern about the extent to which the elderly, lonely, sick or distressed feel themselves subject to pressure, whether real or imagined (1994: §239).

Another problem with a one-sided stress on autonomy is that it is radically asocial, even anti-social: all that matters is that I get my own way. But we are social creatures and human freedom is always exercised within a web of relationships. Christ does not attempt to go to his Passion alone: he takes his best friends with him to the garden and asks them to watch and pray with him. We too have to respect others; we have to consider the implications of our choices for their lives and for the common good. If we want to be 'put out of our misery' someone else must be involved: so someone else's 'autonomy' is unavoidably affected. So too is the community, for as Donne put it 'No man is an island, entire of itself: every man is a piece of the continent, a part of the main . . . Any man's death diminishes me, because I am involved in mankind.'

The third problem with much autonomy talk is that it fails to situate human freedom within the range of opportunities and values which are the context of human choice. The flip-side of the freedom of the patient to consent or refuse treatment, for instance, is that patients must exercise this freedom reasonably, in pursuit of their own good health and with respect for the good of persons in community. Free will is not mere whimsy, as the agony of Christ in the garden demonstrated so graphically: we are not free to do 'whatever we please' with our bodies, our lives, our opportunities. We have to take into account our calling from God, the intrinsic morality of our choices, and their self-constitutive effects: what they do to us, what they make us, what they say about us. In the face of decisions as momentous as are those over life and death, we should say with Christ 'not my will, Father, but thy will be done'.

MARY STOOD BY THE CROSS: THE DUTY TO CARE

Next in the Passion narrative comes the arrest, trial and execution of Jesus. It presents each of us with the challenge: how do I respond to the suffering and impending death of others? In the garden and the court we see Jesus abandoned by his disciples; on the other hand Simon of Cyrene helps carry the cross and Jesus' mother and friend wait by the foot of the cross – by his bedside, if you will. This points to another basic principle in this area: the duty to care for others. Negatively, this means we may not harm people or treat them negligently or with disrespect ('*primum non nocere*': first do not harm); positively, it refers to our 'Good Samaritan' duties to show kindness to others, especially the most needy, and to our special responsibilities towards dependent persons in our particular care.

Time and again the Scriptures and the Christian tradition call us generously to care for those in need: widow, orphan, alien, sick. Compassion expressed in engagement with people to alleviate their suffering was very much a part of Christ's own mission, and was the standard of judgment he offered: when you saw me hungry, thirsty, sick, imprisoned, in one of the least of these my brethren, did you help? (Mt 25:31–46). But such engagement is not the preserve of Judeo-Christian faith: it is a duty supported by documents ranging from the Koran to the International Covenant on Economic, Social and Cultural Rights. It is almost universally agreed that access to certain basic measures such as food, water, shelter, clothing, sanitation, basic medical and nursing care should be available to all out of respect for their human dignity.

In addition to these common humanitarian duties we all have towards each other, healthcare workers have a special duty to do no harm to, nor take any undue risks with, their patients, but rather to seek to promote the patient's health. The principle that medicine is *therapy* (called in the textbooks 'medical beneficence and non-maleficence') excludes the use of medicine for other purposes such as social engineering, exploitative experimentation, mere profit maximization, etc., and has traditionally excluded euthanasia: killing cures no one, is not nursing care, not therapy. It is normally possible to relieve another's suffering, at least to some extent. There *are* positive alternatives to euthanasia: good therapeutic and palliative care, the expert pain management for which the hospice movement is rightly celebrated; good counselling and chaplaincy; love and support of a thousand different kinds. We should not underestimate the possibilities here nor overestimate the difficulty of realizing those possibilities – both of which proponents of euthanasia are inclined to do.

On the other hand we must face the fact (as opponents of euthanasia sometimes fail to do) that these positive alternatives may not eliminate the suffering. There are some problems in life which have no morally and practically available 'solution'. Then comes the really hard loving: the loving of a family surrounding a comatose boy, of a husband whose wife's Alzheimer's disease means she no longer recognizes him, of siblings playing patiently with their profoundly handicapped brother, of a mother watching patiently at the foot of her dying son's cross. Sometimes the best we can do is to invest ourselves – our time, companionship, prayer and hope – in the suffering, the comatose and the dying. By so supporting these people we affirm that bodily life is not merely an instrumental good distinct from the human person, but basic to humanity; we meet our fundamental duty of respect and care for every human life however wounded or handicapped; and we express our love for a particular person, maintaining our human solidarity or communion with that person as best we can. This is a kind of respecting and loving which no one should pretend is easy. The temptation is always to look for a quick-fix, to do anything to make the problem go away, and if not, to desert, to join Peter and the boys fleeing from the scene, abandoning not just another human being but one to whom they had pledged their lives.

Pain and death, we know, will not be eliminated in this life. Suffering must be faced head-on, against the pervasive temptation to demand an immediate technological fix for every discomfort, and to marginalize those who suffer so that the rest can withdraw undisturbed. Faith recalls the profounder possibilities for good occasioned by illness and pain: for the sufferer, re-evaluation, conversion, growth in virtue, setting things right with God and others; for onlookers, compassion and selfless behaviour. The crucified God gives new significance to these redemptive possibilities in suffering; contemplation of the cross and uniting oneself with Christ's passion make possible greater endurance, assist in our redemption (e.g. Mt 27:34; Rom 8:17–18), and overcome temptations to a counterfeit mercy. We are promised the Holy Spirit to help us in our weakness (Rom 8:26). But death remains our last enemy and it cannot be tamed or befriended, only conquered by Christ (1 Cor 15:26). In the end as we humbly admit our incomprehension before these mysteries, we take confidence in the knowledge that Christ has gone before us through pain and death into new life, and in the hope that we will share with him an eternity without sickness or pain.[13]

In medical situations there are many opportunities to save life; there are likewise many ways to abandon people and even to kill them. I have argued elsewhere that active and passive euthanasia are morally equivalent, simply a matter of strategy, and I will not rehearse that argument here.[14] Suffice it here to say that passive euthanasia – intentional killing by means of dehydration, starvation, failure to perform necessary operations or to give appropriate drugs – is far more common in hospitals than killing by more active means. Thus I am advised that infants with certain handicaps are less likely to survive hospitalization today than they were a decade ago, despite advances in medicine. Two recent English cases of what was arguably passive euthanasia of older handicapped persons were those of Tony Bland and 'S'. Both young men were more or less permanently unconscious and their assisted feeding was discontinued on the basis (*a*) that this was in accord with responsible medical opinion, (*b*) continued tube-feeding (and by implication, continued living) were not in the patients' best interests, and (*c*) their continued feeding (and living) were not in other people's interests.[15] One might argue that assisted feeding is an inappropriate 'treatment' for the persistently unconscious, and should be withdrawn, without intending their deaths.[16] But in both these cases the *intention* was apparently to hasten the young men's deaths, to kill by omitting to care, and the courts approved. Most countries have had similar cases in recent years.

Medical abandonment and killing by deliberate neglect, sanctioned by gradual erosion of the common law and gradual change in medical practice, is the most likely way for euthanasia to become widespread. In many places there is already considerable lobbying for the legalization of 'benign neglect by physician' and this is well supported by some medical professional bodies and judicial fiats. Once again we must face the fact that to allow such 'benign neglect' would be to compromise one of the most basic principles of ethics, both religious and secular, a principle common to society generally and (at least historically) to the healthcare professions in particular: the duty of care for others.

DID GOD KILL JESUS? THE LIMITS TO THE DUTY OF CARE

There are, of course, limits to the duty of care as there are to every positive duty. Catholic faith and common morality recognize that while one may never intentionally kill, one need not strive relentlessly to preserve the last vestiges of life. The sanctity of life principle does not require 'survival no matter what'. Indeed, a survival-at-any-cost approach may well be due to therapeutic obstinacy, a refusal to face up to the limitations of healthcare and to human mortality, a product of despair rather than respect for life. Death is always an evil, but not the greatest evil; for many people it is a merciful release, the natural end to a life-story well written and, as believers claim, the door to eternal life.

At some point in most people's life death becomes, as it were, 'inevitable'. If there is an opportunity to do so, it is important to compose oneself to die well – a need which can be frustrated by too strenuous an effort to prolong life. While one should always value life as a gift, one may not be obliged to prolong it by means of highly intrusive or 'extraordinary' treatments. Care and respect for the dying often requires palliative and hospice care, and if this is to be applied it will be necessary for people to accept that death is near and that there is little more that human effort can properly do to postpone it. Thus traditional medical ethics and Catholic morality counsel against over-treatment as well as under-treatment, and allow that some treatments will be withheld or withdrawn for good therapeutic reasons: their continued use may be futile or they may impose such a burden (in terms of pain, indignity, disruption, confinement, risk, cost, etc.) that those concerned judge it disproportionate to the benefit gained (e.g. *Catechism*, 1994: §2278; CDF, 1980; Lords, 1994: §§240, 252–253).

Jesus as he hung upon the cross cried out and he was offered pain-relief, an anaesthetic, vinegar (Mt 27:48 *et par*). Christian tradition teaches that the taking of pain relief may be reasonable even if this has the foreseen side-effect of shortening life (CDF, 1980; *Catechism*, 1994: §2279). The same is true where treatments are withheld or withdrawn for good reasons. This is the so-called doctrine of double-effect. Put simply it is this: when healthcare professionals do some otherwise good thing (e.g. give a pain-relieving drug, withhold or withdraw some treatment) and death results earlier than it might otherwise have done, hastening death need not be why they chose such a course of action. Accelerating death is often no part of the healthcare worker's reason for such conduct; death may or may not be foreseen, but it is not intended; it belongs neither to her ultimate purpose, nor is it the means used to achieve that purpose.[17] On the other hand, a healthcare professional might give a pain-relieving drug or fail to treat because she believes the patient would be 'better off dead', or that others would be better off were the patient dead, etc. In this case hastening the patient's death is certainly part or the whole of the reason for the healthcare worker's chosen conduct and the course of action is immoral. Thus the judgment that a treatment is too burdensome ('extraordinary') or that pain relief should be given is *not* the same as a judgment that a life is too burdensome: it does *not* involve any arbitrary judgments of 'quality of life', 'best interests' or 'well-being' such that a person's life is judged to lack overall value.

When we ask about intentions we are getting to the heart of our moral character: who we are and what we are about. The difference between intending-and-causing and foreseeing-but-not-intending is not always easy to discern, and people's intentions are often as confused as their motives are mixed. But for the most part what is intentional is not in doubt, and various questions and what-if tests can be used to clarify intentions. We do not hold that the martyrs committed suicide even though they foresaw their deaths would 'result from' taking the stands they did. Likewise with Jesus' death. Jesus could have evaded his captors yet again; God could have intervened and saved him. Yet God kept Jesus' executioners in being and grace sufficient to do their dastardly deed. Yet still we say: God did not kill Jesus; we killed Jesus. God's will in this was permissive only, as it is whenever we choose to do evil; he is never the active agent of evil. Likewise with double effect in our choices: there are often undesired side-effects from our morally reasonable choices which we permit but do not will, do not 'purpose'.[18]

JESUS IS TRIED BY THE IDEOLOGIES OF OUR AGE

Finally, if we look back a little in our Passion narrative we will find Jesus tried by the ideologies of *our* own age. First, there is Caiaphas, the model of consequentialist reasoning, who declares: 'better that one man should die for the people . . . ' (Jn 11:50; 18:1) just as some contemporary high priests of bioethics would make new exceptions to the precept against killing as a matter of 'mercy', 'best-interests' or for some 'greater social good'. Here common morality and its Catholic variant replies insistently: 'The end does not justify the means', 'Do not do evil that good may come'.[19] Next there is Pilate who, though staring Truth in the face, shows himself the very model of modern liberal nihilism: 'Truth: what is that? (Jn 18:38). Many of the governors of our age are equally inclined to dodge difficult ethical questions, to pretend that medical ethics is all a matter of private opinion, so that all standards are 'up for grabs' as long as people are 'civil', 'kindly' and 'respectable'. To this common morality responds: of course we should seek by whatever means are morally and practically available to ease people's suffering. But beware: in hard cases sympathy and compassion will tempt us to compromise our basic norms and to fudge our laws. The temptation, one we all know in our moral lives, is to think that what is right is so complex and difficult and relative to each situation that we can allow just one, or a few, exceptions and still hold the line 'as a general rule'. But rational reflection and human experience suggest that the implications of such exceptions go far wider than the relief of hard cases.

Apart from the intrinsic evil of killing people, medical killing changes us individually, as healthcare professionals, and as a society. Even discounting the person killed, euthanasia is not 'victimless' because the person who carries it out is also significantly harmed in the process, as is the wider community. The healthcare professional's character will be very significantly shaped by killing a patient, however noble her motivation. Such an action will change her attitudes, dispositions, taboos. A healthcare worker who has decided that some patients may be killed, has, however well-meaningly, seriously undermined in herself a disposition indispensable to the practice of good medicine: respect for the life and health of every patient. So too with any community. Ethically, psychologically and sociologically, euthanasia invites further extension of 'therapeutic killing', whether by the same healthcare worker or by others. Euthanasia also discourages alternative responses to suffering, such as research into cures and the provision of good palliative care and pain management.

There are many other problems with the euthanasia answer which I have no space to explore here: so I might just flag a few. How are we to interpret the plea of patients or bystanders for euthanasia? Is it really a plea for death or a plea for better pain-relief, better support, comfort and love? What effect will medical killing have on the doctor–patient relationship and medical ethics? How soon would licence for euthanasia become a duty to take part in it, and how soon would we slip from voluntary to non-voluntary euthanasia?[20] There is also the spectre of the economic pressure, in a rapidly aging society in which healthcare costs are escalating, to keep extending the occasions for medical killing as a cost-cutting measure. In all, the House of Lords Committee (1994: §238) was right to conclude that 'these dangers are such that we believe any decriminalization of voluntary euthanasia would give rise to more, and more grave, problems than those it sought to address.'

For all the polemics about 'well-being', 'dignity' and 'mercy' used both by the euthanasia movement and now even by our institutions, we can forget that dignity is not recognized by telling the old, infirm or comatose how undignified their condition is, or how they would be better off dead – as when judges called Tony Bland 'grotesquely alive', 'an object of pity', 'the living dead', called 'S' a mere body for whom starving to death would be 'no ill effect', and called some handicapped children 'cabbages'. For all the special pleading by the Caiaphases and Pilates of our age, well-being and mercy are not served by medical abandonment, by standing by while people starve to death or by intervening to kill them. The so-called mercy killer adds the final rejection to the many already heaped upon the sick and dying by our community.[21] Dignity in old age, handicap, unconsciousness, and suffering are above all recognized by our showing the infirm love and respect. Surely we can find more creative ways of responding to suffering than killing?[22]

REFERENCES

Anscombe, G. E. M. 1963. *Intention*, 2nd ed. Oxford: Blackwell.

Aquinas, St Thomas. *Summa Theologiæ*.

Ashley, B. and O'Rourke, K. 1989. *Healthcare Ethics: A Theological Analysis*, 3rd ed. St Louis: Catholic Health Association.

Bailey, L. 1979. *Biblical Perspectives on Death*. Fortress Press.

Boyle, J. 1980. Toward understanding the principle of double effect. *Ethics* 90: 527–538.

Boyle, J. 1989. Sanctity of life and suicide: tensions and developments within common morality. In *Suicide and Euthanasia*, ed. B. Brody, pp. 221–250. Dordrecht: Kluwer.

Casey, J. 1991. *Food for the Journey*. St. Louis: Catholic Health Association.

Cassidy, S. 1994. *Light from the Dark Valley*. London: DLT.

Catechism of the Catholic Church ('Catechism'). 1994. English trans. London: Chapman.

Clouser, K. D. 1973. The sanctity of life: analysis of a concept. *Annals of Internal Medicine* 78: 119–125.

Congregation for the Doctrine of the Faith ('CDF'). 1974. *Quæstio de abortu: Declaration on Procured Abortion*.

CDF. 1980. *Jura et Bona: Declaration on Euthanasia*.

CDF. 1987. *Donum vitæ: Instruction on Respect for Human Life in its Origins*.

Delhaye, P. 1968. *The Christian Conscience*. New York: Desclee.

Donagan, A. 1977. *The Theory of Morality*. Chicago: Chicago University Press.

Dougherty, F. (ed.) 1982. *The Meaning of Suffering*. New York: Human Sciences Press.

Dworkin, R. 1993. *Life's Dominion*. London: Harper Collins.

Emanuel, E. 1991. *The Ends of Human Life*. Cambridge, MA: Harvard University Press.

'English Bishops'. House of Bishops of the Church of England and the Catholic Bishops' Conference of England and Wales. 1993. *Euthanasia – No! Submission to the House of Lords Select Committee on Medical Ethics*. London: Catholic Truth Society.

Finnis, J. 1980 *Natural Law and Natural Rights*. Oxford: Oxford University Press.

Finnis, J. 1993. *Bland*: crossing the Rubicon? *Law Quarterly Review* 109: 329–337.

Finnis, J. and Fisher, A. 1993. Theology and the four principles: a Roman Catholic view. In *Principles of Health Care Ethics*, ed. R. Gillon, pp. 31–44. London: John Wiley.

Fisher, A. 1993*a*. On not starving the unconscious. *New Blackfriars* 74: 130–145.

Fisher, A. 1993*b*. Old law and new ethics: *Bland's Case* and not feeding the comatose.

Law and Justice 116/117: 4–18.
Fisher, A. 1993*c*. Killing and letting die: what's the difference? *Signum* 21(16): 1–11.
Fisher, A. 1994. Consciousness: the new test of life. *Catholic Herald* [4 March]: 5.
Glover, J. 1977. *Causing Death and Saving Lives*. Harmondsworth: Penguin.
Gormally, L. 1993*a*. Against voluntary euthanasia. In *Principles of Health Care Ethics*, ed. R. Gillon, pp. 763–/74. London: John Wiley.
Gormally, L. 1993*b*. Definitions of personhood: implications for the care of PVS patients. *Catholic Medical Quarterly* 44(4): 7–12.
Gormally, L. (ed.) 1994. *Euthanasia, Clinical Practice and the Law*. London: Linacre Centre.
Grisez, G. 1983. *Christian Moral Principles*. Chicago: Franciscan Herald Press.
Grisez, G. 1993. *Living a Christian Life*. Quincy, IL: Franciscan Press.
Grisez, G. and Boyle, J. 1979. *Life and Death with Liberty and Justice: A Contribution to the Euthanasia Debate*. Notre Dame: Notre Dame University Press.
Hellwig, M. 1985. *Jesus: The Compassion of God*. Wilmington: Michael Glazier.
John Paul II. 1985. Apostolic Letter on the Christian Significance of Human Suffering. In *Divine Providence and Human Suffering*, ed. J. Wealsh and P. Walsh. Wilmington: Michael Glazier.
'Lords'. Select Committee of the House of Lords on Medical Ethics. 1994. *Report of the Select Committee on Medical Ethics*, vol. 1. London: HMSO.
May, W. 1977. *Human Existence, Medicine and Ethics*. Chicago: Franciscan Herald Press.
May, W. 1978. Double effect, principle of. In *Encyclopedia of Bioethics*. New York: Macmillan.
O'Rourke, K. and Boyle, P. 1989. *Medical Ethics: Sources of Catholic Teachings*. St Louis: Catholic Health Association.
Pollard, B. 1989. *Euthanasia: Should We Kill the Dying?* Sydney: Mount Press.
Sena, P. 1981. Biblical teaching on life and death. In *Moral Responsibility in Prolonging Life Decisions*, ed. D. McCarthy and A. Moraczewski, pp. 3–19. St Louis: Pope John Center.
Soelle, D. 1975. *Suffering*. Philadelphia: Fortress Press.
Stone, J. 1994. Withholding life-sustaining treatment: the ultimate decision. *New Law Journal* [11 Feb]: 205–206.
Vatican Council II. 1965. *Gaudium et Spes: Pastoral Constitution on the Church in the Modern World*.
Warnock, M. 1992. *The Uses of Philosophy*. Oxford: Blackwell.

NOTES

My particular thanks to Fr Robert Ombres, O.P., who helped me with this piece.

1 Unlike Abimelech's armour-bearer who slew him at his request, lest he suffer the humiliation of death at the hands of a woman: Judges 9:50–57. Other scriptural examples of suicide include: Saul's armour-bearer (1 Chron 10:5), Ahithophel (2 Sam 17:23), Zimri (1 Kings 16:18–19) and Judas (Mt 27:5; Acts 1:18).

2 A fuller treatment of responsibility and sin in this area would require consideration of the nature of conscience, and especially of the 'vexed' and the 'erroneous' conscience, and of the implications for responsibility of passions (such as overwhelming sympathy) and moral climate (such as upbringing in a pro-euthanasia society). See

O'Rourke and Boyle, 1989: chap. 2, who refer liberally to the teachings of Vatican II on the dignity of conscience; and Delhaye, 1968: 36–99 on the scriptural and patristic sources that underlie the teachings on conscience found in Aquinas and in Vatican documents. The *Catechism*, 1994: §2282, notes that 'grave psychological disturbances, anguish or grave fear of hardship, suffering or torture can diminish the responsibility of the one committing suicide'. On the other hand it also insists (§2277) that killing in response to an error of judgment made in good faith is nonetheless objectively evil.

3 See Boyle, 1989; *Catechism*, 1994: §§2258–2283; Clouser, 1973; Donagan, 1977.

4 CDF, 1987: 'Human life is sacred because from its beginning it involves the creative action of God and it remains for ever in a special relationship with the Creator, who is its sole end. God alone is the Lord of life from its beginning until its end: no one can under any circumstance claim for himself the right directly to destroy an innocent human being' (Quoted also in *Catechism* 1994: §2258). See also: Bailey, 1979; Sena, 1981.

5 CDF, 1974: §5: 'Human life, even on this earth, is precious. Infused by the creator, life is again taken back by him (cf. Gen 2:7; Wis 15:11). It remains under his protection: man's blood cries out to him (cf. Gen 4:10) and he will demand an account of it, "for in the image of God man was made" (Gen 9:5–6). The commandment of God is formal: "You shall not kill" (Ex 20:13). Life is at the same time a gift and a responsibility. It is received as a "talent" (cf. Mt 25:14–30); it must be put to proper use.' Vatican Council II, 1965: §27: 'The varieties of crime are numerous. They include all offenses against life itself, such as murder (*cuiusvis generis homicidia*), genocide, abortion, euthanasia and suicide . . . all these and the like are criminal: they poison civilization; they debase the perpetrators even more than the victims; and they offend against the honour of the Creator'.

6 Likewise CDF, 1980: 'Human life is the basis of all goods, and is the necessary source and condition of every human activity and of all society . . . No one can make an attempt on the life of an innocent person without opposing God's love for that person, without violating a fundamental right, and therefore without committing a crime of the utmost gravity . . . It is necessary to state firmly once more that nothing and no one can in any way permit the killing of an innocent human being, whether a foetus or an embryo, an infant or an adult, an old person or one suffering from an incurable disease, or a person who is dying.' I have not been able to review here the development of the tradition behind this teaching through the fathers, the scholastics and the papal magisterium. CDF, 1980, includes references to some of Pius XII's teaching in this area; O'Rourke and Boyle, 1989: 111–115, include some texts from John Paul II. An example of a recent episcopal statement is English Bishops, 1993.

7 *Catechism*, 1994: §2277: 'an act or omission which, of itself or by intention, causes death in order to eliminate suffering constitutes a murder gravely contrary to the dignity of the human person and to the respect due to the living God, his Creator. The error of judgment into which one can fall in good faith does not change the nature of this murderous act, which must always be forbidden and excluded.'

8 I qualify the prohibition of intentionally killing with 'innocent' here in line with common morality which has traditionally recognized a right (and sometimes a duty) to render unjust aggressors unable to inflict harm, even with lethal force. This might include justifiable capital punishment and war, but obviously not euthanasia. On the justification for the 'exceptions' see Fisher, 1993*a* and *Catechism*, 1994: §2263–2267, 2321 and the sources in each. Hereafter I use the terms person, victim and life presuming (or at least allowing) the traditional qualification 'innocent'.

9 Cf. Ashley and O'Rourke, 1989: chap. 13; Donagan, 1977; Finnis, 1980; Grisez, 1983:

chap. 5, 7, 9; Grisez, 1993: chap. 8; Grisez and Boyle, 1979; May, 1977: chap. 6; Pollard, 1989.

10 *R* v. *Cox* (1992) 12 BMLR 38; likewise: *R* v. *Adams* [1957] Crim LR 365; *R* v. *Arthur* (1981) 12 BMLR 1. In many places there is considerable lobbying for the legalization of 'physician aid-in-dying' as practised in Holland.

11 My thought in this area has been much influenced by Gormally, 1993*a*, *b*, 1994.

12 This was the crucial qualification in the mind of the judges in *Airedale NHS Trust* v. *Bland* [1993] AC 789 ('*Bland's Case*'), so much so that they were sometimes unclear about whether Anthony Bland was really a living human being. Similar reasoning is to be found in the works of Warnock, 1992 and Dworkin, 1993, among others, and has been very effectively rebutted in Gormally, 1994.

13 For some reflections on suffering and death as they are understood in the Judeo-Christian tradition see: Ashley and O'Rourke, 1989: 47–49, 197–199; Casey, 1991: chaps. 4, 5; Cassidy, 1994; *Catechism*, 1994: §§988–1019, 1500–1510, 1521; Dougherty, 1982; Hellwig, 1985; John Paul II, 1985; Soelle, 1975.

14 See Fisher, 1993*c* and Finnis, 1980: 176–177, 195 (*contra* Glover, 1977 and so many since), on where action and omission are morally different and where they are morally equivalent. The law recognizes the equivalence of action and omission in some cases. Thus people have been convicted for killing by omission: *R* v. *Marriott* (1838) 8 C & P 425; *R* v. *Bubb* (1850) 4 Cox CC 455; *R* v. *Nicholls* (1874) 13 Cox CC 75; *R* v. *Istan* [1893] 1 QB 450; *R* v. *Gibbons & Proctor* (1918) 13 Cr App Rep 134; *R* v. *Stone & Dobinson* [1977] QB 354; *R* v. *Unnamed 44 year old man* (Judge Geoffrey Grigson in Old Bailey, 7 March 1994); *Bland's Case per* Lord Keith at 858, Lord Browne-Wilkinson at 881 and Lord Mustill at 893; Smith & Hogan, *Criminal Law* (7th ed, 1992) at 47–50.

15 *Bland's Case*, regarding which see: Finnis, 1993 and Fisher, 1993*a*, *b*. *Frenchay Healthcare NHS Trust* v. *S* ([1994] 1 WLR 601), regarding which see: Fisher, 1994, and Stone, 1994.

16 Though I have argued to the contrary in Fisher, 1993*a*. A good case could certainly have been made, however, for not intervening surgically and with aggressive antibiotics. It is mysterious that such intervention occurred in the last year of Anthony Bland's life, when it might have been withheld without ethical or legal difficulties.

17 'Intentional' here is a term of ethical art. It refers to what one does, identified by reference to one's chosen purpose in acting and the means which are chosen precisely because of their relevance to that project. When death is foreseen but not intended, its causation does not feature among the reasons one has for acting; it is unintended, perhaps even regretted. Some people treat intentional and foreseen-but-unintended causation as morally equivalent, but this would mean one could never build roads, engage in high-risk sports, perform high-risk surgery, give analgesics for pain control which might reduce life span, withhold treatment, and so on, while being opposed to killing.

18 Scriptural examples of just acts involving risk of death to the actor are the deaths of Samson (Judges 16:23–31) and Eleazar (1 Macc 6:43–46). For helpful accounts of intention and double effect: Anscombe, 1963; Aquinas, *S Th*, IIa IIæ 8–21, 79; Boyle, 1980; *Catechism*, 1994: §§1737, 2283; May, 1978.

19 See Finnis and Fisher, 1993 and sources therein for reasons why any comparison which hopes to guide moral judgment by an overall 'weighing' of the goods and evils at stake in morally significant options is always made by feelings, not rational commensuration, and will ultimately be only rationalization.

20 Lords, 1994: §238: 'we do not think it possible to set secure limits on voluntary euthanasia . . . it would not be possible to frame adequate safeguards against non-voluntary euthanasia if voluntary euthanasia were to be legalised . . . Moreover to

create an exception to the general prohibition on intentional killing would inevitably open the way to its further erosion whether by design, by inadvertence, or by the human tendency to test the limits of any regulation'.

21 Lords, 1994: §239: 'We believe that the message which society sends to vulnerable and disadvantaged people should not, however obliquely, encourage them to seek death, but should assure them of our care and support in life'.

22 After the preparation of this chapter Pope John Paul II published *The Gospel of Life: Encyclical on the Value and Inviolability of Human Life (Evangelium Vitae*, 25 March 1995, London: CTS). This is undoubtedly the most authoritative statement of Christian bioethics to date, and it therefore warrants an extended note here. (Numbers in brackets refer to paragraph numbers of the encyclical.)

The object of the letter is 'to be a precise and vigorous reaffirmation of the value of human life and its inviolability, and at the same time a pressing appeal addressed to each and every person, in the name of God: respect, protect, love and serve life, every human life!' (5) It begins with an analysis of the contemporary scene. While the Pope focuses particularly on attacks upon life in its earliest and final stages, he situates these within the broader perspective of the 'extraordinary increase and gravity of threats to the life of individuals and peoples, especially where life is weak and defenceless' (3). He has in mind 'murder, war, slaughter and genocide . . . the violence . . . [of] poverty, malnutrition and hunger because of an unjust distribution of resources . . . the violence inherent not only in wars as such but in the scandalous arms trade . . . the spreading of death caused by reckless tampering with the world's ecological balance, by the criminal spread of drugs, or by the promotion of certain kinds of sexual activity . . . '(10)

In Chapter I the Pope identifies a range of factors contributing to this spiral of violence: new technologies, interpersonal difficulties and crises of family and culture, widespread ethical scepticism, anonymous cities full of marginalized people, the complicity of medical professionals, legal institutions and governments. In a strongly worded critique of contemporary social trends he argues that there has emerged in the West 'a culture which denies solidarity and in many cases takes the form of a veritable *culture of death*. This culture is activity fostered by powerful cultural, economic and political currents . . . a kind of *conspiracy against life*' (12). Fundamental to this cultural shift have been three ideologies: *individualism* (which exaggerates the importance of individual automony and freedom from suffering and fails in solidarity or concern for individual others and the community), *utilitarianism* (which glorifies economic efficiency and devalues the unproductive and burdensome) and *hedonism* (which seeks to 'censor' out suffering at any cost and interprets 'quality of life' in terms of 'consumerism, physical beauty and pleasure, to the neglect of the more profound dimensions – interpersonal, spiritual and religious – of existence').

Against this background, the encyclical offers further insights into the special factors which contribute to the call for euthanasia: 'In the sick person the sense of anguish, of severe discomfort, and even of desperation brought on by intense and prolonged suffering can be a decisive factor. Such a situation can threaten the already fragile equilibrium of an individual's personal and family life, with the result that, on the one hand, the sick person, despite the help of increasingly effective medical and social assistance, risks feeling overwhelmed by his or her own frailty; and on the other hand, those close to the sick person can be moved by an understandable even if misplaced compassion. All this is aggravated by a cultural climate which fails to perceive any meaning or value in suffering, but rather considers suffering the epitome of evil, to be eliminated at all costs . . . [and assumes] a certain Promethean attitude which leads people to think that they can control life and death by taking the decisions about them into their own hands . . . As well as for reasons of a misguided pity at the sight of the patient's suffering, euthanasia is sometimes justified by the utilitarian motive of avoiding costs which bring no return and which weigh heavily on society. Thus it is proposed to eliminate malformed babies, the severely handicapped, the disabled, the elderly, especially when they are not self-sufficient, and the terminally ill.' (15; cf. 64)

In Chapter II John Paul draws upon natural law and a broad range of sources from the Christian tradition, in support of the proposition that 'life is always a good,' indeed one of 'great and inestimable value'. The theological source of human dignity is shown to be the divine origins and destiny of the human being. Parallel to the philosophical affirmation of the inviolability of the basic human good of life is the theological affirmation that God is the sole Lord of life and that he commands reverence and love for the life of every person. This prophetic Gospel of Life not only condemns offences against life but awakens 'hope for a new principle of life', for renewed relationships of reciprocity and care, and for an understanding of the crucial links between life, freedom and (moral) truth.

After detailing the long and unbroken history of teaching on the absolute inviolability of innocent human life, from the Scriptures (which particularly inform this document), through the fathers and scholastics, to more recent conciliar, papal, curial and episcopal texts, the Pope dogmatically defines (or 'confirms') as a matter of Christian faith 'that the direct and voluntary killing of an innocent human being is always gravely immoral' (57). From this 'infallible' proposition he concludes that 'the deliberate decision to deprive an innocent human being of his life is always morally evil and can never be licit either as an end in itself or as a means to a good end. It is in fact a grave act of disobedience to the moral law, and indeed to God himself, the author and guarantor of that law; it contradicts the fundamental virtues of justice and charity . . . Before the moral norm which prohibits the direct taking of the life of an innocent human being there are no privileges or exceptions for anyone. It makes no difference whether one is the master of the world or the "poorest of the poor" on the face of the earth. Before the demands of morality we are all absolutely equal.' (57)

The implications of this for the euthanasia issue should be obvious enough, but John Paul patiently lays them open to our purview. He makes the necessary distinctions between euthanasia ('an action or omission which of itself and by intention causes death, with the purpose of eliminating all suffering') and the appropriate refusal, withholding or withdrawing of aggressive treatments which are 'disproportionate to any expected results' or which 'impose an excessive burden on the patient and his family', especially when death is clearly imminent and inevitable. He supports the use of appropriate palliative care, even when this results (unintentionally, if predictably) in decreased consciousness or a shortening of life. He recognizes that those who seek euthanasia may do so out of anguish, desperation or conditioning, thus lessening or removing subjective responsibility (15; 66); and that those who engage in euthanasia are not necessarily motivated by a selfish refusal to be burdened with the life of someone who is suffering (66). He then declares: 'Taking into account these distinctions, in harmony with the Magisterium of my Predecessors and in communion with the Bishops of the Catholic Church, *I confirm that euthanasia is a grave violation of the law of God*, since it is the deliberate and morally unacceptable killing of a human person. This doctrine is based upon the natural law and upon the written word of God, is transmitted by the Church's Tradition and taught by the ordinary and universal Magisterium. Depending on the circumstances, this practice involves the malice proper to suicide or murder.' (65)

The Pope argues that euthanasia is 'false mercy', indeed 'a disturbing perversion of mercy': 'True *compassion* leads to sharing another's pain; it does not kill the person whose suffering we cannot bear. Moreover, the act of euthanasia appears all the more perverse if it is carried out by those, like relatives, who are supposed to treat a family member with patience and love, or by those, such as doctors, who by virtue of their specific profession are supposed to care for the sick person even in the most painful terminal stages . . . The height of arbitrariness and injustice is reached when certain people, such as physicians or legislators, arrogate to themselves the power to decide who ought to live and who ought to die . . . Thus the life of the person who is weak is put into the hands of the one who is strong; in society the sense of justice is lost, and mutual trust, the basis of every authentic interpersonal relationship, is undermined at its root' (66). He contrasts this with the 'the way of love and true mercy' which recognizes that 'the request which arises from the human heart in the supreme confrontation with suffering and death, especially when faced with the temptation to give up in utter desperation, is above all a request for companionship, sympathy and support in the time of trial. It is a plea for help to keep on hoping when all human hopes fail.' And he reiterates Christ's promise of resurrection, and His call in the meantime to 'live to the Lord' (recognizing that suffering, while an evil and a trial, can become a source of good if it is experienced for and with love through sharing in Christ's suffering) and to 'die to the Lord' (being ready to meet death in obedience at the 'hour' willed and chosen by God) (67). The encyclical then offers some reflections on the appropriate response of law-makers and citizens.

The encyclical though critical is not without hope. It identifies conflicting tendencies in contemporary societies. Against the 'culture of death' there are many individuals, families, voluntary groups and institutions which reverence, defend and serve human life; there is a growing sensitivity towards human rights, quality of life and ecology, and opposition to war and capital punishment; growing numbers of people are willing to embrace 'the inescapable responsibility of choosing to be unconditionally pro-life' (26–27). Building upon this, Chapter IV of *Evangelium Vitae* proposes positive strategies 'to ensure that justice and solidarity will increase and that a new culture of human life will be affirmed, for the building of an authentic civilization of truth and love'. As part of this multi-faceted programme, he proposes that 'special attention must be given to the elderly . . . Neglect of the elderly or their outright rejection are intolerable . . . It is therefore important to preserve, or to re-establish where it has been lost, a sort of "covenant" between generations. In this way parents, in their later years, can receive from their children the acceptance and solidarity which they themselves gave to their children when they brought them into the world . . . The elderly are not only to be considered the object of our concern, closeness and service. They themselves have a valuable contribution to make to the Gospel of life. Thanks to the rich treasury of experiences they have acquired through the years, the elderly can and must be sources of wisdom and witnesses of hope and love.' (94;cf. 46) The Pope exhorts Christians to 'preach the Gospel of life, to celebrate it in the Liturgy and in our whole existence, and to serve it with the various programmes and structures which support and promote life' (79).

Index